Review for USMLE

United States Medical Licensing Examination

Step   3

The National Medical Series for Independent Study

Review for USMLE

United States
Medical Licensing
Examination

Step **3**

Mitchell H. Rosner, MD
Staff Nephrologist
Medical Associates of Savannah
Savannah, Georgia

and

Andrew E. Lazar, MD
Chief Resident, Internal Medicine
University of Virginia
Fellow, Division of Nephrology
Case Western Reserve University

LIPPINCOTT WILLIAMS & WILKINS
A **Wolters Kluwer** Company
Philadelphia • Baltimore • New York • London
Buenos Aires • Hong Kong • Sydney • Tokyo

Editor: Neil Marquardt
Development Editor: Karla Schroeder
Managing Editors: Carol Loyd and Anjou K. Dargar
Marketing Manager: Scott Lavine
Production Editor: Bill Cady
Compositor: Peirce Graphic Services
Printer: DRC

351 West Camden Street
Baltimore, MD 21201

530 Walnut Street
Philadelphia, PA 19106

Printed in the United States of America

Library of Congress Cataloging-in-Publication Data

Lazar, Andrew E.
   Review for USMLE : United States Medical Licensing Examination, step 3 / Mitchell H. Rosner and Andrew E. Lazar.
      p. cm. — (The national medical series for independent study)
   Includes bibliographical references.
   ISBN 0-7817-3201-8
      1. Medicine—Examinations, questions, etc. 2. Medicine—Outlines, syllabi, etc. I. Lazar, Andrew E. II. Title. III. Series.

R834.5 .L38
610.76—dc21

2002072495

To purchase additional copies of this book, call our customer service department at **(800) 638-3030** or fax orders to **(301) 824-7390.** International customers should call **(301) 714-2324.**

Visit Lippincott Williams & Wilkins on the Internet: http://www.LWW.com. Lippincott Williams & Wilkins customer service representatives are available from 8:30 am to 6:00 pm, EST.

04 05 06
3 4 5 6 7 8 9 10

To my Mom and Dad and, most of all, to Michelle, for their never-ending support and encouragement.

Mitchell H. Rosner

To Lisa, Samantha, and Joshua, for tolerating my life as a physician.

Andrew E. Lazar

Preface

Medicine is an ever-changing subject, and in response, the format of the United States Medical Licensing Examination (USMLE) Step 3 has changed. In 1999, the National Board of Medical Examiners implemented a computer-based examination for USMLE Step 3. In addition, the examination now focuses on "clinical encounter frames" that ask the test taker to function as a nonspecialized general physician in a variety of different practice settings. These clinical encounter frames include the following:

- Initial workups, which stress the initial assessment and management of patients that the physician is seeing for the first time; the range of possible clinical problems that may be presented is broad and may include undifferentiated symptoms, chronic illnesses, and emotional problems
- Continued care, which stresses the continuing management of previously diagnosed diseases
- Urgent care, which stresses the management of life-threatening emergencies

These encounters may occur in a variety of practice settings: a satellite health center, a general practitioner's office, an emergency department, and an inpatient facility.

Furthermore, the examination now focuses on a core group of physician tasks that the test taker must master. These tasks include:

- Obtaining a history and performing a physical examination
- Using laboratory and diagnostic studies
- Formulating a likely diagnosis
- Evaluating the severity of a patient's problems
- Managing patients, including health maintenance, clinical intervention, clinical therapeutics, and legal or ethical issues
- Applying scientific concepts

This review book is designed to be an examination preparation guide modeled after the USMLE Step 3 examination content. It exposes the reader to all of the practice settings and physician tasks tested on the examination. Topics of discussion include relevant subject material in internal medicine, general surgery, psychiatry, pediatrics, neurology, and obstetrics/gynecology.

The book is divided into five composite examinations, with detailed explanations of the answers to the multiple-choice questions. The questions and explanations can be used in several ways:

- As a diagnostic tool to assess competency in particular subject areas and identify areas in which further review is needed
- As a postreview test to assess whether core material has been mastered
- As a primary means of review

We believe this book provides a comprehensive review of the relevant topics expected to be mastered on the USMLE, presented in a format that maximizes learning.

Mitchell H. Rosner, MD
Andrew E. Lazar, MD

Permissions

Test I

The figure in questions 19–21 has been reprinted with permission from Brant WE, Helms CA. *Fundamentals of Diagnostic Radiology.* 2nd ed. Philadelphia: Lippincott Williams & Wilkins, 1999:588.

The figure in question 22 has been reprinted with permission from O'Connor BH. *A Color Atlas and Instruction Manual of Peripheral Blood Cell Morphology.* Baltimore: Williams & Wilkins, 1984:192.

The figure in questions 86–88 has been reprinted with permission from Brant WE, Helms CA. *Fundamentals of Diagnostic Radiology.* 2nd ed. Philadelphia: Lippincott Williams & Wilkins, 1999:1019.

The figure in questions 89–90 has been reprinted with permission from Collins J, Stern EJ. *Chest Radiology: The Essentials.* Philadelphia: Lippincott Williams & Wilkins, 1999:5.

The figure in questions 102–107 has been reprinted with permission from O'Connor BH. *A Color Atlas and Instruction Manual of Peripheral Blood Cell Morphology.* Baltimore: Williams & Wilkins, 1984:245.

The figure in questions 108–109 has been reprinted with permission from O'Connor BH. *A Color Atlas and Instruction Manual of Peripheral Blood Cell Morphology.* Baltimore: Williams & Wilkins, 1984:195.

The figure in question 109 has been reprinted with permission from O'Connor BH. *A Color Atlas and Instruction Manual of Peripheral Blood Cell Morphology.* Baltimore: Williams & Wilkins, 1984:179.

Test II

The figure in question 13 has been reprinted with permission from O'Connor BH. *A Color Atlas and Instruction Manual of Peripheral Blood Cell Morphology.* Baltimore: Williams & Wilkins, 1984:184.

The figure in question 25 has been reprinted with permission from Collins J, Stern EJ. *Chest Radiology: The Essentials.* Philadelphia: Lippincott Williams & Wilkins, 1999:92.

The figure in question 52 has been reprinted with permission from Brant WE, Helms CA. *Fundamentals of Diagnostic Radiology.* 2nd ed. Philadelphia: Lippincott Williams & Wilkins, 1999:1125.

The figure in question 69 has been reprinted with permission from Frankel DH. *Field Guide to Clinical Dermatology.* Philadelphia: Lippincott Williams & Wilkins, 1999:69.

The figure in questions 93–94 has been reprinted with permission from Goodheart HP. *A Photoguide of Common Skin Disorders: Diagnosis and Management.* Baltimore: Williams & Wilkins, 1999:112.

The figure in questions 103–104 has been reprinted with permission from Brant WE, Helms CA. *Fundamentals of Diagnostic Radiology.* 2nd ed. Philadelphia: Lippincott Williams & Wilkins, 1999:660.

The figure in question 133 has been reprinted with permission from Goodheart HP. *A Photoguide of Common Skin Disorders: Diagnosis and Management.* Baltimore: Williams & Wilkins, 1999:246.

The figure in questions 143–145 has been reprinted with permission from Fowler NO. *Clinical Electrocardiographic Diagnosis: A Problem-Based Approach.* Philadelphia: Lippincott Williams & Wilkins, 2000:109.

The figure in question 147 has been reprinted with permission from Goodheart HP. *A Photoguide of Common Skin Disorders: Diagnosis and Management.* Baltimore: Williams & Wilkins, 1999:295.

Test IV

The figure in questions 1–3 has been reprinted with permission from Fowler NO. *Clinical Electrocardiographic Diagnosis: A Problem-Based Approach.* Philadelphia: Lippincott Williams & Wilkins, 2000:42.

The figure in questions 111–113 has been reprinted with permission from Wright KW. *Textbook of Ophthalmology.* Baltimore: Williams & Wilkins, 1997:155.

Test V

The figure in question 83 has been reprinted with permission from Brant WE, Helms CA. *Fundamentals of Diagnostic Radiology.* 2nd ed. Philadelphia: Lippincott Williams & Wilkins, 1999:1009.

The figure in question 84 has been reprinted with permission from Brant WE, Helms CA. *Fundamentals of Diagnostic Radiology.* 2nd ed. Philadelphia: Lippincott Williams & Wilkins, 1999:1006.

The figure in questions 98–99 has been reprinted with permission from Fowler NO. *Clinical Electrocardiographic Diagnosis: A Problem-Based Approach.* Philadelphia: Lippincott Williams & Wilkins, 2000:46.

The figure in question 107 has been reprinted with permission from Collins J, Stern EJ. *Chest Radiology: The Essentials.* Philadelphia: Lippincott Williams & Wilkins, 1999:269.

The figure in questions 108–112 has been reprinted with permission from Fowler NO. *Clinical Electrocardiographic Diagnosis: A Problem-Based Approach.* Philadelphia: Lippincott Williams & Wilkins, 2000:64.

The figure in question 123 has been reprinted with permission from Goodheart HP. *A Photoguide of Common Skin Disorders: Diagnosis and Management.* Baltimore: Williams & Wilkins, 1999:96.

Contents

Examination Preparation Guide

You're going to war. The results of the campaign can affect your future. You need a strategy and knowledge of the enemy and the fighting conditions. The USMLE Step 3 is a necessary battle in your crusade toward professional success; you need to pass, and the results might affect your future fellowship and employment opportunities. How can you best prepare yourself for battle?

1. Develop a Plan.

Your strategy for success requires a complete and realistic plan. Be honest with yourself. Set aside as many weeks as you feel you need. During a typical intern year, lack of time might lead to procrastination. Fight it. Make your plan at least 3 months prior to the examination. We recommend that you divide your preparation into sections, including internal medicine, surgery, obstetrics and gynecology, neurology, pediatrics, dermatology, radiology, psychiatry, family practice, ethics, and any other topics you plan to cover. Make a calendar and fill in each available time slot with a topic. Cover each topic, spending the most time on your weaker subjects.

2. Work on Your Weaker Subjects.

There is always a temptation to spend time on the subjects that you have mastered. When you go to the golf range, do you take out the club that you need the most work on, or do you take out the driver and hit the long ball because it's more satisfying and reassuring? Be honest with yourself. Have confidence in what you know, and spend time on your weaknesses; this approach will reap benefits.

3. Peak at the Appropriate Time.

There is such a thing as "peaking" for the examination. You want to do your best on the day of the examination—not the day before, not the day after. Pace yourself as you get close to the examination; don't burn out. Take a break if you feel your performance peaking too early.

4. Choose Team or Solo Preparation.

Decide early whether you like the team approach. Residents have less time for a team approach to USMLE Step 3 preparation than the students preparing for USMLE Steps 1 and 2. Nonetheless, some will attempt a team approach and derive benefit from it. Many use the team approach to help avoid procrastination and for motivational purposes. Are you one of those people? Should you follow the team approach, be sure that each member of the team is contributing equally; don't allow others to hold you back.

If you like to work alone, don't be intimidated by the preparation plans of others. Go with what has worked for you. You've been a success, having made it this far.

5. Get Inside the Head of Your Enemy.

Go into battle with knowledge of your enemy. Prepare mock tests. Simulate the examination and test-taking environment. Time yourself in the same manner as you will be timed on the big day, using an accurate timepiece. After the mock examination, follow up on your shortcomings to maximize the benefits of your preparatory efforts.

6. Hone Your Test-Taking Skills.

You've made it to USMLE 3, achieving success on MCAT, USMLE 1, and USMLE 2 along the way. You have good test-taking skills; now hone them further. Question books prepare one more appropriately for test taking. Remember, part of your performance will depend on your test-taking skills. As with most things, practice is necessary. Questions provide the means for honing these test-taking skills while reviewing the high-yield medical topics.

Note that the examination's passages will be long and often contain many red herrings. A vignette may contain a long description of signs and symptoms, only to tell you the disease process before asking you a seemingly unrelated question. Look at the question at the end of each passage first. This might facilitate a more efficient analysis of the passage and enable you to focus on the true question.

Time management is important for everyone, but some find it more difficult than others. You might only have 1 minute per question, so pace yourself. Make sure that you are on pace to finish on time. Check every 10 minutes to assess whether you need to speed up. Time yourself during your mock examinations.

Be alert for words like "ALWAYS" and "MOST LIKELY"; the test writers use these words to support the correct answer. Be careful with words like "NOT," "EXCEPT," and "LEAST." Don't let them throw you off; instead, use them to your advantage, as they may immediately limit the number of possible correct choices.

If you encounter a cluster of questions pertaining to one vignette, answer the questions in order. Earlier questions might direct subsequent questions.

Know yourself as a test taker. Do you get test anxiety? It is a common phenomenon and, unfortunately, can affect your performance. Mock examinations help you prepare for this; strong review and emotional preparation may help prevent it.

Give yourself a pep talk, if necessary. Remember, you're going to war! These skills will help you stay in control.

7. Know the Terrain.

You MUST be familiar with the new computer-testing environment. For many, this will be your first experience taking a test on a computer. As with anything else, you are at a disadvantage when you have little experience. You will be sent a disk when you register for the test. Practice until you feel comfortable.

The examination will take place at a learning center with many computers. The computers will likely be separated by small dividers. Earplugs are available. Each day is divided into a morning and afternoon session. Each session consists of approximately four blocks of 30 to 50 typical, multiple-choice questions based on clinical vignettes. The computer monitors your time. You are given the option of taking a break between each block, and the option of taking a 45-minute lunch break after block four. (In theory, you could take all eight blocks on your first day without a break and be finished early.) On the second day, the first four blocks are similar to the eight blocks of the first day. The "afternoon" section of the second day consists of nine cases that are interactive in nature. These problems are described by the USMLE:

"You may request information from the history and physical examination; order laboratory studies, procedures, and consultants; and start medications and other therapies. Any of the thousands of possible entries that you type on the 'order sheet' are processed and verified by the 'clerk'. When you have confirmed that there is nothing further you wish to do, you decide when to reevaluate the patient by advancing time. As time passes, the patient's condition changes based on the underlying problem and your interventions; results of tests are reported and results of interventions must be monitored. You suspend the movement of time as you consider next steps. While you cannot go back in time, you can change your orders to reflect your updated management plan.

The patient's chart contains, in addition to the order sheet, the reports resulting from your orders. By selecting the appropriate chart tabs, you can review vital signs, progress notes, nurses' notes, and test results. You may care for and move the patient among the office, home, emergency department, intensive care unit, and hospital ward.

You decide which diagnostic information to obtain and how to treat and monitor the patient's progress. The computer records each step you take in caring for the patient and scores your overall performance. This format permits assessment of clinical decision-making skills in a more realistic and integrated manner than other available formats."

The USMLE Step 3 is specifically aimed at assessing your ability to apply the medical knowledge essential for the **unsupervised** practice of medicine, with emphasis on the ambulatory setting. The patient encounters will range from life-threatening emergency situations to continuity care and ethical situations. The USMLE describes the breakdown as follows:

Clinical Encounter Frame
- 20–30% Initial care
- 55–65% Continued care
- 10–20% Emergency care

Physician Task
- 8–12% Obtaining history and performing physical examination
- 8–12% Using laboratory and diagnostic studies
- 8–12% Formulating most likely diagnosis
- 8–12% Evaluating severity of patient's problems
- 8–12% Applying scientific concepts and mechanisms of disease
- 45–55% Managing the patient
  —Health maintenance
  —Clinical intervention
  —Clinical therapeutics
  —Legal and ethical issues

8. Use Your Experience.

You've been a success. What habits have contributed to this success? This is no time to rework things. Use your materials (notes, outlines, etc.) whenever possible. You organized them in a manner sensible to you. Decide if you like review books. Some students prefer not to use them, but others find that review books provide a sense of "completeness" because one book may cover all areas of interest. Again, do what has worked for you in the past.

Without a doubt, 5 years of training hard will best prepare you for the mission ahead, but we hope that this guide and the cases that follow will help you meet the challenge and emerge victorious.

Mitchell H. Rosner, MD
Andrew E. Lazar, MD

Test I

QUESTIONS

DIRECTIONS: For each question, select the letter corresponding to the best answer. All questions have only one correct answer.

Setting: Office

Questions 1–5

A 29-year-old Caucasian woman from out of town presents with concerns about discharge from her right nipple. She states that she had a normal examination at her gynecologist's office 6 weeks ago. She describes the discharge, which has been present for approximately 3 days, as dark in color. Recently she discovered a lump in the same (right) breast. She has no family history of breast cancer, and her menstrual periods began at 13 years of age. On examination, you find "lumpy," diffusely tender breasts bilaterally, as well as a 1-cm movable mass in the right outer/upper quadrant of the right breast. There is no skin dimpling.

1. Which of the following conditions is the most likely cause of the nipple discharge?

(A) Fibroadenoma
(B) Fibrocystic change
(C) Mastitis
(D) Intraductal carcinoma
(E) Intraductal papilloma

2. Which of the following options regarding management of the nipple discharge would you recommend?

(A) Cytologic studies
(B) Culture studies
(C) Mammography
(D) Excisional biopsy
(E) Reexamination in 2 to 4 weeks

3. Which of the following conditions is the most likely cause of the breast mass?

(A) Fibroadenoma
(B) Lobular carcinoma in situ
(C) Fibrocystic change
(D) Adenocarcinoma
(E) Ductal carcinoma in situ

4. Which of the following procedures for management of the breast mass would you recommend?

(A) Mammography
(B) Excisional biopsy
(C) Fine needle aspiration
(D) Incisional biopsy
(E) Reexamination in 2 to 4 weeks

5. The same woman returns to your clinic 1 year later, while in town visiting her sister. Her primary complaint is lower back pain. She reports the presence of a lump in her other (left) breast that has been unchanged for the past 3 months. On examination you find a 1-cm, smooth, mobile, marble-like, nontender mass. Which of the following procedures do you recommend?

(A) Ultrasound
(B) Mammography
(C) Aspiration
(D) Excisional biopsy
(E) Reexamination in 2 to 4 weeks

Setting: Hospital

Questions 6–9

An 11-year-old girl, who has been healthy, is admitted to the hospital after 2 days of polyuria, polydipsia, nausea, vomiting, and abdominal pain. On admission, her vital signs are temperature, 37°C; blood pressure, 100/62 mm Hg; heart rate, 110 beats/minute; and respirations, 30/minute. Physical examination reveals a lethargic girl in no distress, but, with poor skin turgor and mild, diffuse, abdominal tenderness to deep palpation. Bowel sounds are normal, and no rebound or guarding is apparent. The remainder of the physical examination is within normal limits. Laboratory studies reveal:

Glucose	534 mg/dL
Electrolytes	
Sodium	137 mEq/L
Potassium	5.9 mEq/L
Bicarbonate	8 mEq/L
Chloride	100 mEq/L
White blood cell (WBC) count	16,000/mm^3
Arterial blood gas analysis	
pH	7.13
P_{CO_2}	20 mm Hg
P_{O_2}	90 mm Hg

6. During treatment with intravenous fluids and insulin, which of the following electrolyte disturbances is most likely to occur?

(A) Hyperkalemia
(B) Hypokalemia
(C) Hyperphosphatemia
(D) Hypercalcemia
(E) Hypocalcemia

7. To ensure improvement in the girl's condition, which of the following parameters is the most appropriate to monitor?

(A) Anion gap
(B) Serum bicarbonate
(C) Urinary ketones
(D) Serum glucose
(E) Serum ketones

8. After receiving an intravenous insulin infusion and intravenous fluids, the girl initially improves. However, 3 hours after her arrival, she begins to complain of severe muscle pain, weakness, and shortness of breath. Which of the following conditions most likely explains this development?

(A) Hypocalcemia
(B) Hypokalemia
(C) Hypophosphatemia
(D) Hypoglycemia
(E) Metabolic alkalosis

9. For the first 9 hours of therapy, the girl received 3 L of normal saline, followed by 5,500 mL of 0.5 normal saline with 20 mEq/L of potassium chloride. Her electrolyte abnormalities have resolved, and her anion gap has decreased from 29 to 15. She is now complaining of a severe diffuse headache, and she becomes stuporous within minutes. Which of the following interventions is most appropriate?

(A) Emergent head computed tomography (CT) scan
(B) Intravenous mannitol infusion
(C) Intravenous naloxone
(D) Aspirin
(E) Intravenous heparin

Setting: Emergency Department

Questions 10–12

A 33-year-old African American woman, who is G_4P_3 at 36 weeks' gestation, presents with complaints of worsening shortness of breath and fatigue of 2 weeks' duration. She has noticed swelling in her legs and exacerbation of the dyspnea when she lies flat. On examination, you detect an extra heart sound following S_2 at the apex, jugular venous distension, and bilateral basilar rales.

10. Which of the following factors is NOT a risk factor for the disease that is the most likely diagnosis?

(A) Race
(B) Multiparity
(C) Multiple gestations
(D) First pregnancy
(E) Third trimester of pregnancy

11. Which of the following tests, if abnormal, most likely supports the diagnosis?

(A) Complete blood count (CBC)
(B) Chest radiograph
(C) Echocardiogram
(D) Lower extremity ultrasound
(E) Ventilation-perfusion ($\dot{V}/\dot{Q}$) scan

12. In the process of making your diagnosis, you learn that a screening test for a particular condition has a specificity of 85%. Which of the following statements concerning this test is true?

(A) It has a 15% false-negative rate
(B) It misses only 15% of cases
(C) If it is positive, 85% of tested individuals have the condition
(D) 85% of patients with the condition have a positive test result
(E) 85% of individuals without the condition have a negative test result

Setting: Satellite Clinic

Questions 13–14

A 6-year-old boy is brought to the clinic by his parents who are concerned about possible lead poisoning. Since the age of 3, their son has played at the home of a friend at which lead paint has recently been discovered. The boy has no medical history.

13. Which of the following symptoms is NOT expected in lead poisoning?

(A) Nausea and vomiting
(B) Ataxia
(C) Headaches
(D) Crampy, abdominal pain
(E) Cyanosis

14. Which of the following laboratory abnormalities is NOT present with lead poisoning?

(A) Basophilic stippling on the peripheral smear
(B) Proteinuria
(C) Microcytic anemia
(D) Elevated alkaline phosphatase
(E) Elevated erythrocyte protoporphyrin

Setting: Emergency Department

Questions 15–18

A 47-year-old man with a history of depression, alcohol abuse, and hypertension is transported to the emergency department (ED) after a suicide attempt.

15. Which of the following historical findings is NOT typical?

(A) Family history of suicide
(B) Use of a pistol in the suicide attempt
(C) Employment as a physician
(D) Low socioeconomic class
(E) A previous suicide attempt

16. Which of the following options is the next management step?

(A) Hospitalization
(B) Immediate initiation of a selective serotonin reuptake inhibitor
(C) Electroconvulsive therapy
(D) Discharge, if the patient has good social support
(E) Outpatient group therapy

17. When family members arrive, they claim that the man swallowed most of the tablets from a bottle of acetaminophen 4 to 10 hours ago. Which of the following measures is the next most appropriate step?

(A) Dialysis
(B) Waiting for an acetaminophen level
(C) *N*-Acetylcysteine administration
(D) Sodium bicarbonate administration
(E) Phenytoin loading

18. All of the following agents/conditions are likely to exacerbate acetaminophen toxicity EXCEPT

(A) chronic alcoholism
(B) malnutrition
(C) phenobarbital
(D) cimetidine
(E) isoniazid

Setting: Office

Questions 19–21

A 67-year-old man comes for an initial visit. He has a history of hyperlipidemia; hypertension; coronary artery disease, with a three-vessel coronary artery bypass graft 3 years ago; and peripheral vascular disease. On examination, an abdominal mass is evident. Computed tomography (CT) of the abdomen is necessary.

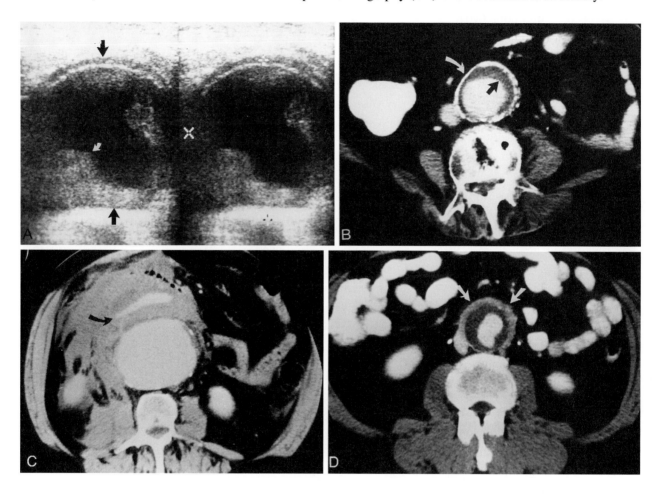

19. The mass is likely to be located between which of the following two structures?

(A) The celiac trunk and the superior mesenteric artery
(B) The inferior mesenteric artery and the aortic bifurcation
(C) The phrenic arteries and the celiac trunk
(D) The superior mesenteric artery and the renal arteries
(E) The superior mesenteric artery and the inferior mesenteric artery

20. For a 6-cm aneurysm, the next most appropriate step is

(A) clinical follow-up
(B) surgical repair
(C) serial ultrasound
(D) angiography
(E) magnetic resonance imaging (MRI)

21. Which of the following conditions is the most common cause of death after elective, abdominal, aortic aneurysm (AAA) repair?

(A) Renal failure
(B) Multiple organ failure
(C) Acute respiratory distress syndrome (ARDS)
(D) Myocardial infarction (MI)
(E) Cerebrovascular accident

Setting: Office

22. A 7-year-old boy with hereditary anemia is brought to the clinic with low-grade fever, lethargy, and shortness of breath. His peripheral blood smear (*below*) is typical of this type of anemia.

A complete blood count (CBC) yields the following values:

Hemoglobin	3 g/dL
Reticulocyte count	1.6%
White blood cell (WBC) count	6,000 cells/mm^3, with 75% neutrophils, 20% lymphocytes
Platelet count	310,000/mm^3

Which of the following conditions is the most likely diagnosis?
(A) Iron deficiency anemia
(B) Splenic sequestration syndrome
(C) Aplastic crisis
(D) β-Thalassemia
(E) Hemolytic crisis

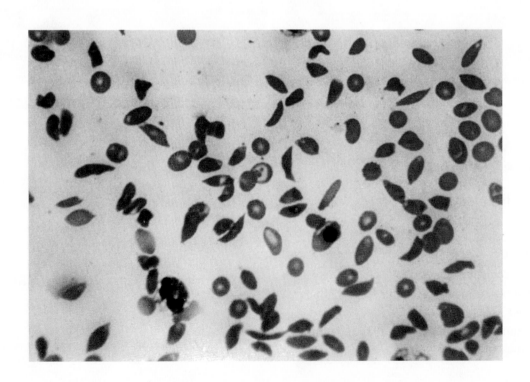

Setting: Emergency Department

Questions 23–29

A 34-year-old woman, who is G_4P_4, complains of abdominal pain. She has a history of asthma, tobacco and alcohol abuse, and sexually transmitted disease. She had a cholecystectomy 8 months ago and a tubal ligation after the birth of her fourth child. On examination, the pain is primarily located in the right lower quadrant; it increases when a hand is quickly removed from the abdomen. The patient has a positive Rovsing sign.

23. Which of the following tests/procedures is most appropriate to conduct next?

(A) Abdominal radiograph (plain film)
(B) Serum β-human chorionic gonadotropin (β-hCG) test
(C) Ultrasound
(D) Complete blood count (CBC)
(E) Pelvic examination

24. All of the following conditions are common in extrauterine pregnancy EXCEPT

(A) abdominal pain
(B) vaginal bleeding
(C) amenorrhea
(D) dizziness
(E) nausea

25. All of the following factors increase the risk of an ectopic pregnancy EXCEPT

(A) increased age
(B) history of salpingitis
(C) history of ectopic pregnancy
(D) oral contraceptive use
(E) African American race

26. The most common location of an extrauterine pregnancy is the

(A) isthmus
(B) ampulla
(C) interstitium
(D) fimbria
(E) peritoneum

27. Which of the following conditions is NOT an indication for admission in the setting of pelvic inflammatory disease (PID)?

(A) Tubo-ovarian abscess
(B) Patient noncompliance
(C) Pregnancy
(D) Ileus
(E) Temperature >38°C

28. Which of the following findings is least sensitive in supporting the diagnosis of appendicitis?

(A) Leukocytosis
(B) Rebound tenderness
(C) Fever
(D) Vomiting
(E) None of the above responses

29. Which of the following findings would you expect on abdominal radiography in the setting of a mechanical, small bowel obstruction?

(A) Dilated loops of bowel with continuous circular folds
(B) Dilated loops of bowel with evidence of haustra
(C) Dilated loops of bowel with air in the rectum
(D) A "sentinel" dilated loop of bowel
(E) Air beneath the diaphragm on an upright chest radiograph

Setting: Office

Questions 30–34

A 53-year-old woman comes in for a routine annual examination. Her complaints are occasional sweating and a sensation of warmth. She has a history of hypothyroidism and mild depression. Her current medications include L-thyroxine and fluoxetine.

30. On further questioning, you may discover which of the following additional complaints?

(A) Increased vaginal secretions
(B) Palpitations
(C) Urinary incontinence
(D) Tremor
(E) Weight loss

31. Which of the following estrogens is predominant at this time in the woman's life?

(A) Androstenedione
(B) Estradiol
(C) Estrone
(D) Estriol
(E) Estrane

32. Measurement of which of the following substances would most likely support the diagnosis?

(A) Thyroid-stimulating hormone (TSH)
(B) Follicle-stimulating hormone (FSH) and luteinizing hormone (LH)
(C) Urinary catecholamines
(D) Free thyroxine (T_4)
(E) β-Human chorionic gonadotropin (β-hCG)

33. Which of the following treatments would be most appropriate at this time?

(A) Increased thyroid replacement
(B) Conjugated estrogens
(C) Aromatase inhibitors
(D) Propylthiouracil (PTU)
(E) Tamoxifen

34. Which of the following factors would put the patient at increased risk for osteoporosis?

(A) Late menopause
(B) Obesity
(C) Multiparity
(D) Early menarche
(E) Cigarette smoking

Setting: Office

35. In the dark, a patient's right pupil is 3 mm greater in diameter than the left pupil. In bright light, the right pupil is only 1 mm larger than the left pupil. Which of the following nervous system pathways contains the lesion?

(A) Afferent sympathetic
(B) Efferent sympathetic
(C) Afferent parasympathetic
(D) Efferent parasympathetic
(E) None of the above responses

Setting: Office

Questions 36–37

A 4-year-old girl presents with several days of worsening lower extremity and facial edema. Her parents have noted that she has worsening fatigue, some mild diarrhea, and loss of appetite. Except for multiple food allergies, her medical history is unremarkable. Physical examination reveals a blood pressure of 100/60 mm Hg and periorbital and lower extremity edema. The remainder of the examination is within normal limits. Laboratory tests reveal:

Serum chemistries	Within normal limits
Serum albumin	2.5 g/dL
Complete blood count (CBC)	Within normal limits
Urinalysis	4+ proteinuria
	No red blood cells (RBCs)
	No white blood cells (WBCs)

36. The most appropriate therapy would be

(A) cyclosporine
(B) prednisone
(C) chlorambucil
(D) methotrexate
(E) azathioprine

37. Which of the following organisms would pose the greatest risk of life-threatening infection (before treatment)?

(A) Cytomegalovirus
(B) *Pneumocystis carinii*
(C) Hepatitis B virus
(D) *Streptococcus pneumoniae*
(E) *Candida albicans*

Setting: Office

38. A 13-month-old male infant is brought in for a routine checkup. His mother reports that he has not been eating as much as usual and is somewhat less active than usual. Otherwise, she has no complaints. On physical examination, the infant is alert and interactive, with language and motor skills appropriate for his age. Chest and cardiac examinations are within normal limits. Abdominal examination indicates a large mass on the left side. The mass is deep and firm, and its margins are not palpable. Laboratory tests, including a complete blood count (CBC) and chemistries, are within normal limits. A CT scan of the abdomen is ordered. Which of the following diagnoses is most likely?

(A) Wilms tumor
(B) Splenic rupture
(C) Hodgkin disease
(D) Leukemic infiltration
(E) Meckel diverticulum

Setting: Office

Questions 39–46

A 58-year-old man with a history of alcoholism, tobacco abuse, and hypertension presents to a general surgery clinic, where he has been referred for further workup of blood in his stool. He reports occasional abdominal pain that is relieved transiently with food; one episode of vomiting occurred with the pain. Recently, his stools have been black. His medications include hydrochlorothiazide and a multivitamin. Examination reveals a few spider angioma, but no palmar erythema, gynecomastia, or hepatosplenomegaly.

39. Which of the following conditions represents the most likely cause of the man's bleeding?

(A) Esophageal varices
(B) Duodenal ulcer
(C) Mallory-Weiss tear
(D) Angiodysplasia
(E) Diverticulosis

40. On leaving, the man complains of difficulty with his "privates." Further discussion reveals erectile dysfunction. All of the following interventions are necessary in evaluating or treating this complaint EXCEPT

(A) alcohol cessation
(B) testosterone level
(C) diabetes screening
(D) prolactin level
(E) follicle-stimulating hormone (FSH) and luteinizing hormone (LH) levels

41. At a later date, the man begins taking sildenafil, which acts most directly on which of the following substances?

(A) Cyclic adenosine monophosphate (cAMP)
(B) Acetylcholine
(C) Norepinephrine
(D) Cyclic guanosine monophosphate (cGMP)
(E) Nitric oxide

42. Six weeks later, the man calls the office asking for an immediate appointment; this time, concerning ankle pain. On examination, the ankle is red, swollen, and extremely tender to even light touch. The patient is afebrile and otherwise unchanged. Which of the following procedures/modes of treatment is the next most appropriate step?

(A) Joint aspiration
(B) Radiography
(C) Colchicine
(D) Uric acid level
(E) Antibiotics

43. All of the following adjunctive measures may help EXCEPT

(A) smoking cessation
(B) alcohol cessation
(C) medication change
(D) steroid therapy
(E) nonsteroidal anti-inflammatory drugs (NSAIDs)

44. Three months later, the man presents to the ED with bright red blood per rectum. His blood pressure is 110/80 mm Hg supine and 85/60 mm Hg sitting. Laboratory studies reveal:

White blood cell (WBC) count	8,000/mm^3
Hemoglobin	11.5 g/dL
Hematocrit	34%
Platelet count	102,000/mm^3
Mean corpuscular volume	90 fL

Which of the following conditions is probably present?

(A) Esophageal perforation
(B) Variceal hemorrhage
(C) Gastroduodenal artery bleeding
(D) Arteriovenous malformation
(E) Diverticular hemorrhage

45. The man undergoes surgery. Two weeks later, he complains of sweating, dizziness, palpitations, and abdominal pain after meals. Which of the following conditions is the most likely explanation?

(A) Malabsorption
(B) Dumping syndrome
(C) Short-bowel syndrome
(D) Afferent loop syndrome
(E) Gastroparesis

46. Which of the following treatments would you recommend for these complaints?

(A) Billroth I conversion
(B) Roux-en-Y anastomosis
(C) Vagotomy
(D) Octreotide
(E) Dietary changes

Setting: Emergency Department

Questions 47–49

A 9-year-old girl has become increasingly weak during the past 48 hours. Initially, her hands and feet felt heavy, but the girl states she now has trouble lifting her legs and is unable to lift her arms to brush her hair. Recently, she was ill with crampy abdominal pain with associated nausea, vomiting, and diarrhea for 5 days. The symptoms resolved approximately 9 days ago. Along with weakness, she has been complaining of tingling and burning in her feet. She denies any difficulty breathing. Except for her recent illness, she has been healthy. Physical examination reveals an ill-appearing girl in no acute distress and the following findings:

Vital signs	Temperature: 37°C
	Blood pressure: 100/65 mm Hg
	Heart rate: 110/min
	Respiratory rate: 12/min
Oropharynx	Normal
Chest	Clear to auscultation
Heart	Regular rate and rhythm; no murmurs
Abdomen	Soft; normal bowel sounds; no organomegaly
Neurologic	Cranial nerves II–XII: within normal limits
	Motor: 4/5 proximal upper and lower extremity weakness with 3/5 distal upper and lower extremity weakness
	Deep tendon reflexes: absent
	Sensory: within normal limits to pinprick
	Anal sphincter tone: normal

47. Which of the following conditions should NOT be considered in the differential diagnosis of this patient?

(A) Guillain-Barré syndrome
(B) Tick paralysis
(C) Porphyria
(D) Neuroblastoma
(E) Poliomyelitis

48. Which of the following cerebrospinal fluid (CSF) patterns are most characteristic of Guillain-Barré syndrome?

	White Blood Cells (WBCs)	Red Blood Cells (RBCs)	Protein	Glucose
(A)	Elevated	Elevated	Elevated	Decreased
(B)	Normal	Normal	Elevated	Normal
(C)	Normal	Elevated	Elevated	Normal
(D)	Elevated	Normal	Elevated	Normal
(E)	Elevated	Normal	Elevated	Decreased

49. Several hours later, the girl begins to complain of shortness of breath, and a bedside vital capacity reveals a significant decline in ventilatory muscle strength. Which of the following treatments is most appropriate?

(A) Plasmapheresis
(B) Cyclophosphamide
(C) Prednisone
(D) Broad-spectrum antibiotics
(E) Cyclosporine

Setting: Satellite Clinic

Questions 50–52

You are evaluating a new serum diagnostic test for Lyme disease that claims a sensitivity of 90% and a specificity of 95%. In the late spring, the prevalence of Lyme disease is 10% in the study of patients who present with fever, arthralgias, and rash.

50. If you use this test in 100 patients, false-negative results will occur in how many patients?

(A) 1
(B) 9
(C) 10
(D) 40
(E) 45

51. For this test, which of the following percentages is the positive predictive value (i.e., if the test is positive, what percentage of patients actually have the disease)?

(A) 33%
(B) 67%
(C) 90%
(D) 95%
(E) 99%

52. If the prevalence of the disease increases to 50%, and a patient has a positive test, the new positive predictive value is

(A) 33%
(B) 67%
(C) 90%
(D) 95%
(E) 100%

Setting: Office

Questions 53–58

A 47-year-old woman, who has not been to see you in approximately 2 years, comes in for a routine examination. She has been "surfing" the Internet, where she has found recent American Cancer Society recommendations for annual screening mammography. A friend of hers recently died from breast cancer.

53. The woman asks you, "If I have breast cancer, what is the chance that a screening mammogram will detect it?" Which of the following test characteristics do you discuss with her?

(A) Specificity
(B) Positive predictive value
(C) Sensitivity
(D) Odds ratio
(E) Negative predictive value

54. The woman has a background in mathematics. She asks about the effectiveness of a mammogram. You give her the example of a test with a sensitivity of 90% and specificity of 75%. What is the positive predictive value of this test?

(A) 10%
(B) 25%
(C) 75%
(D) 90%
(E) Cannot be determined

55. Which of the following statements regarding mammography is true?

(A) Adipose tissue appears dark
(B) It is more sensitive in premenopausal patients
(C) Lobular carcinoma in situ is readily apparent
(D) Malignancy appears dark
(E) Glandular tissue appears dark

56. Toward the end of your conversation, the woman starts to cry. Apparently, the loss of her friend has upset her severely. She has had significant anhedonia, feels that her support system is gone, and has had spontaneous crying spells. She is having difficulty working and sleeping. Which of the following responses is best?

(A) "Call me any time if you need help"
(B) "Try to keep busy with friends and family"
(C) "We'll do the mammogram today if it will make you feel better"
(D) "Have you considered taking your own life?"
(E) "We should meet again tomorrow to see how you are doing"

57. In addition to counseling, you consider using medication. Which of the following agents is most appropriate?

(A) Amitriptyline hydrochloride
(B) Paroxetine
(C) Haloperidol
(D) Buspirone hydrochloride
(E) Clozapine

58. Which of the following side effects is most likely to occur with selective serotonin reuptake inhibitors?

(A) Dry mouth
(B) Diaphoresis
(C) Urinary retention
(D) Weight loss
(E) Anorgasmia

Setting: Office

59. A 9-year-old girl with nearly persistent complaints of sinus pain and purulent nasal discharge is referred to you for evaluation of recurrent pneumonia and sinus infection. She has received treatment for three to four episodes of pneumonia per year during the past 2 years. Her primary physician became worried when the girl developed hemoptysis that resolved spontaneously during her last bout of pneumonia. The girl has had the recent onset of multiple, loose, foul-smelling, bowel movements a day. During the past year, she missed significant amounts of school, and she has not participated in physical education because of severe fatigue and shortness of breath. She uses an albuterol inhaler and a saline nasal spray, and takes loratadine tablets 10 mg once a day.

Physical examination reveals a chronically ill-appearing, thin girl. Chest examination indicates diffuse rhonchi with scattered wheezes. The right maxillary sinus is tender to percussion, with a single, right, nasal polyp. You strongly suspect a certain diagnosis and order the appropriate laboratory tests. Which of the following statements concerning the girl's condition is true?

(A) Inheritance is autosomally dominant
(B) Boys have normal fertility
(C) Liver disease, including cirrhosis, is the most common manifestation
(D) Kidney stones consisting of calcium oxalate may be present
(E) Meconium ileus occurs in nearly all affected infants

Setting: Emergency Department

Questions 60–61

A 15-year-old boy presents with several days of a severe sore throat, fevers, and generalized malaise. He has no significant medical history and denies drug use and sexual activity. On physical examination, he is ill-appearing, with a temperature of 39.5°C and a blood pressure of 96/50 mm Hg. A diffuse exudate on both tonsils is present, with a petechial rash at the junction of the hard and soft palate. Shotty, tender, cervical lymphadenopathy is evident. The chest and cardiovascular examination is normal. Palpable splenomegaly, normal bowel sounds, and mild hepatomegaly are evident. Laboratory studies reveal:

White blood cell (WBC) count	12,000/mm^3 (50% neutrophils, 12% monocytes, 38% lymphocytes)
Aspartate aminotransferase (AST)	Twice upper limit of normal
Serum chemistries	Normal
Rapid pharyngeal streptococcal screen	Negative

60. To confirm the likely diagnosis, which of the following studies is the next appropriate test?

(A) Hepatitis panel
(B) Ultrasound of the spleen
(C) Examination of the peripheral smear to investigate for leukemia
(D) Heterophile antibody screen
(E) Human immunodeficiency virus (HIV) antibody test

61. Which of the following conditions is NOT a possible complication?

(A) Splenic rupture

(B) Guillain-Barré syndrome

(C) Jaundice

(D) Diffuse maculopapular rash after treatment with ampicillin

(E) Increased risk of hepatocellular carcinoma

Setting: Office

Questions 62–66

A 65-year-old obese woman, with a history of hypertension, diabetes mellitus, cigarette smoking, and depression, presents for routine follow-up. Her medications include pentoxifylline, aspirin, hydrochlorothiazide, metformin, sertraline, and insulin. Her last glycosylated hemoglobin was 9.2%. Her complaints today are vague epigastric pain and new, low back pain. She has no fever, weight loss, diarrhea, or other complaints.

62. Which of the following physical findings is most diagnostic?

(A) Murphy sign

(B) Dullness to percussion at the left lung base

(C) Costovertebral angle tenderness

(D) Pulsatile abdominal mass

(E) Iliopsoas sign

63. Which of the following diagnostic tests is indicated?

(A) Angiogram

(B) CT scan

(C) Ultrasound

(D) Intravenous pyelogram

(E) Chest radiograph

64. Which of the following health maintenance procedures would you recommend?

(A) Ophthalmologic examination every 3 to 5 years

(B) Pneumococcal vaccine every 4 to 6 years

(C) Urine test for microalbumin

(D) Mammogram every 2 years

(E) Flexible sigmoidoscopy every 10 years

65. Which of the following drugs might prove a better blood pressure medication for this woman?

(A) Captopril

(B) Nifedipine

(C) Propranolol hydrochloride

(D) Verapamil

(E) Diltiazem hydrochloride

66. Based on the recommendations of the Sixth Report of the Joint National Committee on Detection, Evaluation and Treatment of High Blood Pressure (JNC VI) and without the results of further laboratory tests, this woman's blood pressure (in mm Hg) should be

(A) <125/75

(B) <130/85

(C) <140/85

(D) <140/90

(E) <150/90

Setting: Emergency Department

Questions 67–71

A 24-year-old man, with a history of bipolar disorder, is brought to the hospital by a friend who found him lying on his bathroom floor with vomitus on his clothing. She reports that he has been particularly agitated lately. He is afebrile, with a blood pressure of 160/85 mm Hg, a heart rate of 95 beats/minute, and respiratory rate of 16/minute. On examination, he has difficulty walking and has a mild tremor. He is alert but confused.

67. Which of the following statements regarding bipolar disorder is true?

(A) There is no known familial disposition
(B) Depressive episodes predominate in youth; mania predominates in adulthood
(C) Women experience more severe mania than men
(D) Alcohol use occurs in >50% of cases
(E) Onset at 40 to 50 years of age is average

68. After further questioning, which of the following conditions would you be most surprised to discover?

(A) Occasional delusions
(B) Excessive sleepiness
(C) Recent unrestrained spending
(D) Suicidal ideation
(E) Lower socioeconomic status

69. Which of the following conditions is the likely cause of this man's presenting symptoms?

(A) Subdural hematoma
(B) Hypernatremia
(C) Hypocalcemia
(D) Medication toxicity
(E) Status epilepticus

70. Which of the following studies is least important at this time?

(A) Electrocardiogram (ECG)
(B) Carbamazepine level
(C) Blood chemistry
(D) Lithium level
(E) Arterial blood gas measurements

71. Which of the following ECG findings is most characteristic of carbamazepine toxicity?

(A) QRS duration of 0.160 msec
(B) PR interval of 0.210 msec
(C) Peaked T waves
(D) QT interval of 310 msec
(E) ST elevation

Setting: Office

Questions 72–73

A 32-year-old healthy woman presents with a bloody discharge from her left nipple of 2 weeks' duration. Initially, the discharge was clear but, recently, it has become bloody. The patient, who performs monthly breast self-examinations, has never felt a mass. Currently, she does not feel anything in the left breast that seems abnormal. Her family history is negative for any malignancies. She is taking no medications. On physical examination, the breasts are symmetrical, and no dimpling or retraction of the skin is apparent. No abnormalities are palpable in either breast; only a scant, clear discharge can be expressed from the left nipple. There is no lymphadenopathy.

72. Your next step should be

(A) referral to a surgeon for exploration
(B) ultrasound of the left breast
(C) reassurance, with routine breast cancer surveillance
(D) mammography
(E) obtaining a sample of the bloody fluid for cytology

73. The most likely diagnosis is

(A) breast carcinoma
(B) fibroadenoma
(C) mastitis
(D) fat necrosis
(E) intraductal papilloma

Setting: Hospital

Questions 74–75

A 45-year-old man, who is infected with HIV, is admitted to your service with 1 week of headaches and difficulty performing his activities of daily living. He reports poor control of the use of his left hand, and he feels as if he no longer knows how to dress himself. In addition, he has trouble remembering things. His medical history is significant for an episode of *Pneumocystis carinii* pneumonia 6 weeks ago and recurrent herpes zoster. At present, he is taking trimethoprim-sulfamethoxazole; he has decided against antiretroviral therapy.

Physical examination reveals a cachectic man in no acute distress. Results indicate:

Vital signs	Temperature: 37.6°C
	Blood pressure: 100/65 mm Hg
	Heart rate: 100 beats/min
	Respirations: 20/min
Oropharynx	Thrush
Chest	Clear to auscultation
Heart	Regular rate, no murmurs
Abdomen	No masses, nontender, normal bowel sounds
Neurologic	Left-sided hemiparesis with weakness greater in arm than leg
	Left-sided homonymous hemianopsia with left-sided neglect

74. You order a CT scan of the brain with contrast. While waiting for the scan result, your medical student asks you where the lesion is most likely to be. Your answer is the

(A) right parietal lobe
(B) left parietal lobe
(C) right internal capsule
(D) right mid-pons
(E) right occipital cortex

75. The CT scan reveals a ring-enhancing lesion in the brain. All of the following are possible causes for this lesion EXCEPT

(A) toxoplasmosis
(B) lymphoma
(C) bacterial abscess
(D) progressive multifocal leukoencephalopathy
(E) metastatic cancer

Setting: Hospital

Questions 76–79

76. You are asked to see a patient for gastrointestinal (GI) bleeding on postoperative day 1 after repair of an abdominal aortic aneurysm (AAA). Which of the following conditions represents the likely cause?

(A) Diverticulosis
(B) Gastric ulcer
(C) Angiodysplasia
(D) Colonic ischemia
(E) Stress gastritis

77. What is the diagnostic study of choice?

(A) Esophagogastroduodenoscopy
(B) Barium enema
(C) Colonoscopy
(D) CT of the abdomen
(E) Upper GI series

78. During this episode of severe GI bleeding, serious hypotension developed, and the patient underwent a significant decline in mental status. In which of the following locations might you expect CT findings?

(A) Bilateral cortex
(B) Brainstem
(C) Cerebellum
(D) Internal capsule
(E) Basal ganglia

79. Which of the following criteria is NOT required for confirmation of brain death?

(A) Absence of sedative drug intoxication
(B) Six hours of absent brain function with a confirmatory flat electroencephalogram (EEG)
(C) Presence of pupillary reflexes
(D) Normothermia
(E) Unresponsiveness to sensory input

Setting: Emergency Department

80. You are asked to evaluate a 14-month-old female infant who has become lethargic during the past 4 hours. Her parents state that she has a fever (temperature, 40°C) and a rash. She has no medical history and has reached all appropriate growth and developmental milestones. On examination, her anterior fontanelle feels full, and a diffuse petechial rash is evident. The most appropriate initial step is

(A) administration of acetaminophen
(B) administration of antibiotics and dexamethasone
(C) blood culture followed by immediate administration of antibiotics
(D) blood culture and lumbar puncture
(E) dermatologic consult for biopsy of the skin lesions

Setting: Emergency Department

81. A 3-year-old girl, recently emigrated from Russia, is brought to the ED by her foster parents after the abrupt onset of a fever (temperature to 40°C), respiratory distress, and stridor. On examination, the girl appears acutely ill. She is sitting, leaning forward with her mouth open, and drooling. Her foster parents do not know her medical history. Which of the following therapeutic steps is most appropriate initially?

(A) Obtain lateral neck views with plain radiography
(B) Culture the oropharynx and then begin intravenous antibiotics
(C) Give racemic epinephrine by inhalation
(D) Administer intravenous corticosteroids and intravenous third-generation cephalosporin
(E) Administer emergent intubation and intravenous third-generation cephalosporin

Setting: Satellite Clinic

Questions 82–84

A 34-year-old woman, who is G_3P_2, presents to the clinic with complaints of jitteriness and nervousness. On examination, her reflexes are mildly increased diffusely. Laboratory studies reveal:

Hemoglobin	11.5 g/dL
Hematocrit	34%
Platelet count	350,000/mm³
Thyroxine, total (T_4)	15 μg/dL

82. Which of the following procedures/treatments is the most appropriate next step?

(A) Start methimazole
(B) Start propylthiouracil (PTU)
(C) Order triiodothyronine (T_3) resin uptake
(D) Order thyroid uptake scans
(E) Radioactive ablation

83. Which of the following disorders is the most common cause of thyrotoxicosis in pregnancy?

(A) Subacute thyroiditis
(B) Hydatidiform mole
(C) Thyrotoxicosis factitia
(D) Toxic diffuse goiter
(E) Choriocarcinoma

84. Which of the following changes would be most consistent with the diagnosis of choriocarcinoma?

(A) Increased β-human chorionic gonadotropin (β-hCG)
(B) Increased α-fetoprotein (AFP)
(C) Increased thyroid-stimulating hormone (TSH)
(D) Decreased AFP
(E) Decreased thyroxine (T_4)

Setting: Emergency Department

85. A 36-year-old woman with systemic lupus erythematosus has right-sided loss of pain and temperature from the umbilical level downward. The lesion is at which of the following sites?

(A) Left lateral spinothalamic tract at T9
(B) Right lateral spinothalamic tract at T10
(C) Right gracile fasciculus at T10
(D) Left thalamus
(E) Right precentral gyrus

Setting: Emergency Department

Questions 86–88

A 19-year-old man presents for evaluation of a painful right leg after a motorcycle accident approximately 6 hours earlier. He claims that because his leg did not become extremely painful until 30 minutes ago, he did not think it was broken. Radiography indicates the presence of a fracture.

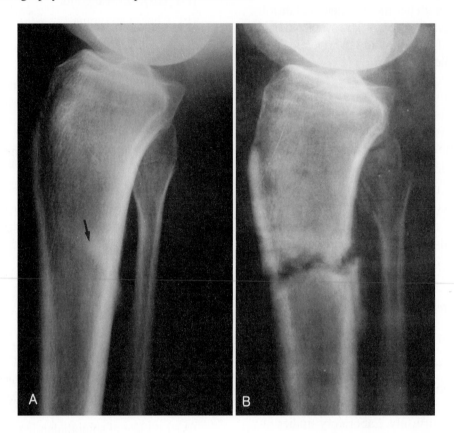

86. Which of the following procedures is the most appropriate next step?

(A) MRI
(B) Ultrasound with Doppler
(C) Blood cultures
(D) Immobilization with casting
(E) Intrafascial pressure measurement

87. Which of the following therapies is the most appropriate treatment?

(A) Embolectomy
(B) Fasciotomy
(C) Antibiotics
(D) Tissue plasminogen activator (tPA)
(E) Hyperbaric oxygen

88. The man's mother voices concern that her son may be abusing alcohol. She asks what the most successful means of cessation might be. Of the following measures, which one should be your answer?

(A) Group therapy
(B) Aversion therapy
(C) Naltrexone
(D) Psychotherapy
(E) Disulfiram

Setting: Office

Questions 89–90

A 33-year-old woman presents with a dry, hacking cough of 6 months' duration. The cough initially began after an upper respiratory tract infection but has never completely improved. It is particularly bad at night and in the early morning. The woman does not complain of rhinorrhea, shortness of breath, fatigue, fevers, or weight loss. Her medical history is significant only for an appendectomy at age 12. Her family history is significant, with lung cancer in her father and maternal grandfather. She does not smoke, and she works as a secretary for a software manufacturer. Over-the-counter cough syrups have provided only minimal relief. The physical examination is within normal limits. The chest radiograph is shown below:

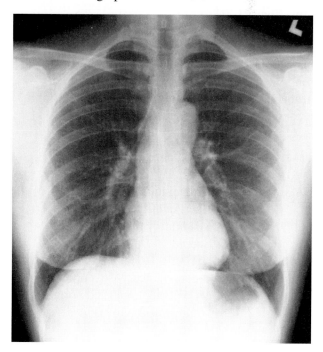

89. Which of the following procedures/modes of therapy would you perform first?

(A) Pulmonary function tests
(B) Chest CT
(C) Purified protein derivative skin testing for tuberculosis exposure
(D) Trial of antihistamine or decongestant with intranasal steroid
(E) Upper endoscopy

90. The woman returns after a 6-week trial of this therapy, reporting no improvement. In fact, she believes that her cough may have worsened. Once again, she has no other complaints other than her cough. Which of the following management steps should be next?

(A) Pulmonary function tests
(B) Chest CT
(C) Purified protein derivative skin testing for tuberculosis exposure
(D) Trial of antihistamine/decongestant with intranasal steroid
(E) Upper endoscopy

Setting: Satellite Clinic

Questions 91–94

A 56-year-old African American woman, with a history of hypertension and diabetes mellitus, presents with complaints of nausea, vomiting, and headache. She has no chest pain or shortness of breath. Examination reveals:

Vital signs	Blood pressure: 185/110 mm Hg
	Temperature: 37.8°C
	Heart rate: 105 beats/min
	Respiratory rate: 18/min
Neck	Supple
Cardiovascular	Tachycardia, with S_4 heart sound; otherwise, normal
Eyes	Mild photophobia and normal movement of eyes in all directions
	Right eye is erythematous and painful, with blurred vision
	Pupil size: right, 3 mm; left, 4 mm
	Pupillary response to light: left > right
Urinalysis	Normal

91. Which of the following physical examination features would you expect to be present in this case?

(A) Kernig sign
(B) Flame-shaped hemorrhages
(C) Pain on light reflex testing
(D) Fixed pupil
(E) Chemosis

92. Which of the following interventions might allow you to make a definitive diagnosis?

(A) Measurement of intracranial pressure
(B) Lumbar puncture
(C) Fluorescein angiography
(D) Pilocarpine drops
(E) Atropine drops

93. Which of the following conditions is the likely diagnosis?

(A) Posterior uveitis
(B) Conjunctivitis
(C) Glaucoma
(D) Hypertensive emergency
(E) Meningitis

94. Which of the following modes of treatment is definitive therapy for this disease?

(A) Antihypertensive agents
(B) Laser surgery
(C) Corticosteroids
(D) Miotic eyedrops
(E) Intravenous antibiotics

Setting: Hospital

Questions 95–98

A 48-year-old woman with a history of intravenous drug abuse has fevers, chills, cough, and pleuritic chest pain of several days' duration. On the morning of admission, she had one episode of hemoptysis. She states that she has recently injected cocaine. Her medical history is significant for multiple admissions for detoxification, multiple skin abscesses, and gonorrhea. Physical examination reveals:

Vital signs	Temperature: 39°C
	Blood pressure: 100/60 mm Hg
	Heart rate: 110 beats/min
	Respiratory rate: 24/min
Chest	Scattered rales but no dullness to percussion and no egophony
Heart	II/VI systolic murmur at lower left sternal border that increases with inspiration
Other notable features	Multiple injection sites on arms without evidence of infection
Chest radiograph	Multiple, bilateral, nodular densities

95. The cardiac murmur is most consistent with

(A) mitral regurgitation
(B) mitral stenosis
(C) aortic stenosis
(D) tricuspid regurgitation
(E) pulmonic insufficiency

96. The organism most likely to be identified from blood cultures is

(A) *Streptococcus viridans*
(B) *Staphylococcus aureus*
(C) *Candida* species
(D) *Coxiella burnetii*
(E) polymicrobial infection

97. After being successfully treated with intravenous antibiotics, the woman is discharged. Two days later, she presents to the ED after having a generalized tonic-clonic seizure. She has a blood pressure of 190/100 mm Hg, a heart rate of 140 beats/minute, and a respiratory rate of 30/minute. After administration of intravenous diazepam, her heart rate is 95 beats/minute with a blood pressure of 170/90 mm Hg. A drug screen performed at admission is most likely to find which of the following substances?

(A) Opiates
(B) Cocaine
(C) Δ-9-Tetrahydrocannabinol
(D) Ethanol
(E) Phencyclidine

98. Which of the following techniques is most likely to aid in producing long-term drug abstinence?

(A) Pharmacologic therapy for drug dependence
(B) Incarceration
(C) Peer assistance groups with psychotherapy
(D) Behavioral modification therapy
(E) Removal of the patient from the current environment

Setting: Office

99. A 5-year-old boy was bitten on his arm by his dog. The dog is a healthy animal that has had all vaccinations. The next day, the boy's parents notice that the area surrounding the bite has become erythematous, painful, and warm. Which of the following antibiotic agents is the best choice in this situation?

(A) Amoxicillin-clavulanate
(B) Penicillin
(C) Metronidazole
(D) Tetracycline
(E) Ciprofloxacin hydrochloride

Setting: Emergency Department

Questions 100–101

An obese 42-year-old man presents with the acute onset of severe pain in the left knee, which seems swollen and red. He states that the pain awakens him from sleep and that severe pain results from the slightest movement or touch. His medical history is significant for obesity, hypertension, and alcohol abuse, and his only current medication is hydrochlorothiazide. On examination, the patient has a temperature of 38°C and a swollen left knee, with surrounding erythema. Because of the severity of the pain, only a limited examination is possible.

100. The most appropriate next management step is

(A) empiric treatment for gout with indomethacin
(B) radiographs of the knee to rule out trauma
(C) ceftriaxone disodium, while routine laboratory work is pending
(D) joint aspiration with Gram's stain and inspection under a polarizing microscope
(E) orthopedic consult in the ED

101. As the result of appropriate treatment, the man's pain improves during the next few days. He now presents to your clinic and wants to know how he can avoid future attacks such as the one he just experienced. The best advice involves

(A) long-term colchicine therapy
(B) long-term use of nonsteroidal anti-inflammatory drugs (NSAIDs)
(C) weight loss and abstinence from alcohol
(D) regular exercise
(E) intra-articular injections of corticosteroids

Setting: Hospital

Questions 102–107

A 4-year-old boy is admitted to the hospital with pallor, fatigue, easy bruising, and fever (temperature to 38.9°C). Physical examination reveals cervical lymphadenopathy, a palpable spleen tip, and petechiae on both lower extremities. He is unable to abduct his right eye. Laboratory analysis includes a peripheral blood smear (*below*). After you make a definitive diagnosis, you initiate treatment. Within 36 hours, the patient complains of numbness and tingling around the mouth.

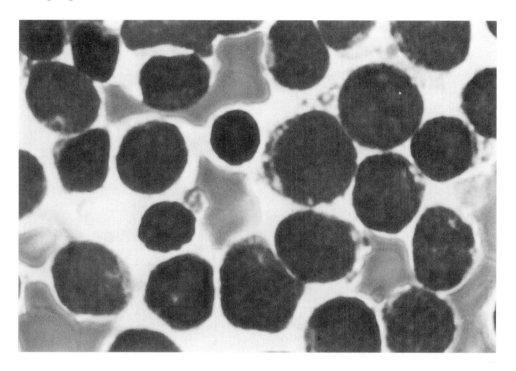

102. What is the diagnosis?

(A) Acute lymphoblastic leukemia
(B) Hairy cell leukemia
(C) Chronic myelogenous leukemia
(D) Acute myelogenous leukemia
(E) Waldenström macroglobulinemia

103. To make the definitive diagnosis, which of the following procedures is necessary?

(A) CT of the abdomen
(B) Bone marrow biopsy
(C) Liver biopsy
(D) Blood cultures
(E) Complete blood count (CBC)

104. Which of the following abnormalities is NOT associated with this disorder or its treatment?

(A) Hypokalemia
(B) Hyperphosphatemia
(C) Hyperuricemia
(D) Hypercalcemia
(E) Hyperkalemia

105. Which of the following prophylactic treatments would have been beneficial?

(A) Probenecid
(B) Allopurinol
(C) Sulfinpyrazone
(D) Acidification of the urine
(E) Colchicine

106. Which of the following agents does this patient need immediately?

(A) Potassium chloride

(B) Sodium phosphate

(C) Magnesium phosphate

(D) Allopurinol

(E) Calcium gluconate

107. An ECG is performed. What changes might be apparent as a result of this patient's treatment?

(A) Short QT interval, wide QRS complex, peaked T waves

(B) Short PR interval, wide QRS complex, peaked T waves

(C) Flattened P wave, wide QRS complex, peaked T waves

(D) Long PR interval, narrow QRS complex, peaked U waves

(E) Long QT interval, wide QRS complex, flat U waves

Setting: Hospital

Questions 108–109

A 63-year-old African American man is having a preoperative evaluation before elective arthroscopy of the shoulder. He has no complaints other than mild dyspnea on extreme exertion and occasional epigastric discomfort, which are easily relieved by antacids. His medical history is notable for mild asthma (forced expiratory volume in 1 second/forced vital capacity [FEV_1/FVC] ratio: 72%) and chronic left shoulder pain. His only medication is an albuterol inhaler, which he uses infrequently. Physical examination and vital signs are within normal limits. Laboratory studies reveal:

Hemoglobin	10 g/dL
Mean corpuscular volume	70 fL
Mean corpuscular hemoglobin concentration	28 g/dL
White blood cell (WBC) count	4,500/mm^3
Platelet count	600,000/mm^3

Analysis also includes a peripheral blood smear (*below*).

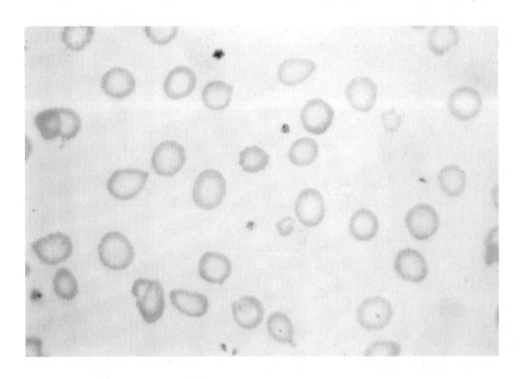

108. The next diagnostic step is

(A) colonoscopy
(B) vitamin B$_{12}$ levels
(C) hemoglobin electrophoresis
(D) reticulocyte count
(E) protoporphyrin levels

109. The man responds to the therapy. Several years later, he complains of numbness and tingling of the feet. Since you have last seen him, his wife has died and he has become a recluse. He states that his appetite is poor and that he "has lost the taste for food." His physical examination is notable for a cachectic man with a depressed affect. Laboratory studies reveal a hemoglobin level of 10 g/dL and a peripheral smear (*below*).

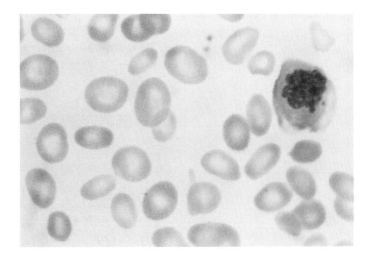

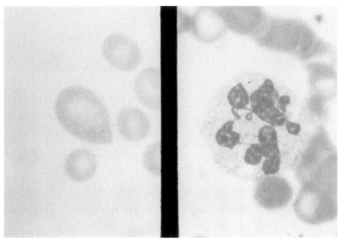

Which of the following features would you expect to find on neurologic examination?
(A) Decreased proximal muscle strength
(B) Slow relaxation phase of the deep tendon reflexes
(C) Decreased vibratory sensation
(D) Restricted peripheral visual fields
(E) Muscle atrophy and decreased tone

Setting: Office

Questions 110–113

A 28-year-old woman, who is G_2P_1 at 26 weeks' gestation, comes to your office for routine care. Her pregnancy has been without complications. She feels consistent fetal movement, has had no contractions, and has experienced no bleeding. She complains of burning chest pain that worsens at night and after meals. Laboratory tests reveal:

Aspartate aminotransferase (AST)	50 U/L
Alanine aminotransferase (ALT)	55 U/L
Alkaline phosphatase	125 U/L
Albumin	3.5 g/dL
CHEM-7	Within normal limits

110. Which of the following steps is the next most appropriate?

(A) Right upper quadrant ultrasound
(B) Esophagogastroduodenoscopy
(C) Reassurance
(D) Endoscopic retrograde pancreaticoduodenoscopy
(E) Computed tomography (CT) of the abdomen

111. Which of the following interventions is advisable at this time?

(A) Cholecystectomy
(B) Dietary changes
(C) Sphincterotomy
(D) Cholestyramine
(E) Omeprazole

112. The woman returns 3 weeks later complaining of occasional shortness of breath. A nurse practitioner performs pulmonary function tests in the office. What changes might you expect?

(A) Increased tidal volume
(B) Decreased minute ventilation
(C) Decreased inspiratory capacity
(D) Increased residual volume
(E) Increased total lung capacity

113. The expected results of arterial blood gas are

	pH	PCO_2 (mm Hg)	PO_2 (mm Hg)	HCO_3 (mEq/L)
(A)	7.30	50	75	20
(B)	7.35	40	90	26
(C)	7.42	36	95	22
(D)	7.46	30	65	28
(E)	7.60	46	85	34

Setting: Office

Questions 114–116

A 23-year-old woman, who is G_1P_0, is screened for gestational diabetes mellitus (GDM).

114. The best time for GDM screening is at

(A) 14 weeks' gestation
(B) 18 weeks' gestation
(C) 22 weeks' gestation
(D) 28 weeks' gestation
(E) 32 weeks' gestation

115. The woman's GDM screening test is positive. A 3-hour glucose tolerance test also yields consistent results. Which of the following series of glucose levels (0-, 1-, 2-, and 3-hour plasma glucose levels after 100 g of Glucola) is consistent with the diagnosis of GDM?

(A) 90, 180, 140, 130 mg/dL
(B) 105, 185, 150, 140 mg/dL
(C) 105, 190, 165, 145 mg/dL
(D) 105, 205, 160, 140 mg/dL
(E) 130, 185, 170, 145 mg/dL

116. All of the following statements regarding GDM are true EXCEPT

(A) there is an increased risk for respiratory distress syndrome
(B) there is no increased risk of postpartum diabetes mellitus for the mother if the GDM is well controlled
(C) there is increased risk for neonatal hypoglycemia
(D) there is increased risk for polyhydramnios
(E) there is no increased risk of spontaneous abortion if GDM is well controlled

Setting: Emergency Department

Questions 117–122

A 22-year-old woman presents with complaints of difficulty climbing stairs. On review of symptoms, she reports a recent fever with diarrhea after a family picnic, as well as headache and occasional depression. On examination, decreased lower extremity reflexes bilaterally and lower extremity weakness are present.

117. Lumbar puncture is likely to find a(an)

(A) elevated white blood cell (WBC) count
(B) decreased glucose
(C) oligoclonal bands
(D) elevated protein
(E) decreased protein

118. Nerve conduction studies are likely to find

(A) shortened F-wave latencies
(B) decreased conduction velocity
(C) decreased amplitude
(D) muscle grouping
(E) smaller motor units

119. The likely cause of the woman's diarrhea is

(A) *Staphylococcus aureus*
(B) *Vibrio parahaemolyticus*
(C) *Shigella sonnei*
(D) *Campylobacter jejuni*
(E) *Salmonella typhi*

120. Which of the following modes of therapy is the treatment of choice?

(A) Intravenous immunoglobulin
(B) Plasmapheresis
(C) Corticosteroids
(D) Antibiotics
(E) Riluzole

121. You are called to see the woman about mild dyspnea. The most useful study is

(A) peak flow
(B) chest radiography
(C) vital capacity
(D) ventilation-perfusion ($\dot{V}/\dot{Q}$) scan
(E) minute ventilation

122. Several hours later, you are called to the woman's bedside to evaluate a decline in mental status. During the evaluation, an arterial blood gas is performed. Which of the following results would you expect?

	pH	P_{CO_2} (mm Hg)	P_{O_2} (mm Hg)
(A)	7.08	80	45
(B)	7.14	60	75
(C)	7.30	50	80
(D)	7.45	35	65
(E)	7.54	30	50

Setting: Hospital

Questions 123–125

At 2:00 AM, you are called emergently to the bedside of a 79-year-old man with severe coronary artery disease. He was admitted earlier in the day with chest pain and shortness of breath. The nurse reports that no pulse could be obtained. The cardiac monitor shows ventricular fibrillation. The nurse has begun cardiopulmonary resuscitation, and another resident is preparing to intubate the patient. Intravenous access is available from a central line placed in the right subclavian vein approximately 20 minutes ago in preparation for pulmonary artery catheterization.

123. You should

(A) give magnesium sulfate 1 g intravenous push
(B) give lidocaine 1.5 mg/kg intravenous push
(C) give epinephrine 1 mg intravenous push
(D) give epinephrine 3 mg intravenous push
(E) defibrillate up to 3 times at increasing power

124. After your intervention, the cardiac monitor shows sinus rhythm at 120 beats/minute. However, no pulse or blood pressure is obtainable. Which of the following examination procedures is most likely to yield the correct diagnosis and guide therapy?

(A) Careful inspection and examination of the abdomen
(B) Auscultation of the heart
(C) Auscultation of the lungs
(D) Careful examination of the head and neck
(E) Funduscopic examination

125. Based on your physical examination findings, which of the following interventions is most likely to be lifesaving?

(A) Emergent paracentesis
(B) Emergent pericardiocentesis
(C) Placement of a large-bore angiography catheter into the pleural space on the right side of the chest
(D) Administration of bicarbonate, insulin, and glucose intravenously
(E) Administration of atropine

Setting: Emergency Department

Questions 126–130

A 20-year-old woman, who is G_1P_0 at 12 weeks' gestation with an intrauterine pregnancy, complains of burning when she urinates. She also reports increased urgency and frequency.

126. What physical examination finding is most useful in this setting?

(A) Suprapubic tenderness
(B) Costovertebral angle tenderness
(C) Murphy sign
(D) Rebound tenderness
(E) Cervical motion tenderness

127. A urine dipstick finds leukocyte esterase and a small amount of blood. Which of the following steps should be next?

(A) Urine microscopy
(B) Antibiotics
(C) Urine culture
(D) Complete blood count (CBC)
(E) Pelvic examination

128. Which of the following pathogens is most likely?

(A) *Chlamydia trachomatis*
(B) *Staphylococcus saprophyticus*
(C) *Candida albicans*
(D) *Escherichia coli*
(E) *Proteus mirabilis*

129. All of the following are reasonable treatment choices EXCEPT

(A) ciprofloxacin hydrochloride
(B) sulfisoxazole
(C) nitrofurantoin
(D) ampicillin
(E) cefuroxime

130. At 38 weeks' gestation, the woman returns to the ED with findings consistent with a urinary tract infection. At birth, her child is found to have hyperbilirubinemia with a normal hematocrit. The mother probably received treatment for the urinary tract infection with

(A) ciprofloxacin
(B) sulfisoxazole
(C) nitrofurantoin
(D) ampicillin
(E) cefuroxime

Setting: Office

Questions 131–133

A 14-year-old girl presents with severe, cramping, abdominal pain and associated diarrhea of 2 weeks' duration. She had a similar episode 6 weeks ago that spontaneously resolved. The diarrhea is often bloody, and bowel movements are accompanied by severe, diffuse cramping. She complains of some painful oral lesions, which have been present for 2 to 3 days. Her medical history is unremarkable. Her family history is notable for a grandfather who had a colostomy and died from gastrointestinal (GI) disorder. Physical examination reveals a thin girl in no distress.
Results indicate:

Vital signs	Normal
Oropharynx	Three, small, aphthous ulcers with clean bases
Chest and cardiovascular	Normal
Abdomen	Hyperactive bowel sounds with mild, diffuse, tenderness
	Indistinct fullness in left lower quadrant with overlying tenderness
Rectum	Tender
	Gross blood
	No fissures or hemorrhoids

131. Which of the following conditions should NOT be considered in the differential diagnosis?

(A) Crohn disease
(B) *Entamoeba* infection
(C) Henoch-Schönlein purpura
(D) *Giardia* infection
(E) *Shigella* infection

132. A colonoscopy with biopsy is performed. The results show transmural inflammation with skip areas of involvement, granulomas, and fibrosis. The extraintestinal manifestations of this condition include all of the following EXCEPT

(A) erythema nodosum
(B) uveitis
(C) arthritis
(D) kidney stones
(E) GI lymphoma

133. All of the following therapies are effective for this condition EXCEPT

(A) prednisone
(B) mesalamine
(C) monoclonal antibodies to tumor necrosis factor
(D) 6-mercaptopurine
(E) neomycin sulfate

Setting: Office

134. A 28-year-old woman with epilepsy that is controlled with phenytoin asks your advice about pregnancy. She wants to know if she can continue taking phenytoin and if this drug poses some risk to the fetus. Which of the following statements regarding epilepsy and pregnancy is true?

(A) The risk of congenital malformations in offspring is increased in women who have epilepsy
(B) The period of maximal risk of congenital malformations is in the second trimester
(C) Valproic acid is safe during pregnancy
(D) Orofacial malformations in the offspring are least commonly seen
(E) No attempt should be made to withdraw medications from patients who have been seizure-free for several years

Setting: Office

135. A 38-year-old woman with chronic migraine headaches presents for evaluation. She states that she has suffered from headaches since she was 16 years of age and that her headaches have become more frequent and more severe during the past 3 to 4 years. She reports that the headaches begin as visual phenomena (sparkling lights or visual field deficits) that lead to severe, throbbing headaches located over the left eye. Often, nausea and vomiting occur. The woman has two or three headaches per week and has to leave work when they occur. Attempts at dietary manipulation and herbal remedies have not been successful. She asks for your advice concerning how she can reduce the frequency of attacks. Which of the following medications can be used prophylactically to decrease the occurrence of the headaches?

(A) Sumatriptan
(B) Metoclopramide hydrochloride
(C) Dihydroergotamine
(D) Meperidine hydrochloride
(E) Amitriptyline hydrochloride

Setting: Outpatient Clinic

136. A 12-year-old boy presents with several days of generalized malaise, painful joints (especially his knees), nodular swellings over his elbows, low-grade fever, and a rash on his chest. Several weeks earlier, he had been seen for a sore throat; no rapid streptococcal antigen test was performed, and he was not treated. Which of the following conditions is the most likely diagnosis?

(A) Systemic lupus erythematosus
(B) Rheumatic fever
(C) Rheumatoid arthritis
(D) Reiter syndrome
(E) Scarlet fever

Setting: Office

137. A 6-year-old boy is brought to see you for his first visit. His parents note that he seems to tire easily and complains of weakness in his legs. They have attributed this to his shyness and his preference for watching videos rather than playing outside. Physical examination reveals a healthy-appearing boy, with a blood pressure of 138/94 mm Hg in his right arm. His lower extremities are slightly atrophic and mottled-appearing. Which of the following other physical and laboratory findings are most likely NOT to be present?

(A) Diminished lower extremity pulses
(B) Cyanosis of the toes
(C) A bicuspid aortic valve on echocardiography
(D) Rib notching on chest radiography
(E) Left ventricular hypertrophy on ECG

Setting: Office

138. A 1-year-old boy has tetralogy of Fallot characterized by bouts of irritability, cyanosis, tachypnea, and, on one occasion, syncope. Based on the pathophysiology of this disorder, which of the following maneuvers is the best treatment for these episodes?

(A) Providing reassurance; the episodes are self-limited
(B) Raising the lower extremities
(C) Lowering the lower extremities
(D) Placing the child with the knees up to the chest
(E) Placing the child in the Trendelenburg position

Setting: Office

Questions 139–141

A 54-year-old African American man with type 2 diabetes mellitus and hypertension, for whom you have been caring for the past 5 years, presents for a routine office visit. His blood pressure is 150/94 mm Hg, his weight is 90 kg, and his height is 5′11″. Physical examination reveals some background diabetic retinopathy, a right carotid bruit, an S_4 cardiac sound, and 1+ lower extremity edema. His only complaint is that his blood sugar levels have been falling below 50 mg/dL more frequently. He believes this is due to his new job; he does not have time to eat a regular lunch. Laboratory work reveals:

Serum creatinine	1.4 mg/dL
Urinalysis	1+ proteinuria
Serum cholesterol	156 mg/dL
High-density lipoprotein (HDL)	35 mg/dL
Electrocardiogram (ECG)	Left ventricular hypertrophy
Average blood sugar based on hemoglobin$_{A1C}$	160 mg/dL

139. The man has been reluctant to take any medications except oral hypoglycemic medication (glipizide, 10 mg/day). He agrees to one additional medication at this visit. Which of the following agents would offer the patient the greatest benefit?

(A) Long-acting insulin
(B) Metoprolol
(C) Amlodipine
(D) Ramipril
(E) Vitamin E and folic acid

140. Which of the following agents would NOT be expected to increase the patient's high-density lipoprotein (HDL) fraction?

(A) Simvastatin
(B) Niacin
(C) Gemfibrozil
(D) Alcohol
(E) Vitamin E

141. Which of the following agents may worsen the patient's glycemic control?

(A) Niacin
(B) Metoprolol
(C) Verapamil
(D) Ramipril
(E) Amoxicillin

Setting: Satellite Clinic

Questions 142–145

A 12-year-old girl is brought to the clinic by her parents because she is experiencing vomiting and diarrhea. She has no fever but complains of intermittent, cramping, abdominal pain. They just returned from a family picnic where, apparently, other people have been sick as well. The girl ate potato salad and chicken approximately 90 minutes before the onset of her symptoms. The parents believe it is unlikely that her symptoms are due to infection because she has been taking antibiotics for an ear infection for the past 5 days.

142. Which of the following pathogens is the most likely cause of the patient's diarrhea?

(A) *Campylobacter jejuni*
(B) *Entamoeba histolytica*
(C) *Salmonella paratyphi*
(D) *Staphylococcus aureus*
(E) *Clostridium difficile*

143. Which of the following measures is the most appropriate next step?

(A) Stool cultures
(B) Enzyme-linked immunosorbent assay (ELISA) test for *C. difficile* toxin
(C) Stool examination for ova and parasites
(D) Liver function studies
(E) Supportive therapy

144. If a methylene blue stool study is positive, all of the following organisms are possible causes EXCEPT

(A) *Campylobacter jejuni*
(B) *Shigella sonnei*
(C) *Salmonella paratyphi*
(D) *Vibrio cholerae*
(E) *Yersinia enterocolitica*

145. A recent paper describes a clinical prediction scoring system that can be used to determine a pretest likelihood of *C. difficile* colitis. You want to determine the posttest probability after using this predictive tool combined with the *C. difficile* toxin assay (ELISA test). Which of the following characteristics of the ELISA test is needed to determine posttest probability?

(A) Odds ratio
(B) Sensitivity
(C) Sensitivity and specificity
(D) Prevalence of disease
(E) Positive predictive value

Setting: Hospital

146. A 45-year-old alcoholic man is admitted to the intensive care unit with severe pancreatitis. In the first 24 hours after admission, severe hypoxemia that requires ventilatory support and high concentrations of inspired oxygen develop. Which of the following conditions is the most likely cause of the respiratory compromise?

(A) Congestive heart failure
(B) Pneumonia
(C) Aspiration
(D) Acute respiratory distress syndrome (ARDS)
(E) Pneumothorax

Setting: Office

147. A 59-year-old woman complains of dyspnea on exertion. She is otherwise healthy but has noticed that during the past year she has limited her activity because of shortness of breath. One year ago, she could walk up four to five flights of stairs; however, she now has to stop twice on a single flight. She does not have chest pain but does complain of a dry cough. She does not smoke, and she works as a secretary at an insurance firm. The following pulmonary function tests are obtained as part of her workup:

	Normal	Observed	Predicted (%)
Spirometry			
Forced vital capacity (FVC) [L]	6.01	1.12	19
Forced expiratory volume in 1 second (FEV$_1$) [L]	4.89	1.04	21
FEV$_1$/FVC	81	93	
Volumes			
Total lung capacity (TLC) [L]	7.45	2.09	28
Residual volume (RV)/TLC (%)	19	17	
Diffusion capacity (DLCO) [mL/m per mm Hg]	35	9	26

Which of the following best describes the pulmonary process?

(A) Restrictive lung disease
(B) Obstructive lung disease
(C) A combination of restrictive and obstructive disease
(D) Extrathoracic obstructive disease
(E) Neuromuscular disease

Setting: Office

Questions 148–150

A 49-year-old man visits the office for an annual physical examination. He has had hypertension for the past 6 years. Social history reveals consumption of 6 to 8 beers/day for the past 25 years plus 50 pack-years of cigarette use. The man works as a pipe fitter. On review of symptoms, he complains of frequent urination. Today his major complaint is numbness and pain in the lower extremities. On examination, he has 5-/5 strength in plantar and dorsiflexion, with diminished light touch distally.

148. Which of the following conditions is the likely cause of his complaint?

(A) Diabetes mellitus
(B) Alcohol abuse
(C) Hypothyroidism
(D) Tobacco abuse
(E) Asbestosis

149. Which of the following tests is least necessary at this time?

(A) Glycosylated hemoglobin
(B) Thyroid-stimulating hormone (TSH) level
(C) Complete blood count (CBC)
(D) Serum protein electrophoresis
(E) Liver function studies

150. The patient's records show:

White blood cell (WBC) count	7,400/mm^3
Hemoglobin	11.6 g/dL
Hematocrit	34.1%
Mean corpuscular volume	103 fL
Platelet count	146,000/mm^3

All of the following conditions are consistent with these findings EXCEPT

(A) vitamin B_{12} deficiency
(B) alcohol abuse
(C) hypothyroidism
(D) anemia of chronic disease
(E) folate deficiency

ANSWER KEY

1-E	31-C	61-E	91-D	121-C
2-D	32-B	62-D	92-D	122-A
3-C	33-B	63-C	93-C	123-E
4-E	34-E	64-C	94-B	124-C
5-C	35-B	65-A	95-D	125-C
6-B	36-B	66-B	96-B	126-B
7-A	37-D	67-D	97-B	127-A
8-C	38-A	68-B	98-C	128-D
9-B	39-B	69-D	99-A	129-A
10-D	40-E	70-E	100-D	130-B
11-C	41-D	71-A	101-C	131-D
12-E	42-A	72-D	102-A	132-E
13-E	43-A	73-E	103-B	133-E
14-D	44-C	74-A	104-D	134-A
15-D	45-B	75-D	105-B	135-E
16-A	46-E	76-D	106-E	136-B
17-C	47-D	77-C	107-C	137-B
18-D	48-B	78-A	108-A	138-D
19-E	49-A	79-C	109-C	139-D
20-B	50-A	80-C	110-C	140-E
21-D	51-B	81-E	111-B	141-A
22-C	52-D	82-C	112-A	142-D
23-B	53-C	83-D	113-C	143-E
24-E	54-E	84-A	114-D	144-D
25-D	55-A	85-A	115-E	145-C
26-B	56-D	86-E	116-B	146-D
27-E	57-B	87-B	117-D	147-A
28-D	58-E	88-A	118-B	148-B
29-A	59-D	89-D	119-D	149-D
30-C	60-D	90-A	120-A	150-D

ANSWERS AND EXPLANATIONS

1–5. The answers are: 1-E, 2-D, 3-C, 4-E, 5-C. *(Obstetrics/gynecology)*
Breast cancer eventually affects one of eight women in the United States. The disease is the second leading cause of cancer death among women, with more than 180,000 new cases and more than 40,000 deaths per year. The fear of breast cancer is prominent in women with breast-related complaints, although most of these conditions are benign.

Intraductal papillomas, benign polypoid epithelial tumors that occur in the ducts of the breast, are the most common cause of bloody discharge from the nipple. These fibrovascular tumors, which are covered by benign ductal epithelium, are typically not palpable and may be 1 to 5 mm in size. They manifest as serosanguinous or bloody nipple discharge that may be recurrent or persistent. Excisional biopsy must be used to exclude the possibility of intraductal papillary carcinoma. Mastitis, which occurs in 1% to 3% of all nursing mothers, is characterized by painful erythema of the skin overlying the breast. Often there is accompanying fever and, occasionally, abscess formation. *Staphylococcus aureus* is usually the offending organism, and systemic antibiotic therapy is required.

When evaluating a breast mass, a physician must assess the patient's risk of breast cancer by noting the existence of certain risk factors. These risk factors include family history of breast cancer (female relative, such as mother or sister), previous history of breast cancer, early menarche (age <12 years) or late menopause (age >55 years) (i.e., longer period of estrogen exposure), nulliparity, first delivery at >35 years, fibrocystic changes, and history of radiation treatment (e.g., Hodgkin disease treatment). Whether oral contraceptives and hormone replacement therapy pose risks is controversial and each study varies. The risk is likely minimal; however, The Women's Health Initiative, a multicenter study of thousands of women, which should be completed in the next decade, will elucidate this issue. In this case, the patient has no family history of breast cancer and few high-risk factors. In young women such as this one, the two most common causes of a breast mass are fibrocystic changes and fibroadenomas.

Fibrocystic changes, the most common cause of benign breast masses, are essentially an exaggerated response to hormones. The three histologic states characteristic of this process include stromal proliferation; adenosis, consisting of ductal proliferation; and the occurrence of less painful, larger cysts. Clinically, patients have cyclical, bilateral mastalgia and engorgement. Fibrocystic changes are a risk factor for future breast cancer.

Fibroadenomas, the second most common cause of benign breast disease, consist of firm, painless, freely moveable masses of 2 to 3 cm in size that do not change with the menstrual cycle. Usually solitary, they are multiple in 15% to 20% of cases. Fibroadenomas are not a risk factor for future breast cancer.

In the absence of any worrisome physical findings (e.g., skin dimpling, fixed mass, erythema, peau d'orange), the physician should reassess this patient's mass in 2 to 4 weeks for cyclical change. This is appropriate because the most likely cause of the mass is fibrocystic disease in the setting of mastalgia and the "lumpy" consistency of her breasts. Note that the mass is unlikely to be an intraductal papilloma because this mass is usually not palpable. The follicular phase of the menstrual cycle, days 5 to 7, is often best for evaluation of a potentially dominant breast mass.

When the patient returns with a mass consistent with a fibroadenoma, aspiration of the mass is the first necessary procedure. If the mass is solid, mammography is generally warranted. If the mammogram has suspicious features, an excisional biopsy is in order. If the mammogram has benign features, one might consider observation. In this age group, some experts believe that a mammogram is unnecessary and choose to perform excisional biopsies on all solid masses, unless there are features that suggest breast cancer.

6–9. The answers are: 6-B, 7-A, 8-C, 9-B. *(Pediatrics)*
Diabetic ketoacidosis results from the absolute deficiency of insulin (rarely, it may occur in patients with a relative lack of insulin) in combination with a surge in the counterregulatory hormones glucagon, growth hormone, and catecholamine. The result is hyperglycemia and ketonemia. These metabolic effects ultimately result in polyuria, dehydration, and metabolic acidosis. In evaluating patients who present with diabetic ketoacidosis, several key features of the pathogenesis of this disorder must be kept in mind. Furthermore, it is

critical to determine whether any predisposing factors, such as infection, medical noncompliance, or abdominal processes (e.g., pancreatitis), may have caused this condition.

Hypokalemia is one of the common electrolyte disturbances during the early stages of treatment for diabetic ketoacidosis. Typically, patients with this condition have total body potassium depletion secondary to urinary loss. However, on presentation, serum potassium levels are typically in normal ranges or elevated due to the accompanying metabolic acidosis. A shift of potassium out of cells into the extracellular compartment accompanies an intracellular shift of hydrogen ions into cells. During treatment, two processes occur, causing a rapid fall in serum potassium: (1) insulin therapy drives the intracellular movement of potassium, and (2) correction of metabolic acidosis leads to a reversal of intracellular ion shifts, with intracellular movement of potassium. It is essential to anticipate this change in serum potassium during treatment, and once urine output is adequate (>30 mL/hour), addition of potassium into the intravenous replacement fluids is appropriate.

Successful treatment of diabetic ketoacidosis requires meticulous attention to serum chemistries and electrolyte replacement. During treatment, it is essential to follow the anion gap, the most important indication of improvement. Serum bicarbonate values can be misleading because, during the course of successful treatment, non–anion gap (hyperchloremic) acidosis may occur. This is secondary to loss of potential bicarbonate in the urine in the form of ketones. Thus, the serum bicarbonate may not rise, but the anion gap will decrease. Following the level of ketones in either the blood or urine is misleading because the assay for ketones detects acetone and acetoacetate. However, the predominant ketone in diabetic ketoacidosis is β-hydroxybutyrate. During treatment, β-hydroxybutyrate is converted to acetoacetate; this may give a false impression of worsening ketonemia despite adequate treatment.

Hypophosphatemia is another electrolyte disturbance that may occur during the treatment of diabetic ketoacidosis. On presentation, patients typically have total body phosphate depletion. Treatment with insulin drives the intracellular movement of phosphate, lowering the serum level. When hypophosphatemia is severe, it may lead to muscle weakness, rhabdomyolysis, and hemolysis. The other answer choices in question 8 generally do not occur during the treatment of diabetic ketoacidosis.

Cerebral edema is a feared complication of diabetic ketoacidosis treatment in children. The pathogenesis of this condition is ill-defined but correlates with aggressive fluid replacement, especially with hypotonic fluids. Typically, children have headaches that progress to obtundation and coma. Focal neurologic deficits are rare. To be successful, therapy must be initiated immediately—before any diagnostic tests, including computed tomography (CT) scanning. The mainstay of treatment is reduction of the intracranial pressure, which may involve osmotic agents such as mannitol, raising the head of the bed, hyperventilation and, if needed, neurosurgical decompression. Aspirin and, possibly, heparin are indicated for a thrombotic stroke. Thrombotic events may occur in older patients but would not be likely with this girl's symptom complex. Naloxone, which is used in the treatment of opioid overdose, has no role in diabetic ketoacidosis therapy.

10–12. The answers are: 10-D, 11-C, 12-E. (*Obstetrics/gynecology, emergency medicine, statistics*)

Both the patient's risk factors and the signs and symptoms suggest a diagnosis of peripartum cardiomyopathy, a condition seen commonly from the last month of pregnancy until 6 months' postpartum, with a peak incidence at 2 months' postpartum. The condition occurs more frequently with increasing age, multiparity, African American race, hypertension, and multiple gestation.

Cardiovascular disease is the fourth leading cause of maternal death. The demands on the heart increase as pregnancy progresses. By 20 weeks' gestation, cardiac output increases 30% to 50%, and the demands on the heart increase further during labor and in the puerperium. After expulsion of the placenta, the maternal circulation receives a 500-mL blood "transfusion." In pregnant women with cardiac disease, these changes are problematic.

Management of peripartum cardiomyopathy consists of bed rest, digitalis, diuretics, sodium restriction, and angiotensin-converting enzyme (ACE) inhibitors. Persistent cardiomegaly after 6 months' postpartum has a higher than 50% mortality within 5 years. Subsequent pregnancies carry a 10% to 15% mortality if heart size normalized and a 40% to 80% mortality if persistent cardiomegaly occurred.

In the setting of shortness of breath in pregnant women, the physician must always consider thromboembolism. In this case, an echocardiogram is most likely to support the diagnosis. The patient has an extra heart sound, an S_3, and she likely has pulmonary edema. As anemia could potentially cause shortness of breath as cardiac output increases later in pregnancy, a complete blood count (CBC) would be a reasonable study. A chest radiograph would be supportive and should be ordered, but the physician should not use it in place of an echocardiogram to make a definitive diagnosis. A lower extremity ultrasound and a ventilation-perfusion (V/Q) scan may be helpful if a high clinical suspicion exists.

Specificity refers to the percentage of cases *without* disease that will have a *negative* test. Sensitivity refers to the percentage of cases *with* disease that will have a *positive* test.

13–14. The answers are: 13-E, 14-D. (*Pediatrics*)
Lead poisoning in children remains a public health concern, with numerous, potential, environmental sources of lead, including paints, plaster, and pipes. Lead principally affects the following: the brain, the peripheral nervous system, the bone marrow, and the kidneys. The peripheral nerves show a patchy demyelination. Lead blocks several steps in the pathway of heme synthesis, leading to microcytic anemia with basophilic stippling (representing clumping of microsomes). In the kidney, tubule damage occurs and can lead to glycosuria, proteinuria, and aminoaciduria.

The signs and symptoms of lead poisoning are not specific but, in the proper clinical circumstances, should lead to the consideration of the diagnosis. Some general signs include anorexia, nausea and vomiting, constipation, diarrhea, irritability, ataxia, sleep disturbances, headaches, sedation, limb pain, abdominal pain, peripheral neuropathy, and convulsions. In the most severe cases, encephalopathy with increased intracranial pressure may be present. Typically, cyanosis is not a feature of lead poisoning.

Suggestive laboratory features include glycosuria, proteinuria, microcytic anemia with basophilic stippling, and elevated levels of protoporphyrins (secondary to the lead-induced block in heme synthesis). Radiographic films of long bones may show lead lines in preschool children, and this suggests more long-term exposure. Blood lead levels are diagnostic, with a normal level below 10 μg/dL or less. Levels above 25 μg/dL are often an indication for chelation therapy.

15–18. The answers are: 15-D, 16-A, 17-C, 18-D. (*Emergency medicine, psychiatry*)
Suicide is the eighth leading cause of death in the United States. Several factors contribute to the risk of suicide, including family history, age, sex, marital status, socioeconomic class, ethnic background, and profession. Suicide is more likely to occur in first-degree relatives of those who have attempted suicide; in middle-aged adults (men older than 45 years, women older than 55 years); in men, who are more successful at completing suicide because they use more violent means (shooting, hanging, jumping); in children of divorced parents; in individuals of higher socioeconomic classes; in whites; and in physicians, dentists, lawyers, and law enforcement agents. Marriage is a protective factor.

The majority of suicide victims are mentally ill. Actively suicidal patients require hospitalization in a locked ward, and lethal items should be taken from patients. Concomitant treatment for the underlying illness is necessary; including electroconvulsive therapy, antidepressants, or antipsychotics or mood stabilizers for psychotic patients.

After acetaminophen ingestion, the treatment of choice is *N*-acetylcysteine, which contains many sulfhydryl groups and maintains glutathione in its reduced state to act on the potentially dangerous intermediary. Acetaminophen is broken down to a nontoxic substance by the process of glucuronidation. Alternatively, the cytochrome P-450 system acts on a small portion (of acetaminophen) to make a toxic intermediary that cell proteins use to make a hepatotoxic chemical, or, via a glutathione-dependent mechanism, a nontoxic chemical. Dialysis, sodium bicarbonate, and phenytoin have no role in management unless renal failure develops.

If the patient arrives at the ED within 2 hours of acetaminophen ingestion, gastric lavage with activated charcoal is appropriate. *N*-Acetylcysteine should be administered immediately if significant ingestion is suspected. Much controversy surrounds the issue of enteral versus parenteral administration of *N*-acetylcysteine. In theory, the oral form may have advantages that relate to its accumulation in the liver via the portal system.

Cimetidine can protect against hepatic centrilobular necrosis because it reduces cytochrome P-450 levels. Chronic alcohol use leads to depleted stores of glutathione, resulting in increased risk of hepatotoxicity from acetaminophen overdose. Chronic alcohol use also induces the cytochrome P-450 system, which forms more of the toxic intermediary. Paradoxically, acute alcohol ingestion may provide protection from acetaminophen toxicity by competing for the cytochrome P-450 system. Malnutrition may lead to decreased glutathione stores, increasing the toxicity of acetaminophen. Phenobarbital and isoniazid, which are classic examples of cytochrome P-450 inducers, can increase the risk of hepatotoxicity.

19–21. The answers are: 19-E, 20-B, 21-D. (*Internal medicine, surgery*)
Vascular anatomy, from rostral to caudal, proceeds as follows: inferior phrenic arteries, middle suprarenal arteries, superior mesenteric artery, renal arteries, inferior mesenteric artery, and aortic bifurcation. The majority (75% to 95%) of abdominal aortic aneurysms (AAAs) are infrarenal and most likely to be located between the renal arteries (or superior mesenteric artery) and the inferior mesenteric artery.

After an AAA is found, the primary concern is rupture. The risk of rupture increases significantly when the aneurysm is greater than 5 cm in diameter. One recent study, conducted at the Mayo Clinic, found that the estimated risk of AAA rupture is 0% per year if the diameter is less than 4 cm, 1% per year if it is 4.0 to 4.9 cm, 11% per year if it is 5.0 to 5.9 cm, and 25% per year if it is greater than 6 cm.

For individuals with significant medical comorbidity, such as this patient, the threshold for surgical repair is 6 cm. Other important treatments include smoking cessation and hypertension control. Had this patient had an AAA with a diameter of 4 cm, serial ultrasound every 6 months would be the approach of choice.

Because most AAAs are secondary to atherosclerosis, the most common cause of postoperative death is myocardial infarction (MI). Renal failure may develop in 1% to 10% of cases but, in itself, does not lead to death. Multiple organ failure and acute respiratory distress syndrome (ARDS) may be seen in complicated postoperative courses, especially with sepsis. Strokes are less common after AAA repair.

22. The answer is C. (*Pediatrics*)
This patient suffers from sickle cell anemia, as typified by the sickle cells seen in the peripheral smear. Individuals with sickle cell anemia are susceptible to other hematologic problems, including folate deficiency, aplastic crisis, hemolytic crisis, and splenic sequestration syndrome.

Normally, the bone marrow in persons with sickle cell anemia is hypercellular, and red blood cell (RBC) production is higher to compensate for the increased turnover of the sickled red cells; reticulocyte counts typically range from 5% to 15%. The diminished reticulocyte count is indicative of an aplastic crisis, which is often associated with parvovirus B19 infection. Folate deficiency, which is also characterized by a low reticulocyte count, is a slowly progressive disorder and does not present with such a severe anemia. Iron deficiency and thalassemia are both causes of microcytic anemias and are not consistent with the clinical history or blood smear. Splenic sequestration, which occurs in patients with sickle cell disease for unknown reasons, is typified by pooling of large amounts of blood in the spleen. Associated conditions include massive splenomegaly and circulatory collapse. Hemolytic crises are most often found in individuals who have concomitant glucose-6-phosphate dehydrogenase deficiency and receive a drug with oxidant properties (e.g., sulfa-containing medication).

23–29. The answers are: 23-B, 24-E, 25-D, 26-B, 27-E, 28-D, 29-A. (*Emergency medicine, obstetrics/gynecology, surgery*)
Abdominal pain in sexually active women should always raise the suspicion of ectopic pregnancy. Risk factors include a history of salpingitis or ectopic pregnancy, increasing age, multiparity, and African American or Hispanic race. Previous salpingitis carries a sixfold greater risk and previous ectopic pregnancy carries a

tenfold greater risk. Women older than 35 years are three times more likely to have an ectopic pregnancy than women 15 to 24 years of age. Most ectopic pregnancies occur in women who have had three or more pregnancies. A history of tubal ligation may increase risk, but because sterilization failure is so rare, it may offset the risk. Contraception and previous abortion do *not* increase risk.

The classic presentation includes abdominal pain, amenorrhea, and vaginal bleeding. In one study, the frequency of symptoms was abdominal pain, 95% to 100%; vaginal bleeding, 65% to 85%; amenorrhea, 75% to 95%; dizziness, 20% to 35%; syncope, 10% to 18%; and nausea, 15%. The pain, described as colicky, is usually unilateral but not necessarily on the same side as the ectopic pregnancy. With a ruptured ectopic pregnancy, features on presentation and physical examination may vary from mild abdominal pain to hypovolemic shock with peritoneal signs. A temperature higher than 38°C is uncommon and should prompt a search for an infectious cause. Cervical motion tenderness is common secondary to intraperitoneal hemorrhage, and an adnexal mass is present in approximately one third of cases.

The differential diagnosis, which includes pelvic inflammatory disease (PID), appendicitis, abortion, corpus luteum cyst rupture, endometriosis, adnexal torsion, and gastroenteritis, guides the workup. A pregnancy test, using urine or serum, is essential. A 50 mIU/mL threshold test detects β-human chorionic gonadotropin (β-hCG) as early as 14 days after conception; it is positive in more than 90% of cases. (Serum hCG tests detect hCG as early as 5 days after conception.)

In patients with an ectopic pregnancy, quantitative β-hCGs do not increase appropriately (66% every 48 hours in early pregnancy). Pelvic ultrasound can determine whether the pregnancy is intrauterine and ascertain the location of an ectopic pregnancy. The most common location of an ectopic pregnancy is the ampulla (75%), followed by the isthmus (12%), distal fimbria (5%), proximal interstitial portion (2% to 3%), abdomen (1% to 2%), ovary (1%), and cervix (0.5%). Management includes surgical removal or, more recently, the use of methotrexate if the patient is stable. Rh-negative mothers should receive RhoGAM to prevent Rh sensitization.

In the setting of PID, indications for admission include tubo-ovarian abscess, patient noncompliance, ileus, pregnancy, temperature higher than 39°C, severe pain, peritonitis, intrauterine device use, white blood cell (WBC) count higher than 20,000/mm^3, and previous treatment failure. Oral contraceptives actually decrease the incidence of PID by creating a barrier type of mucus.

Appendicitis must be ruled out. A recent study found that the three most sensitive findings in support of appendicitis diagnosis are leukocytosis, fever, and rebound tenderness; however, nausea and vomiting were common as well.

This patient has a history of abdominal surgery, which increases the risk for small bowel obstruction. A plain film would reveal dilated loops of small bowel proximal to the obstruction with distal decompression because of normal peristalsis. The continuous folds of small bowel that travel the circumference of the viscera distinguish it from large bowel. Large bowel has haustra that do not traverse the entire circumference of bowel. A history of abdominal surgery does not lead to a sentinel loop, which is an isolated, dilated loop of bowel occasionally seen in inflammatory conditions, such as pancreatitis. The focal inflammation leads to irritation of the adjacent bowel and subsequent bowel dilation.

30–34. The answers are: 30-C, 31-C, 32-B, 33-B, 34-E. (*Internal medicine, obstetrics/gynecology*)
Menopause is the cessation of menses. Ovarian function ceases by age 55 in 95% of women, with a mean age of 51 years; menopause occurs earlier for smokers. Hot flashes are the first physiologic manifestation of ovarian failure. Most women complain of a sudden sensation of warmth and flushing of the skin, lasting for approximately 90 seconds. This process is the result of declining levels of estradiol-17β secretion by the ovarian follicles.

The frequency of hot flashes increases during the perimenopausal period, as women approach menopause. Other symptoms and sequelae of menopause include difficulty sleeping, vaginal dryness, dyspareunia, dysuria, urinary incontinence secondary to loss of bladder suspension, depression, skin thinning, increasing facial hair, brittle nails, osteoporosis, and cardiovascular lipid changes. Tremor, weight loss, and palpitations are not often associated with ovarian failure.

Under the stimulation of luteinizing hormone (LH), the theca cells of the postmenopausal ovary produce androstenedione and testosterone. Estrone, a product of androstenedione conversion in adipose tissue, is the predominant estrogen in menopause. Estradiol is the most prevalent estrogen in the reproductive years, and estriol is made by the placenta during pregnancy. Estrane is a minor estrogen.

As menopause approaches, the ovarian follicles become more resistant to follicle-stimulating hormone (FSH), which rises in a negative feedback fashion. This is the best laboratory indicator of approaching menopause. It would be appropriate to measure thyroid-stimulating hormone (TSH) and thyroxine (T_4) if hypothyroidism or hyperthyroidism was the suspected cause of the patient's symptoms. However, her symptoms are more consistent with the onset of menopause. Urinary vanillylmandelic acid is a screening test for pheochromocytoma, and β-human chorionic gonadotropin (β-hCG) is a glycoprotein hormone made by the syncytiotrophoblasts of the placenta in pregnancy.

The treatment of choice for menopause is exogenous estrogen replacement therapy (ERT). With ERT, hot flashes generally resolve in 3 to 6 weeks; without ERT, resolution takes approximately 3 years. In addition, patients with osteoporosis clearly benefit from ERT treatment, calcium, and vitamin D. Bone mineral density decreases 1.0% to 2.5% per year in the postmenopausal years, and ERT can prevent this decline. Studies have found that ERT leads to decreased rates of spine and hip fractures, in particular. Other than menopause, risk factors for osteoporosis include low body mass index, family history of osteoporosis, early ovarian failure, low calcium intake, smoking, nulliparity, alcohol, and high caffeine intake. It should be noted that the benefits of ERT are not as compelling in light of new data that question its cardiovascular benefits.

35. The answer is B. (*Neurology*)
The size of the pupils is dependent on the "average" light perceived by both eyes. In other words, if one eye experiences optic nerve damage, the average light "seen" by two eyes will be diminished, and the pupils will dilate in response to the decreased light stimulus. This is consistent with an afferent defect.

Anisocoria is caused by an efferent defect only. The diameter differential in this patient's pupils is greatest in the dark. The sympathetic system is responsible for pupillary dilation in the dark; therefore, this patient has efferent sympathetic dysfunction.

36–37. The answers are: 36-B, 37-D. (*Pediatrics*)
This clinical and laboratory description is most consistent with nephrotic syndrome. In this condition, glomerular injury leads to massive loss of plasma proteins into the urine, resulting in sodium retention, hypoalbuminemia, and edema. Pathologically, no gross light microscopic findings are apparent; however, on electron microscopy, effacement of the podocytes, with loss of the foot processes and charge barrier, is evident. In children, empiric corticosteroid treatment has a high likelihood of success. In adults, the differential diagnosis of nephrotic syndrome is much greater, and often biopsy is necessary to tailor the appropriate therapy. The other agents listed in question 36 may occasionally be used in the management of refractory disease and are subject to numerous side effects.

In children, minimal-change disease accounts for the majority of nephrotic syndrome cases. Interestingly, minimal-change disease in children is associated with allergic diseases, and treatment of the underlying allergy often improves nephrotic syndrome.

Along with the loss of albumin in the urine, patients with nephrotic syndrome lose antibodies. This increases the susceptibility to encapsulated organisms, especially *Streptococcus pneumoniae*. Host defense against fungal and viral pathogens are largely T cell–mediated and are minimally affected by the loss of immunoglobulins in the urine.

38. The answer is A. (*Pediatrics*)
Abdominal masses in children are always worrisome and raise the possibility of underlying malignancy. The differential diagnosis of an abdominal mass depends on the location of palpation and the age of the child. In

infants and young children, the three common causes are Wilms tumor, neuroblastoma, and hepatoblastoma. In older children and adolescents, the three common tumors are non-Hodgkin lymphoma, germ cell tumors, and rhabdomyosarcoma. Only Wilms tumor is a serious possibility in this patient. Splenic rupture occurs in the setting of preceding trauma, and without such a history, consideration is not warranted. Hodgkin disease, which is extremely rare in infants, would not be a consideration. Leukemic infiltration is a rare cause of abdominal mass. Meckel diverticulum is commonly associated with painless gastrointestinal (GI) bleeding, abdominal pain, and intussusception.

Wilms tumors account for approximately 6% of childhood tumors and occur commonly during the first 5 years of life, occurring from neoplastic embryonal renal cells of the metanephros. Presenting symptoms include abdominal mass (more common), hypertension, and hematuria (less common). The tumors may be associated with aniridia and hemihypertrophy. It is postulated that deletion or inactivation of tumor suppressor genes are critical in the development of this tumor (in a manner similar to retinoblastoma). Combined modality therapy using surgery, radiotherapy, and chemotherapy has led to dramatic advances in survival, and patients with localized disease have a 90% chance of survival.

39–46. The answers are: 39-B, 40-E, 41-D, 42-A, 43-A, 44-C, 45-B, 46-E. (*Internal medicine, surgery*)
This patient has upper gastrointestinal (GI) bleeding. The stools are black, suggesting blood in the GI tract that has been acted on by the gut enzymes. Risk factors for upper GI bleeding include alcohol and tobacco abuse, liver disease, nonsteroidal anti-inflammatory drug (NSAID) use, burn or trauma, vomiting, sepsis, esophageal varices, and history of peptic ulcer disease. The occasional abdominal pain and transient relief with food should suggest a duodenal ulcer. The common causes of upper GI bleeding (proximal to the ligament of Treitz), in descending order of frequency, are duodenal ulcer, gastric ulcer, gastritis, esophageal varices, Mallory-Weiss tears, gastric cancer, esophagitis, aortoenteric fistulas, epistaxis, and duodenal diverticulosis.

Most duodenal ulcers are within 2 cm of the pylorus in the duodenal bulb. They occur more commonly in men, primarily between the ages of 20 and 40 years. The patient's history of alcohol abuse with evidence of chronic liver disease (spider angioma) might tempt one to consider esophageal varices as the likely source, but recall that only 20% of alcoholics develop cirrhosis and, of those, only 35% develop esophageal varices. Among those patients with varices, only one third have documented variceal bleeding. Mallory-Weiss tears are proximal stomach or esophageal longitudinal tears that occur after retching. Angiodysplasia and diverticulosis are common causes of lower GI bleeding.

Erectile dysfunction is a common complaint in individuals who abuse alcohol. Other common causes of this condition include diabetes mellitus, peripheral vascular disease, tobacco abuse, prostatectomy, pelvic radiation, medications, and hyperprolactinemia. Reasonable diagnostic tests include glycosylated hemoglobin, testosterone level, and prolactin level, although these are all controversial. Alcohol cessation is important. Smoking cessation is unlikely to have an impact. Follicle-stimulating hormone (FSH) and luteinizing hormone (LH) levels are not part of a standard workup. Treatment includes sildenafil (Viagra), a cyclic guanosine monophosphate (cGMP) phosphodiesterase inhibitor. Studies have demonstrated that the mechanism of sildenafil involves cyclic adenosine monophosphate (cAMP), a second messenger that affects the action of several hormones. Sildenafil does not affect the neurotransmitters acetylcholine and norepinephrine. Nitric oxide, a recently identified substance, participates in numerous physiologic functions, such as vasodilation. Although it may act through cGMP, sildenafil does not act on it directly.

The patient's ankle pain is consistent with acute gouty arthritis. His risk factors include alcohol abuse and the use of hydrochlorothiazide; however, any factor that causes an abrupt increase or decrease in uric acid levels may induce an attack. Provoking factors include stress; trauma; infection; surgery; hospitalization; alcohol abuse; and many medications, including hydrochlorothiazide. The joint is generally swollen with erythema, warmth, and tenderness. Gout is usually a monoarticular arthritis but may be polyarticular, more often in women. The most commonly involved site is the first metacarpophalangeal joint; however, other large joints, such as the knees and ankles, are commonly affected.

For a definitive diagnosis, the joint should be aspirated, and the clinician should look for negatively bire-fringent urate crystals. A radiograph may be useful to assess for possible destructive changes if the gout recurs.

For unclear reasons, alcohol use appears to increase the frequency of gout flares. Therefore, alcohol cessation should aid in decreasing the number of gout attacks. Colchicine and nonsteroidal anti-inflammatory drugs (NSAIDs) are useful acutely, but allopurinol should be avoided. Steroids help with the inflammation but are rarely necessary. A change in blood pressure medication is also reasonable. Smoking has not been linked to gout.

Erosion of the ulcer into the artery, causing massive hemorrhage, is a potential complication because of the proximity of the gastroduodenal artery posteriorly. The acute, life-threatening, GI hemorrhage in a patient with a history of a duodenal ulcer, such as this one, should suggest posterior perforation of the ulcer with ero-sion into the gastroduodenal artery. Esophageal perforation results in severe, acute chest pain and rapid he-modynamic compromise. Variceal hemorrhage has presenting symptoms similar to those of this patient, usu-ally with prominent hematemesis. Arteriovenous malformation and diverticular bleeding tend to result in slow, lower GI bleeding with less severe hemodynamic compromise.

When this patient returned with bleeding into the gastroduodenal artery, he likely underwent a Billroth II procedure (antrectomy with gastrojejunostomy). This procedure has the lowest ulcer recurrence rate but the highest incidence of dumping syndrome. After any procedure that impairs the integrity of the pylorus, there is "free" delivery of hyperosmotic chyme to the small intestine, causing fluid shifts into the intestinal lumen. This distension causes diaphoresis; light-headedness; tachypnea; abdominal pain; flatus; and, occasionally, hypotension. Symptoms occur within 30 minutes of eating a meal.

Afferent loop syndrome is a less common complication seen after a Billroth II operation. Patients experi-ence abdominal pain and bloating 20 minutes to 1 hour after eating, with or without vomiting. The syndrome is caused by distension of an incompletely draining, afferent, intestinal loop (proximal to the anastomosis).

Treatment of short-bowel syndrome involves eating frequent, small meals, eliminating liquids at mealtime, and avoiding liquids that contain simple sugars. In severe cases, a somatostatin analog (octreotide) can be used. Secondary measures to consider if neither dietary changes nor octreotide is successful include Billroth I con-version, roux-en-Y anastomosis, or vagotomy.

47–49. The answers are: 47-D, 48-B, 49-A. (*Pediatrics, emergency medicine, neurology*)
In Guillain-Barré syndrome, also known as acute demyelinating inflammatory polyneuropathy, weakness usu-ally develops for several days, beginning in the distal extremities and ascending proximally. Facial weakness may occur in up to 50% of patients. A viral or gastrointestinal (GI) (especially *Campylobacter*-caused) illness often precedes the development of symptoms by 1 week to several weeks. The greatest danger derives from the possibility of respiratory muscle weakness, not usually apparent at disease onset but occurring at any time, which may require ventilatory support. Autonomic dysfunction may also occur, with episodes of arrhythmia, hypotension, or hypertension. Sensory complaints are often present. Deep tendon reflexes are lost early. Max-imum neurologic deficit usually occurs within 2 weeks.

In diagnosing Guillain-Barré syndrome, several conditions must be considered, including poliomyelitis, tick paralysis, shellfish poisoning, diphtheria, toxic neuropathy, and porphyria. However, each of these con-ditions has distinctive features that make the diagnosis apparent. For example, poliomyelitis is characterized by prominent myalgia, porphyria by prominent abdominal complaints, and diphtheria by involvement of the pharyngeal muscles. Neuroblastoma should not be confused with any of these diagnoses.

A characteristic feature of the cerebrospinal fluid (CSF) in Guillain-Barré syndrome is spinal fluid protein rise in the absence of significant pleocytosis. It is unusual to see abnormal glucose concentrations or red blood cells (RBCs) outside of a traumatic lumbar puncture. An elevated white blood cell (WBC) count and an ele-vated protein value should prompt consideration of meningitis.

Therapy for Guillain-Barré syndrome is primarily supportive; however, in those patients with life-threatening disease, plasmapheresis has been shown to be lifesaving. Plasmapheresis shortens the hospital course, decreases the need for mechanical ventilation, and accelerates the return to normal ambulation. Cyclophosphamide, prednisone, broad-spectrum antibiotics, and cyclosporine are not appropriate; none of these agents have proved effective in Guillain-Barré syndrome.

50–52. The answers are: 50-A, 51-B, 52-D. (*Statistics*)
The outcome of any test may be illustrated schematically.

Disease state

	Present	Absent
Positive	True-positive (a)	False-positive (b)
Negative	False-negative (c)	True-negative (d)

Test result (row label)

If there are 100 patients in the study group and the prevalence of the disease is 10%, then 10 individuals have the disease. The sensitivity is 90%, which means that 9 of 10 patients with the disease test positive. Thus, 1 person falls into the false-negative category.

	Lyme Disease Present	Absent
Positive test	9 (a)	4.5 (b)
Negative test	1 (c)	85.5 (d)
TOTALS	10	90

Sensitivity	a/(a + c)	Specificity	d/(b + d)
False-negative	c/(a + c)	False-positive	b/(b + d)
Positive predictive value	a/(a + b)	Negative predictive value	d/(c + d)

The positive predictive value (i.e., the likelihood that a patient has the disease, given a positive test) is a/(a + b), or 9/(9 + 4.5), which equals 67%.

If the prevalence of the disease increases to 50%, the table must be recomputed:

	Lyme Disease Present	Absent
Positive test	45	2.5
Negative test	5	47.5
TOTALS	50	50

With the increased prevalence of the condition, the positive predictive value now increases to 45/(45 + 2.5), which equals 95%. This is an important example of how the prevalence of a condition significantly influences the operating characteristics of a test.

53–58. The answers are: 53-C, 54-E, 55-A, 56-D, 57-B, 58-E. (*Obstetrics/gynecology, statistics, psychiatry*)

The sensitivity is the percentage of patients *with* disease who have a *positive* test. The specificity is the percentage of patients *without* disease who have a *negative* test. The positive predictive value, which is dependent on the prevalence of disease in a population, is the percentage of patients with a *positive* test who do have disease. The negative predictive value, which is also dependent on disease prevalence, is the percentage of patients with a *negative* test who *do not* have disease. Sensitivity and specificity are operating characteristics of a particular test but, clinically, physicians use predictive values when they use a test result to judge the likelihood of a patient having a particular disease. Sensitivity is important to discuss in this case because it determines the likelihood that a screening mammogram will find breast cancer. The odds ratio, primarily reported in retrospective studies, is the probability of having a risk factor if one has a disease.

As explained in answers 50 to 52, disease prevalence is required to determine predictive value. Therefore, the positive predictive value cannot be determined with the information given in the case for questions 53 to 58.

Mammography is more sensitive in postmenopausal patients because the breast becomes less glandular and more fatty with increasing age. Fat appears dark and glandular tissue and malignant areas appear white. Thus, malignancies are more easily seen in the mammograms of older women. Lobular carcinoma in situ is not readily visible on mammography.

Toward the end of the patient's visit, she displays signs consistent with major depression based on criteria in the *Diagnostic and Statistical Manual of Mental Disorders,* fourth edition (DSM-IV). Her anhedonia and crying spells are particularly worrisome. In such a depressed patient, the physician must always ascertain the risk of suicide.

An antidepressant may be appropriate; however, when choosing such an agent, the clinician should try to avoid unwanted side effects. Many antidepressants have significant anticholinergic effects, including mydriasis, blurred vision, fever, dry skin, flushing, ileus, urinary retention, tachycardia, hypertension, psychosis, and seizures ("hot as a hare, dry as a bone, red as a beet, mad as a hatter"). However, selective serotonin reuptake inhibitors, such as paroxetine, have little or no anticholinergic activity. Paroxetine may cause weight gain and sleepiness, which are less common with fluoxetine. Anorgasmia is a side effect of all selective serotonin reuptake inhibitors. Buspirone hydrochloride is an antianxiety agent whose actions are mediated by serotonin (5-HT_{1A}) receptors. Amitriptyline hydrochloride is a tricyclic antidepressant with significant anticholinergic properties. Haloperidol is a butyrophenone antipsychotic that also has significant anticholinergic effects. Clozapine, a dibenzodiazepine antipsychotic, has less anticholinergic activity, but it is clearly not a good choice for depression without psychosis.

59. The answer is D. (*Pediatrics*)

Many conditions lead to recurrent pneumonia in children, including hypersensitivity pneumonitis; congenital, structural, lung abnormalities (e.g., pulmonary sequestration, bronchial stenosis); recurrent aspiration; tracheoesophageal fistula; immunodeficiency states; and primary ciliary dyskinesias. Cystic fibrosis, which should always be considered a primary cause of associated recurrent pneumonias, diarrhea, and sinusitis in children, is the diagnosis in this case.

Cystic fibrosis, a multisystem disease, is due to an autosomal recessive trait on chromosome 7. The involved gene (*CFTR*), which has been cloned, encodes a large transmembrane channel involved in chloride transport. Pathology generally results from the thick, viscous secretions characteristic of the disease.

The list of clinical manifestations of cystic fibrosis is extensive. Recurrent pneumonia and bronchiectasis that result in respiratory failure are common. Obstruction of the ileum by thick meconium is nearly complete in approximately 10% of infants. Pancreatic insufficiency frequently occurs, leading to chronic malabsorption and steatorrhea. Increased absorption of oxalate from the intestine is secondary to steatorrhea. Normally, oxalate complexes with calcium in the intestine and is excreted in the stool. However, in the presence of steatorrhea, calcium binds to the fatty acids in the stools, leaving free oxalate to be absorbed. This increases the likelihood of kidney stones. Other manifestations of cystic fibrosis include biliary cirrhosis in approximately

2% to 3% of patients, diabetes mellitus secondary to pancreatic insufficiency, impaired infertility in both men and women, and chronic sinusitis.

60–61. The answers are: 60-D, 61-E. (*Pediatrics, emergency medicine*)

This constellation of symptoms should lead to the strong consideration of infectious mononucleosis or Epstein-Barr virus infection. This infection occurs early in life in developing countries; however, in the United States, the age at which infection occurs is related to socioeconomic status. Seropositivity for adolescents is 60% to 80%, with poorer populations being more affected. Transmission of Epstein-Barr virus is by exchange of saliva that harbors the virus. The incubation period is 30 to 60 days, and the onset is insidious; often a prodrome of malaise, fatigue, headache, and nausea or abdominal pain, which lasts for about a week. Fever and a severe sore throat generally ensue, prompting affected individuals to seek medical attention.

Moderate-to-severe pharyngitis with marked tonsillar swelling and occasional exudates generally accompany the sore throat. Petechiae at the junction of the hard and soft palates are often apparent. Other important signs include lymphadenopathy and hepatosplenomegaly. The spleen is generally palpable 2–3 cm below the costal margin. Massive enlargement is uncommon. Elevated liver transaminases may occur in 80% of patients.

It is important to realize that several other conditions can mimic Epstein-Barr virus infection, including acute HIV infection, cytomegalovirus infection, infectious hepatitis, leukemia, malaria, and tuberculosis. In this case, the physician should first obtain a diagnostic test for the most likely condition. The heterophile antibody screen relies on the fact that acute Epstein-Barr virus infection results in the production of a large number of abnormal antibodies that react with either sheep or horse red blood cells (RBCs). The other tests listed as possible answers to question 60 might be used if the heterophile antibody screen was negative.

Infectious mononucleosis has numerous complications. The most serious is splenic rupture, which typically occurs during the second week of infection and is commonly related to trauma. Swelling of the tonsils may be severe enough to cause respiratory compromise. Neurologic involvement may include convulsions, Guillain-Barré syndrome, encephalitis, and transverse myelitis. Other complications include hemolytic anemia, myocarditis, pancreatitis, orchitis, and hepatitis. Interestingly, a maculopapular rash develops in 80% of patients treated with ampicillin. Epstein-Barr virus, an oncogenic virus, has been associated with an increased risk of nasopharyngeal carcinoma and Burkitt lymphoma. However, it is not linked with hepatocellular carcinoma, which is associated with chronic hepatitis B virus infection.

62–66. The answers are: 62-D, 63-C, 64-C, 65-A, 66-B. (*Internal medicine*)

This patient has many risk factors for atherosclerosis, including diabetes, hypertension, cigarette smoking, and pentoxifylline use, which raises the suspicion of peripheral vascular disease. This combination of factors places her at great risk for abdominal aortic aneurysm (AAA). Nearly all AAAs are related to atherosclerotic disease, and 20% of patients with peripheral vascular disease will have an AAA at some time in their lives. The most common risk factors are hypertension, diabetes, smoking, male sex, and advanced age (older than 70 years).

Patients with AAAs are usually asymptomatic but occasionally complain of a strong pulsatile sensation in the abdomen, vague epigastric pain, or low back pain. Approximately 75% to 95% of AAAs are infrarenal. The physician usually detects an AAA incidentally while evaluating another problem. On physical examination, a pulsatile, nontender mass is often palpable. A Murphy sign is seen in acute cholecystitis, costovertebral angle tenderness may occur in either nephrolithiasis or pyelonephritis, and an iliopsoas sign is typically seen in acute appendicitis; all of these signs are highly unlikely in this patient.

The initial study of choice is an abdominal ultrasound because it provides data about the diameter of the aneurysm, which is the most important prognostic indicator in management. Prognosis also correlates with concomitant coronary artery disease. Angiography often underestimates AAA size because of mural thrombosis within the aneurysm. CT scanning and MRI are being used more often; in the future, these techniques will likely become the gold standard for evaluation and follow-up of AAAs. Intravenous pyelography would be helpful if nephrolithiasis was suspected. Cross-table, lateral radiography shows eggshell calcifications in 75% of patients with AAAs.

Regarding health maintenance, a urine test for microalbumin is essential to check for nephropathy in people with diabetes. The American Diabetes Association recommends annual ophthalmology examinations; however, a recent cost analysis suggested that biennial examinations are acceptable in the absence of diabetic retinopathy. All individuals should receive the pneumococcal vaccine at 65 years of age. This vaccine is also recommended for high-risk individuals with chronic disease (e.g., diabetes) or immunosuppression. These high-risk patients should receive a second vaccination at age 65 if they received the first vaccination 3 or more years earlier. Only patients who have undergone splenectomy and those with HIV need vaccinations every 4 to 6 years (according to the Centers for Disease Control and Prevention [CDC]). Based on the recommendations of the American Cancer Society, this woman should have a mammogram every year because she is age 65. Screening for colon cancer with flexible sigmoidoscopy is warranted every 5 years, as recommended by the U.S. Preventative Disease Task Force.

Captopril, an angiotensin-converting enzyme (ACE) inhibitor, is the best choice for this patient's hypertension because this drug, and other ACE inhibitors, reduces the rate of progression to end-stage renal disease in patients with diabetes. Nifedipine, verapamil, and diltiazem hydrochloride, which are all calcium channel blockers, do not limit progression to cardiovascular or renal end points (i.e., coronary artery disease, end-stage renal disease). Propranolol hydrochloride is a good choice in an individual with diabetes because coronary artery disease develops more slowly when patients take β-blockers. There is a risk that β-blockers may exacerbate peripheral vascular disease and depression; however, no studies have shown that the $β_1$-selective blockers worsen depression.

In the setting of a chronic disease such as diabetes mellitus, the Sixth Report of the Joint National Committee on Detection, Evaluation and Treatment of High Blood Pressure (JNC VI) guidelines recommend a systolic blood pressure of less than 130 mm Hg and a diastolic blood pressure of less than 85 mm Hg to decrease the progression of disease. If the patient has proteinuria greater than 1 g/day, the target values decrease to 125 mm Hg and 75 mm Hg, respectively.

67–71. The answers are: 67-D, 68-B, 69-D, 70-E, 71-A. (*Emergency medicine, psychiatry*)

Bipolar disorder is a common disease characterized by unpredictable swings between mania and depression. Some individuals primarily experience depression; some, primarily mania. In general, depressive episodes are more likely to occur in women, and manic episodes are more frequent in men. Manic episodes predominate in younger individuals (20 to 30 years of age), and depressive episodes predominate in older patients (older than 40 years). The most frequent age of onset is between 20 and 30 years of age. Prevalence is similar for men and women. Bipolar disorder is more common among individuals of lower socioeconomic status.

Mania is associated with psychomotor agitation, social extroversion, decreased need for sleep, impairment in judgment, impulsivity, and grandiose or irritable moods. Patients with severe mania experience delusions and paranoid thinking. Two particular concerns are the high incidence of alcohol abuse (>50%) and suicide (10% to 15%).

Given the patient's history of bipolar disorder, medication toxicity is the most likely cause of his symptoms. All of the other choices listed in question 67 may lead to mental status changes. Subdural hematomas, which occur in the context of a fall or in older individuals, are often manifested by confusion and focal neurologic signs. Hypernatremia, usually seen in nursing home residents or patients with diabetes mellitus or insipidus, is also manifested by confusion and stupor. Hypocalcemia produces tetany. Status epilepticus most commonly occurs in individuals with a history of seizures, and patients are not alert at presentation.

Lithium carbonate is the mainstay of treatment; carbamazepine is used as first-line therapy as well. The therapeutic window is small for both medications, however, so levels must be checked. The side effects of lithium, even within the therapeutic window, include nausea, diarrhea, weight gain, alopecia, and nephrogenic diabetes insipidus. Lithium toxicity may cause nausea, vomiting, diarrhea, weakness, ataxia, tremor, seizures, arrhythmias, and hypotension. Diuresis and alkalinization are standard treatment; hemodialysis is reserved for severe toxicity, with levels greater than 3 mmol/L. The physician should obtain an electrolyte panel to look for hypernatremia and other electrolyte changes. Laboratory abnormalities include leukocytosis, hyperglycemia, glycosuria, and hypernatremia. An electrocardiogram (ECG) may show tachycardia, bradycardia, inverted T waves, atrioventricular block, or a prolonged QT interval.

An ECG is an essential part of the initial workup. Carbamazepine, a tricyclic compound, has sodium channel blocking characteristics. With carbamazepine intoxication, QRS duration prolongation and QT interval lengthening, both risk factors for ventricular arrhythmia, are the most characteristic ECG changes. ST elevation, PR lengthening, and peaked T waves are not classic features of carbamazepine (or tricyclic antidepressant) intoxication. Carbamazepine intoxication also causes central nervous system (CNS) depression, cardiotoxicity, seizures, and hypotension.

72–73. The answers are: 72-D, 73-E. (*Obstetrics/gynecology*)
Bloody discharge from the nipple is a worrisome finding in any patient. However, the most common cause (especially in low-risk patients) is intraductal papillomas, which are usually small (2 to 10 mm) lesions that develop in close proximity to the nipple and are rarely palpable. Although they are not associated with an increased risk of malignancy, given the risk of breast carcinoma in this situation, a workup is necessary. A mammogram should be obtained as an initial step and, in some cases, ductography may be performed. Surgery should identify the responsible duct and it can be excised.

Other benign breast conditions include fibroadenomas, mastitis, and fat necrosis. Fibroadenomas, the most common breast masses in adolescents and young children, are firm, well-demarcated, and mobile. They may enlarge, especially just after menarche or just before menopause, and enlarging masses warrant excision. The incidence of breast carcinoma may be slightly increased in women who have had a single fibroadenoma removed.

Mastitis, which may affect lactating women, is commonly secondary to *Staphylococcus aureus*. Intense, painful inflammation and destruction of breast tissue leads to abscess formation. Treatment with drainage and antibiotics is necessary. It is important to view any inflammatory breast changes in postmenopausal women as neoplastic until proven otherwise.

Fat necrosis is secondary to breast trauma, although a substantial proportion of affected women never recall such an event. The sclerotic lesions can lead to a high suspicion for cancer because skin retraction may occur, and mammography can demonstrate worrisome features. Excision is recommended.

74–75. The answers are: 74-A, 75-D. (*Internal medicine, neurology*)
This patient's lesion is localized to the right parietal lobe. The combination of left-sided hemiparesis that is greater in the arm than the leg and contralateral homonymous hemianopsia (affecting the optic radiations) excludes all other locations. A lesion involving the right occipital cortex would lead to homonymous hemianopsia (often with the patient being unaware of the visual deficit) with macula sparing and would not explain the motor difficulties. A lesion in the right internal capsule would likely result in left-sided motor and sensory abnormalities. A lesion in the mid-pons would be characterized by involvement of the abducens nerve (CN VI) and impaired horizontal eye movements.

The appearance of a ring-enhancing lesion on a contrast CT scan of the brain is not specific and may be seen in any condition in which the blood-brain barrier is interrupted. Possibilities include toxoplasmosis, metastatic tumors, brain abscesses, and lymphoma. Progressive multifocal leukoencephalopathy does not cause these lesions. This disorder is thought to be caused by a JC virus, a papovavirus most often seen in patients with advanced AIDS, lymphoma, leukemia, or pharmacologic immunosuppression. The virus causes a subacute infection, with death occurring 3 to 6 months after symptoms begin. Dominant features of the clinical picture are dementia and focal cortical dysfunction. CT scanning reveals low-density areas within the subcortical white matter.

76–79. The answers are: 76-D, 77-C, 78-A, 79-C. (*Surgery, neurology, internal medicine*)
The potential operative complications after abdominal aortic aneurysm (AAA) repair are atheroembolism, declamping hypotension, acute renal failure (acute tubular necrosis), arrhythmias, stroke, gastrointestinal (GI) hemorrhage, and myocardial infarction (MI). The common cause of GI hemorrhage after an AAA repair is colonic ischemia. Stress gastritis may occur postoperatively; however, on postoperative day 1, the problem is likely colonic ischemia. The inferior mesenteric artery is often sacrificed during the procedure. If the patient does not have adequate collaterals from the left colon, ischemia will occur. Colonoscopy is the diagnostic study of choice for colonic ischemia. The other choices are less likely to be temporally related to the procedure.

After significant hypotension has occurred, ischemic change would be expected in the watershed regions of the cerebral cortex where the anterior cerebral artery and the middle cerebral artery overlap, as well as where the middle cerebral artery and the posterior cerebral artery overlap. In addition, a change in level of consciousness would require dysfunction of both cortical hemispheres or the reticular activating system.

Irreversible cessation of all brain function is required for a diagnosis of brain death. First, unresponsiveness to sensory input, including pain and speech, is essential. Second, brainstem reflexes, including pupillary function, corneal reflexes, and oropharyngeal reflexes, must be absent. Respiratory responses should be absent in the setting of a PCO_2 greater than 60 mm Hg. Third, it is imperative to rule out sedative drug intoxication, hypothermia, neuromuscular blockade, and shock. These criteria must persist for more than 6 hours, together with a confirmatory, flat, isoelectric electroencephalogram (EEG), or for more than 12 hours without an EEG.

80. The answer is C. (*Emergency medicine, pediatrics*)
This constellation of symptoms strongly suggests meningococcal meningitis. This rapidly progressive disease is fatal if not recognized early and treated promptly. Thus, the most important initial action is to rapidly obtain blood cultures and institute appropriate antibiotic therapy; a third-generation cephalosporin would be a good choice. In meningococcal meningitis, one of the most important negative predictors of outcome is a delay in providing therapy. Acetaminophen would help alleviate the fever but this is of less importance than the administration of antibiotics. A lumbar puncture can be obtained when the patient is stable. Use of dexamethasone in the treatment of meningitis is controversial; most studies indicate that the agent may be effective in decreasing hearing loss in children with *Haemophilus influenzae* type B infection.

81. The answer is E. (*Emergency medicine, pediatrics*)
This child has epiglottitis, which is typically caused by *Haemophilus influenzae* type B infections. This disorder affects children 2 to 7 years of age. In the United States, the incidence of this disease has dramatically declined secondary to vaccination against the bacterium. However, this patient came to the United States at an early age and may not have received the vaccination.

The onset of epiglottitis is rapid; within 4 to 12 hours, patients are febrile and have dysphagia and respiratory distress with stridor. Children with the disease generally sit forward, with their mouths open, drooling. Diagnosis must be rapid, and care must be taken to minimize anxiety that can lead to respiratory failure. Visualization of the epiglottis with a laryngoscope or bronchoscope should be undertaken only in a setting where rapid cardiorespiratory support is available.

In this patient, who has onset of acute stridor, visualization followed by rapid intubation is essential. In a child who is not acutely ill, lateral neck radiographs may show "thumbprinting" of the epiglottis, which is indicative of swelling and inflammation. Intravenous antibiotic therapy with a third-generation cephalosporin is indicated. Neither racemic epinephrine nor corticosteroids have any role in therapy of acute epiglottitis.

82–84. The answers are: 82-C, 83-D, 84-A. (*Obstetrics/gynecology, internal medicine*)
The complaint of nervousness is a nonspecific symptom and, based on the laboratory results given, one might conclude that the patient has hyperthyroidism. However, the thyroid-binding globulin level is elevated in pregnancy, increasing the total thyroxine (T_4) level. If a triiodothyronine (T_3) resin uptake is ordered, it will *not* be

elevated, as in hyperthyroidism. Measurement of free T_4, which should be normal if the patient is euthyroid, is another option.

Methimazole and propylthiouracil (PTU) decrease the production and release of T_4 and T_3. PTU also inhibits the peripheral conversion of T_4 to T_3. PTU is the treatment of choice for documented hyperthyroidism in pregnancy. However, neither methimazole nor PTU is necessary because a diagnosis of hyperthyroidism has not yet been made. Radioactive iodine (for the purpose of diagnosis) and ablation should be avoided during pregnancy. Propranolol is used to control heart rate and inhibits peripheral conversion of T_4 to T_3.

The common causes of thyrotoxicosis in pregnancy (in decreasing order of frequency) are toxic diffuse goiter (Graves disease), acute thyroiditis, toxic nodular goiter (Plummer disease), and toxic adenoma. Less common causes of thyrotoxicosis are hydatidiform mole, choriocarcinoma, and thyrotoxicosis factitia. Typical presenting features of Graves disease are weight loss, ocular signs, pretibial edema, and nervousness. T_4 and T_3 resin uptakes are elevated. Maternal and fetal prognosis is good in well-controlled hyperthyroidism. However, studies have found an increased stillbirth rate with maternal hyperthyroidism, and the risk of fetal goiter must be recognized.

Gestational trophoblastic disease may involve hydatidiform mole, choriocarcinoma, or placental trophoblastic tumor. Trophoblastic tissue produces β-human chorionic gonadotropin (β-hCG) and, thus, β-hCG levels are elevated in all of these conditions. α-Fetoprotein (AFP) is increased in the neural tube defect setting when screening is performed at 15 to 18 weeks' gestation. AFP may be decreased in Down syndrome.

85. The answer is A. (*Neurology*)
This patient has loss of right-sided pain and temperature sensation. Transmission of right-sided pain and temperature from the umbilical level downward starts with unmyelinated C fibers of free nerve endings at the associated regions. The first-order neurons of these nerves are in the dorsal root ganglia, one to two segments above the region that they innervate. From the dorsal root ganglia, the first-order neurons enter the spinal cord posteriorly and synapse immediately. The second-order neurons are in the dorsal horn of the spinal cord and give rise to axons that decussate in the ventral white commissure anteriorly and ascend in the contralateral spinothalamic tract. These axons synapse in the ventroposterolateral nucleus of the thalamus. Here, the third-order neurons arise and travel through the internal capsule and corona radiata to the postcentral gyrus in the parietal cortex.

The umbilical region is the T10 dermatome. These fibers and those "below" travel up one to two segments before entering the dorsal horn of the spinal cord. Therefore, *right-sided* loss of pain and temperature at the umbilical level and below is best explained by damage to the *left* lateral spinothalamic tract at one to two levels above T10—either at T9 or T8. All pain and temperature sensation below the level of the lesion will be abnormal.

86–88. The answers are: 86-E, 87-B, 88-A. (*Emergency medicine, surgery, psychiatry*)
Because this patient did not have severe pain initially, the later presentation of pain cannot be attributed to the fracture alone. Compartment syndrome has developed. Following fracture, bleeding from the bones and adjacent soft tissues produces a rapidly enlarging hematoma that surrounds the fracture site. Bleeding within a closed structure, such as the fascia, causes an increase in compartment pressure, leading to muscular ischemia and necrosis. The most common sites of this complication are the anterior leg compartment (tibia) and the volar compartment of the forearm (Volkmann contracture of a supracondylar fracture of the humerus). Intrafascial pressure measurement is essential because tissue integrity is at risk if the pressure reaches 30 mm Hg.

Fasciotomy is the treatment of choice. Thrombolytics and embolectomy are not indicated because thrombosis is not the cause of this complication. Antibiotics would be of great importance if an infectious fasciitis was suspected. Even in the setting of infection in a patient with peripheral vascular disease (e.g., diabetes), the value of hyperbaric oxygen is questionable.

Studies have shown that group therapy is the best treatment for alcoholism. Alcoholics Anonymous involves a 12-step process and uses group therapy. Aversion therapy is effective for the short term. For example, disulfiram, an agent of aversion therapy, blocks acetaldehyde breakdown and causes flushing, headache, anxiety, and sweating within 10 minutes of alcohol use. Controlled studies have not shown unequivocally that disulfiram increases duration of sobriety. Naltrexone, an opioid antagonist, reduces alcohol craving and is useful as an adjunct to a formal treatment program. However, most relevant studies have only short follow-up periods. Psychotherapy impedes maintenance of sobriety when used early in treatment, but may be useful in patients with underlying psychosis.

89–90. The answers are: 89-D, 90-A. (*Internal medicine*)
Chronic cough is defined as a cough that persists for more than 3 weeks. Chronic bronchitis from smoking or environmental irritants is the common cause. However, in nonsmoking patients, the common cause of chronic cough is postnasal drip. The workup should include a detailed history, physical examination, and chest radiograph. Historical clues that may indicate postnasal drip syndrome are sensation of nasal drainage, frequent throat clearing, and a cough that worsens at night and in the early morning. Causes include the common cold, allergic rhinitis, vasomotor rhinitis, postinfectious rhinitis, sinusitis, and environmental irritants. Other important causes of chronic cough include asthma, gastroesophageal reflux, bronchiectasis, drugs (e.g., angiotensin-converting enzyme [ACE] inhibitors), and interstitial pulmonary disease.

In this patient, a trial of an antihistamine/decongestant with an intranasal steroid spray is warranted. If the patient does not show improvement, pulmonary function testing is appropriate; the second most common cause of chronic cough is asthma.

91–94. The answers are: 91-D, 92-D, 93-C, 94-B. (*Internal medicine, neurology*)
In this case, the primary presentation is nausea, vomiting, and headache. The pupil generally becomes fixed in midposition and is less reactive to light. Often a vascular prominence of the sclera is evident around the perimeter of the cornea, and the cornea has a "steamy" appearance. Kernig sign is a finding consistent with meningitis. Flame-shaped hemorrhages are seen in hypertensive retinopathy. Pain on light reflex testing is most consistent with iritis. Chemosis can be seen in the setting of any conjunctivitis.

The application of pilocarpine 4% decreases intraocular pressure by constricting the pupil and drastically improves symptoms in 20 to 30 minutes. High intracranial pressures could result in nausea, vomiting, and headache but should not cause this patient's eye findings. A lumbar puncture would be useful if meninigitis was a consideration. Atropine would dilate the pupil and further increase intraocular pressure.

This patient has acute angle-closure glaucoma, which accounts for approximately 5% of glaucoma cases. In this type of glaucoma, the passageway for aqueous outflow, via the Schlemm canal, is abruptly blocked. The primary risk factor for angle-closure glaucoma is a narrow angle containing the Schlemm canal. Dilating the pupil can precipitate an attack by bringing the iris up against the cornea, blocking the Schlemm canal and, therefore, aqueous humor outflow. In some patients, when the pupil is in midposition, the iris comes into close apposition with the lens, preventing the flow of aqueous humor between the posterior and anterior chambers. As pressure builds, it pushes the iris forward, which further contributes to angle closure. Intense pain usually occurs, and the cornea has a hazy appearance. The patient may complain of seeing halos around lights and generally experiences significantly decreased vision.

Coincidentally, this woman has a significant risk factor for open-angle glaucoma, a chronic disease that accounts for approximately 95% of glaucoma cases. It is the single most important cause of blindness in the African American population. Open-angle glaucoma generally results in the insidious onset of peripheral visual loss. There is usually no pain or redness of the eye, and visual acuity remains normal until late in the course of disease. The diagnosis of open-angle glaucoma rests on measuring the intraocular pressure, examining the optic disc, and testing the visual field. Intraocular pressures are 20 to 30 mm Hg, in contrast to the higher values sometimes seen in acute closed-angle glaucoma; the physiologic cup/disc ratio is greater than 0.5; and visual field testing finds prominent loss peripherally.

Uveitis is inflammation of one of the uvea structures, which include the choroid (posterior), iris (anterior), and ciliary bodies (anterior). Uveitis is usually associated with photophobia, particularly when it involves the iris, and often occurs with infection, rheumatologic disease, or allergic disease. Technically, acute angle-closure glaucoma involves the anterior uveal structures and has an anterior uveitis component. The pupils of a patient with uveitis are classically miotic. Conjunctivitis should not cause pupil abnormalities or significant eye pain. With chronic hypertension, a blood pressure of 185/110 mm Hg would be unlikely to cause symptoms. In addition, the patient has no other symptoms of end-organ involvement. Nevertheless, it is an important consideration. Meningitis is always an important consideration in a patient with headache, nausea, vomiting, and diabetes. However, meningitis cannot account for the patient being afebrile and having a red eye. Another consideration would be diabetic ketoacidosis but, again, the red eye and other physical findings would be inconsistent with diabetic ketoacidosis. However, the physician should watch carefully for the development of diabetic ketoacidosis in this setting.

Some experts recommend the administration of intravenous mannitol to further reduce intraocular pressure. Once the attack has been relieved, a peripheral iridectomy may be performed to provide a supplementary route of aqueous humor efflux. This procedure commonly uses a laser; it involves burning a hole in the iris on its peripheral aspect. The chronic administration of pupillary constrictor drops has not been effective in preventing attacks of acute angle-closure glaucoma.

95–98. The answers are: 95-D, 96-B, 97-B, 98-C. (*Internal medicine, psychiatry*)

Initially, this patient presents with classic findings of right-sided endocarditis. This is a common complication of intravenous drug use; before the AIDS epidemic, this condition accounted for 5% to 16% of all hospital admissions for drug abusers.

The tricuspid valve is most commonly involved, and damage may result from multiple injections of talc or other foreign material. The damaged valve is more at risk for bacterial infection. Involvement of the tricuspid valve leads to tricuspid regurgitation, with the characteristic midsystolic murmur heard best at the left lower sternal border. With inspiration, blood flow increases across the valve, and the intensity of the murmur increases. Embolic events from the infected valve can lead to infected pulmonary nodules that may cavitate or result in hemoptysis.

The most common organism isolated is *Staphylococcus aureus* (60% to 90% of cases). It is believed that *S. aureus* is part of the patient's own flora and is introduced from the skin into the bloodstream during injection. Other organisms that may be isolated include streptococci; enterococci; and gram-negative rods, including *Pseudomonas*.

In the ED, the patient's presentation is typical of a cocaine overdose. Pharmacologic effects of cocaine include blockade of cellular membrane transport and prevention of the reuptake of biogenic amines (dopamine, norepinephrine, serotonin). High doses of cocaine lead to hyperpyrexia, hypertension, tachycardia, and tonic-clonic seizures. Opiates and phencyclidine tend to produce respiratory depression at high doses, but can also cause seizures. Δ-9-Tetrahydrocannabinol intoxication and withdrawal are not associated with seizures. Typically, ethanol produces seizures after cessation of use when blood alcohol levels fall.

Treatment of chronic cocaine abuse requires a multidisciplinary approach, with the physician, social worker, and psychiatrist all playing important roles. As of yet, there are no effective pharmacologic agents that lead to abstinence. Behavioral modification therapy and stimulus removal have been largely unsuccessful.

99. The answer is A. (*Pediatrics*)

Animal bites lead to approximately two million ED visits per year. A majority (80%) of these visits are due to dogs and involve bites of the hands or arms. Because of the numerous bacterial species present in the mouth of the animal and the skin of the patient, it is not surprising that the common cause of hospitalization after an animal bite is local infection (cellulitis, lymphangitis) that develops 24 to 36 hours after the bite. Approximately

4% of dog bites and 80% of cat bites become infected. Infections are commonly polymicrobial. The causative organisms include aerobic and anaerobic species; *Pasteurella multocida* is common in dog or cat bites. Initial therapy should be broad. For superficial infections, orally administered amoxicillin-clavulanate is a good choice. Erythromycin can be used for penicillin-allergic patients. Metronidazole provides only adequate anaerobe coverage, and tetracycline and ciprofloxacin hydrochloride lack the necessary anaerobe coverage.

100–101. The answers are: 100-D, 101-C. (*Emergency medicine, internal medicine*)
This represents a classic presentation of gout, which is typically an acute, monoarticular, inflammatory arthritis resulting from the deposition of urate crystals. Hyperuricemia is invariably present and results from either decreased excretion or increased production of uric acid. Causes of increased production include idiopathic factors, obesity, alcohol, hemolytic disease, purine-rich diets, and other conditions that may be associated with rapidly proliferating cells. Causes of decreased excretion include idiopathic factors, renal failure, hypertension, alcohol, and diuretics. This patient has several risk factors for hyperuricemia; however, an infectious cause cannot be excluded. The proper approach to this patient would involve a rapid diagnostic test, such as joint aspiration, Gram's stain, and culture and inspection for urate crystals. Empiric treatment without joint aspiration could miss a potentially joint-threatening infection.

Appropriate treatment for the acute gout flare-up includes colchicine, nonsteroidal anti-inflammatory drugs (NSAIDs), or intra-articular corticosteroids. In high doses, colchicine leads to abdominal pain, diarrhea, and nausea. Before placing this patient on chronic therapy after a single gout attack, the physician should identify and correct any reversible causes of hyperuricemia, if possible. This approach involves weight loss, cessation of alcohol consumption, and a change in the patient's antihypertensive medication from hydrochlorothiazide to another drug. If these strategies are not effective, and the patient continues to suffer from gout attacks, chronic drug therapy may be indicated.

102–107. The answers are: 102-A, 103-B, 104-D, 105-B, 106-E, 107-C. (*Pediatrics*)
This patient has acute lymphoblastic leukemia, which is characterized by the uncontrolled proliferation of immature lymphoblasts with consequent obliteration of the bone marrow and subsequent suppression of normal hematopoiesis. The disease commonly affects men, Caucasians, and individuals of higher socioeconomic status. Peak incidence occurs at approximately 4 years of age.

Leukemic cells are randomly introduced into the blood from the bone marrow. They may divide in the blood or infiltrate organs such as the spleen, liver, or lymph nodes, where they may divide and reenter the blood. The lymphoblasts have a predilection for the reticuloendothelial system; kidneys; brain; testicles; and, occasionally, bone. Acute lymphoblastic leukemia is classified into three types: L1, L2, and L3. Prognosis is best in L1 and worst in L3. The majority of lymphocytic leukemias arise from the clonal proliferation of B-cell progenitors.

Patients with acute lymphoblastic leukemia usually present with nonspecific signs and symptoms, such as fatigue, lethargy, malaise, anorexia, pallor and, occasionally, weight loss. Symptoms of anemia often predominate. Evidence of thrombocytopenia, such as easy bruising, petechiae, or menorrhagia, may be present. Lymphadenopathy in the cervical region is palpable in most patients, and the spleen is palpable in 50% of cases. The liver is infrequently palpable. Fever due to infection occurs in 15% of patients. The most common offenders are *Staphylococcus* species and gram-negative bacteria.

Bone marrow examination is necessary for definitive diagnosis of acute lymphoblastic leukemia, and is used to assess the status of blood cell production and cytogenetic anomalies and to help classify the disease. On bone marrow examination, lymphoblasts predominate, and normal hematopoietic elements are reduced. The normal fat spaces are partially or completely obliterated by the leukemic infiltrate. In addition, because the central nervous system (CNS) is a common sanctuary site for acute lymphoblastic leukemia, evaluation of the cerebrospinal fluid (CSF) is necessary. Cranial nerves VI and VII are most frequently involved.

Most treatment regimens include prophylactic intrathecal chemotherapy, as well as cranial irradiation. Therapy generally includes an intensive initial induction phase with prednisone; asparaginase; and vincristine sulfate, with or without doxorubicin; followed by consolidation therapy and, finally, by maintenance therapy for 2 to 3 years.

Tumor lysis syndrome may develop within 1 to 5 days of the initiation of induction therapy for acute lymphoblastic leukemia. The incidence of the condition correlates with tumor burden and, thus, lactate dehydrogenase (LDH) and white blood cell (WBC) count. It is caused by the mass destruction of a large number of rapidly proliferating neoplastic cells. Most commonly seen in acute lymphoblastic leukemia and Burkitt lymphoma, it rarely occurs in solid tumors. Tumor lysis syndrome is characterized by various combinations of hyperuricemia, hyperkalemia, hyperphosphatemia, hypocalcemia, and lactic acidosis. (Acute lymphoblastic leukemia may be associated with hypokalemia secondary to a renal tubular defect, but this is exclusive of tumor lysis syndrome.) The hypocalcemia may occur acutely and is associated with neuromuscular irritability, tetany, and paresthesia.

In anticipation of tumor lysis syndrome, patients should receive adequate hydration for maintenance of an increased urine output. In addition, they should receive bicarbonate in the intravenous fluids; this, together with increased urine output, may help prevent the precipitation of uric acid crystals. Urine should be maintained at approximately 7.0 to 7.5 pH. Note that alkalinization of the blood can cause an abrupt decrease in free calcium and could exacerbate the hypocalcemia seen in tumor lysis syndrome. Allopurinol at a dosage of approximately 300 mg/m^2 per day should decrease uric acid production. Electrolytes, uric acid, calcium, and phosphate must be watched closely.

Patients with hyperkalemia are at risk for arrhythmias and cardiac arrest. On ECG, early peaking of T waves, flattening of P waves, and late widening of QRS are evident. An early ECG is essential and, if necessary, patients should receive calcium, bicarbonate, glucose, insulin, an inhaled β-agonist, and a potassium-binding resin. If hyperkalemia, hyperuricemia, and hyperphosphatemia persist in the face of decreasing urine output, dialysis may be necessary.

108–109. The answers are 108-A, 109-C. (*Internal medicine, neurology*)
This patient has microcytic, hypochromic anemia, which is clearly visible on his peripheral blood smear, and most likely has iron deficiency anemia. In an older man, the probable cause of this condition is blood loss from the gastrointestinal (GI) tract, and an evaluation with colonoscopy is mandatory. Vitamin B$_{12}$ levels, hemoglobin electrophoresis, a reticulocyte count, and protoporphyrin levels provide no useful information.

The patient's peripheral blood smear now shows macrocytes and hypersegmented neutrophils (more than five lobulations). The differential diagnosis includes vitamin B$_{12}$ and folate deficiency, as well as drugs that either impair vitamin B$_{12}$ or folate metabolism or directly interfere with DNA synthesis (e.g., azathioprine, zidovudine). The common cause of vitamin B$_{12}$ deficiency in temperate climates is pernicious anemia, whereas folate deficiency is more often seen in alcoholism and malnutrition. Anorexia and weight loss are common in vitamin B$_{12}$ deficiency. The clinical distinction between vitamin B$_{12}$ and folate deficiency is sometimes difficult to make and involves laboratory testing. This patient is complaining of numbness and tingling in his feet, so vitamin B$_{12}$ deficiency may be more likely.

The neurologic changes resulting from vitamin B$_{12}$ deficiency begin with demyelination and lead to axonal degeneration and cell death. The commonly affected sites are the peripheral nerves, posterior and lateral columns of the spinal cord, and the cerebrum. On physical examination, reflexes may be either increased or decreased. Romberg and Babinski signs may be positive, and position and vibration sense are usually diminished. Disturbances of thinking may be prominent, with symptoms ranging from mild irritability to dementia and psychosis.

110–113. The answers are: 110-C, 111-B, 112-A, 113-C. (*Obstetrics/gynecology*)
The patient's complaints are most consistent with gastroesophageal reflux. Pregnancy results in decreased gastrointestinal (GI) motility, relaxation of the lower esophageal sphincter, and anatomic displacement of the gastroesophageal junction, which all contribute to the development of reflux. The motility and tone changes are primarily secondary to progesterone.

The key to this case is noting that alkaline phosphatase, an enzyme made primarily by the liver, bone, intestine, and placenta, is normally elevated in pregnancy. Therefore, reassurance is adequate. Alkaline phosphatase may be pathologically elevated with hemolysis, elevated liver enzymes, low platelet count (HELLP) syndrome; cholestasis of pregnancy; and cholecystitis. Cholelithiasis is more common in pregnancy secondary to gallbladder relaxation, with subsequent biliary stasis and stone formation. Bile composition does not change. Aspartate aminotransferase (AST) and alanine aminotransferase (ALT) may be slightly elevated in normal pregnancy as well. Because this patient has no symptoms that suggest cholecystitis or cholelithiasis, right upper quadrant ultrasound is unnecessary at this time. Esophagogastroduodenoscopy would be useful to evaluate for mucosal changes in long-standing reflux, but it is not needed in this setting. Because cholestasis or cholangitis are unlikely, endoscopic retrograde cholangiopancreatography is unnecessary.

Dietary changes are the best recommendation for this progestin-mediated gastroesophageal reflux. Sphincterotomy is necessary for gallstone pancreatitis or cholangitis. Cholestyramine is a bile acid resin primarily used to treat hypercholesterolemia. Omeprazole would improve the patient's symptoms, but it is listed in Food and Drug Administration (FDA) pregnancy category C and may have deleterious effects.

During pregnancy, an increase in minute ventilation occurs secondary to an increase in tidal volume, not respiratory rate. Tidal volume increases 30% to 40%, minute ventilation increases 30%, residual volume decreases by 20%, inspiratory capacity (tidal volume + inspiratory reserve volume) increases by 5%, and total lung capacity decreases by 5%.

The result of the increased minute ventilation is respiratory alkalosis. One would expect renal compensation for this with a decreased bicarbonate. The arterial blood gas shows a mild alkalemia, decreased PCO_2, and normal PO_2 with an appropriately compensated bicarbonate.

114–116. The answers are: 114-D, 115-E, 116-B. (*Obstetrics/gynecology*)

Gestational diabetes mellitus (GDM), which occurs in 3% to 12% of all pregnancies, strictly refers to cases of new glucose intolerance during pregnancy. These cases account for approximately 90% of all diabetes that occurs during pregnancy. Many factors are related to the development of GDM. Human placental lactogen acts as an anti-insulin, increasing lipolysis and decreasing glucose uptake and gluconeogenesis. Insulinase, which is made by the placenta, breaks down insulin. Both estrogen and progesterone interfere with the insulin–glucose relationship.

Gestational diabetes mellitus is associated with an increased risk for congenital malformations and prenatal morbidity and mortality. Glycemic control generally reduces the incidence of both maternal and neonatal complications. Maternal complications include increased rates of preeclampsia and pregnancy-induced hypertension. The most common infantile anomalies are cardiac and limb deformities. Macrosomia (fetal weight greater than 4,500 g) is the more common of these and is associated with fetopelvic disproportion and shoulder dystocia. Gestational diabetes mellitus leads to an increased risk of neonatal hypoglycemia, hyperbilirubinemia, hypocalcemia, and polycythemia. Polyhydramnios, with a subsequent, increased risk of abruptio placentae, preterm labor, and postpartum uterine atony, develops in 10% of pregnant women. The risk of spontaneous abortion is increased if glucose control is poor, as is the risk of intrauterine fetal demise and stillbirth. Last, respiratory distress syndrome occurs more frequently (risk is increased 5 to 6 times).

Screening for GDM should take place at 24 to 28 weeks' gestation for two reasons: (1) glucose intolerance is usually manifested by this time, increasing the sensitivity of the screening test; and (2) good glucose control can still affect outcome. The most commonly used screening modality is plasma glucose testing 1 hour after the ingestion of 50 g of Glucola. A plasma glucose level exceeding 140 mg/dL warrants a 3-hour glucose tolerance test. After 3 days of 150 grams of carbohydrates/day, a fasting plasma glucose is drawn. Then 100 grams of Glucola are ingested, with the subsequent measure of plasma glucose at 1, 2, and 3 hours. The upper limit for normal is 105, 190, 165, and 145 mg/mL for *plasma* glucose, and 90, 165, 145, and 125 mg/mL for *blood* glucose. Two or more abnormal values indicate the presence of GDM.

Regardless of glucose control in pregnancy, diabetes develops later in life in 5% to 30% of these women; therefore, glucose tolerance testing is advocated in the postpartum period.

117–122. The answers are: 117-D, 118-B, 119-D, 120-A, 121-C, 122-A. (*Neurology, internal medicine*)
This patient has signs and symptoms suggestive of Guillain-Barré syndrome. Classic findings include weakness or paralysis (usually symmetrical) associated with the loss of deep tendon reflexes. Guillain-Barré syndrome commonly starts in the lower extremities and ascends. Weakness progresses, with nadir occurring an average of 14 days after the onset of symptoms. Most patients regain the majority of their function in months.

The cerebrospinal fluid (CSF) exhibits a classic "albuminocytologic" dissociation consisting of increased protein without pleocytosis. A low glucose usually occurs in infectious meningitis. Oligoclonal bands are most common in multiple sclerosis.

Histologically, lymphocytic infiltration of the spinal roots and peripheral nerves with macrophage-mediated demyelination is seen. In North America, a minority of cases also have axonal involvement and have a poorer prognosis.

Nerve conduction studies involve stimulating individual nerves with electrodes at two sites and measuring the conduction velocity between them. In general, demyelinating processes cause prominent reductions in conduction velocity, whereas axonal degeneration disproportionately decreases the amplitude of the action potential to the reduction in velocity. F waves, which are elicited during nerve conduction studies, represent the result of antidromic (i.e., toward the spinal cord) impulse travel with subsequent anterior horn cell discharge. They may be prolonged in nerve root disease. Muscle grouping (or fiber-type grouping) is a phenomenon apparent on muscle biopsy in the setting of chronic, ongoing, denervation–reinnervation. However, it is not seen acutely, and nerve conduction studies alone do not illustrate it. The cause of muscle grouping is reinnervation of muscle fibers that were formerly innervated by the now-damaged nerve. Evaluation of motor unit size is apparent on electromyography (EMG). Recall that a motor unit is made up of an anterior horn cell, motor fibers, and the muscles they innervate. In the chronic denervating–reinnervating process, the motor units become larger as healthy nerve fibers "pick up" the denervated muscle fibers.

In at least 60% of cases, Guillain-Barré syndrome follows infection. The best documented antecedents include *Campylobacter jejuni,* Epstein-Barr virus, cytomegalovirus, HIV, and *Mycoplasma*. Guillain-Barré syndrome has been seen after influenza vaccination, particularly after the 1967–1977 swine flu vaccination, and it also occurs in lymphoma and systemic lupus erythematosus.

Intravenous immunoglobulin is the best treatment option. It is at least as effective as plasmapheresis and is less invasive. No data support the use of corticosteroids or antibiotics. Riluzole, a presynaptic inhibitor of glutamate release, may slow disease progression in amyotrophic lateral sclerosis. It is particularly appropriate for those patients with significant bulbar disease.

A major concern in patients with Guillain-Barré syndrome is the development of respiratory failure secondary to respiratory muscle involvement, which may occur acutely. Negative inspiratory force (or pressure) and vital capacity are the best measures of impending muscular failure. Both peak flow and minute ventilation would be diminished; however, neither is a specific test. A chest radiograph would be normal, and a ventilation-perfusion ($\dot{V}/\dot{Q}$) scan would be unnecessary.

In an arterial blood gas analysis, a near-normal alveolar–arterial gradient would be apparent because hypoventilation causes both an increase in carbon dioxide and a decrease in oxygen. One should look for the appropriate decrease of 0.08 pH for each increase of 10 mm Hg in P_{CO_2} that would be representative of acute hypoventilatory failure. Only in option A is there concomitant hypoxia and hypercarbia consistent with alveolar hypoventilation.

123–125. The answers are: 123-E, 124-C, 125-C. (*Internal medicine, critical care medicine*)
The advanced cardiac life support (ACLS) algorithms available for the treatment of cardiac arrest and life-threatening cardiac arrhythmias stress that early defibrillation and cardioversion of patients with cardiopulmonary arrest increase long-term survival. After attention to airway, breathing, and circulation (ABC), rapid defibrillation up to 3 times with increasing energy levels should be attempted before delivery of medications.

In this patient, defibrillation results in pulseless electrical activity. The differential diagnosis of this condition includes hypovolemia, hypoxia, cardiac tamponade, tension pneumothorax, hypothermia, massive pulmonary embolism, drug toxicity, hyperkalemia, acidosis, and massive myocardial infarction (MI). Because this patient has recently had a central line placed in the subclavian vein, tension pneumothorax is a likely possibility. Rapid placement of a large-bore angiography catheter in the chest cavity of a patient with tension pneumothorax decompresses the chest cavity, allowing venous return and rapid restoration of the pulse. Administration of atropine would be helpful for bradycardia; insulin, glucose, and bicarbonate for hyperkalemia; and pericardiocentesis for cardiac tamponade.

126–130. The answers are: 126-B, 127-A, 128-D, 129-A, 130-B. (*Obstetrics/gynecology*)
Urinary tract infections are common in pregnancy because of progesterone-related stasis changes, increased urinary glucose, and anatomic changes. Asymptomatic bacteriuria detection is important because of its association with preterm labor and its progression to acute pyelonephritis in about 20% of cases. Pyelonephritis is associated with sepsis in 3% of cases and respiratory failure in 2% to 8% (secondary to acute respiratory distress syndrome [ARDS]). Asymptomatic bacteriuria is more common with sickle cell trait, diabetes mellitus, multiparity, increasing age, and lower socioeconomic status.

Once cystitis is suspected, the most important next step is to determine whether the infection has progressed to pyelonephritis. Costovertebral angle tenderness may help distinguish between cystitis and pyelonephritis. Suprapubic tenderness is likely to be present in both settings. A positive Murphy sign would be present in the setting of cholecystitis, which does not cause dysuria. Without significant abdominal pain, rebound tenderness is unlikely to be elicited. Cervicitis is unlikely without vaginal discharge; therefore, cervical motion tenderness should not be present.

As part of this patient's workup, a complete blood count (CBC) and urine culture are necessary. Antibiotic administration may begin, but urine microscopy is essential to assess for white blood cell (WBC) casts. It may also suggest an atypical cause of infection. *Escherichia coli* accounts for approximately 85% of cystitis cases in pregnancy, followed by *Proteus mirabilis, Klebsiella* species, *Enterobacter* species, *Staphylococcus saprophyticus,* and group B streptococci.

Acceptable treatment includes ampicillin, cephalosporins, or nitrofurantoin. Sulfa-containing medications should be avoided in the third trimester because of their association with infantile jaundice. Tetracyclines and quinolones should be totally avoided during pregnancy. If the infection does not respond to antibiotics, consideration of urinary calculi is warranted. *Proteus* is likely if the urine is alkaline because of its ability to split urea.

131–133. The answers are: 131-D, 132-E, 133-E. (*Pediatrics*)
This patient has Crohn disease, an inflammatory condition that involves the entire gastrointestinal (GI) tract, which has frequent extraintestinal manifestations. Most affected patients are older than 10 years, and the cause is unknown. Patients typically have abdominal pain and bloody diarrhea. The differential diagnoses must include enteric infection with *Salmonella, Shigella,* and *Entamoeba,* hemolytic uremic syndrome, Henoch-Schönlein purpura, and ulcerative colitis. Infection with *Giardia* (a protozoan parasite), which occurs in the small bowel, leads to cramping, abdominal pain, distension, and watery diarrhea. Bloody diarrhea is rare in *Giardia* infections.

Extraintestinal manifestations of Crohn disease are diverse and include all of the conditions listed in question 132 except for intestinal lymphoma. The risk of intestinal lymphoma is increased in celiac sprue but not in inflammatory bowel disease. Uveitis, arthritis, and erythema nodosum are immunologically mediated. Malabsorption from involvement of the terminal ileum occurs as a result of nephrolithiasis and leads to increased oxalate absorption and kidney stones.

Treatment of Crohn disease centers on suppression of the immune system and the use of 5-aminosalicylate compounds, such as mesalamine. The mechanism of action of the 5-aminosalicylate compounds is not known. One of the newest effective treatments is infliximab, a monoclonal antibody to tumor necrosis factor-α. Neomycin, a nonabsorbable antibiotic, has no role in the treatment of Crohn disease. This agent is useful for bowel decontamination and in the treatment of hepatic encephalopathy.

134. The answer is A. (*Neurology, obstetrics/gynecology*)
Epilepsy is a common disorder that affects women of childbearing age. It is important to realize which anticonvulsants are contraindicated during pregnancy. Among commonly used anticonvulsants, valproic acid is associated with an increased risk of neural tube defects. Phenobarbital, phenytoin, and carbamazepine also pose some teratogenic risk. The period of maximum risk is the first 6 weeks of gestation. Common malformations include orofacial clefts, congenital heart lesions, skeletal abnormalities, and hypospadias. In patients who have been seizure-free for several years, it is reasonable to attempt tapering and withdrawal of therapy. Furthermore, every attempt should be made to treat patients with monotherapy at the lowest effective dosage. Finally, it is important to realize that the enhanced metabolism of pregnancy may lead to lower serum levels of anticonvulsants, so levels must be monitored carefully.

135. The answer is E. (*Neurology, internal medicine*)
In a patient with frequent and debilitating migraine headaches, prophylactic therapy is warranted. It is also appropriate in the patient for whom ergot alkaloids are either contraindicated or poorly tolerated. The mainstays of prophylaxis are amitriptyline, propranolol, and ergonovine. Each agent is effective in a substantial proportion of migraine sufferers—failure of one agent does not predict failure of an agent from a different class. The choice of agent depends on the patient and associated comorbidities. For example, propranolol may be relatively contraindicated in a patient with asthma or diabetes mellitus. Other agents that are effective as prophylactic therapy include calcium channel blockers and nonsteroidal anti-inflammatory drugs (NSAIDs). All of the other medications listed are treatments for acute migraine headaches and are not effective as prophylactic therapy.

136. The answer is B. (*Pediatrics*)
The boy has rheumatic fever, a dreaded complication of streptococcal pharyngitis. It is important to realize that a rapid streptococcal antigen test is not perfect, with sensitivities ranging from 50% to 95% and specificities of 95% to 100%. In the setting of a strong clinical suspicion, a negative rapid antigen test must be confirmed with a culture. It is believed that rheumatic fever is caused by specific strains of group A streptococci that elicit an intense immune response and autoimmunity. The diagnosis of acute rheumatic fever is based on the Jones criteria, which require evidence of a preceding streptococcal infection (positive throat culture and positive rapid antigen test or elevated or rising streptococcal antigen titer) *and* the presence of two major criteria or one major and two minor criteria:

Major Criteria	Minor Criteria
Carditis	Arthralgias
Polyarthritis	Fever
Chorea	Laboratory findings: elevated
Erythema marginatum	erythrocyte sedimentation rate (ESR)
Subcutaneous nodules	or C-reactive protein
	Prolonged P-R interval

It is important to recognize rheumatic fever because prophylaxis against further streptococcal infection is necessary in affected patients until 20 years of age and 5 years after their last attack (longer with carditis).

This patient does not have systemic lupus erythematosus, which is more common in young women and marked by multisystem involvement, including malar rash, fever, arthritis, hair loss, thrombocytopenia, urinary abnormalities (hematuria and proteinuria), and a positive antinuclear antibody. Rheumatoid arthritis is also unlikely and is more often seen in middle-aged women with deforming, symmetrical, polyarthritis. Reiter syndrome generally leads to a combination of arthritis, conjunctivitis, and urethritis. Scarlet fever is seen early in *Streptococcus pyogenes* infection and consists of fever with a sandpaper-like rash.

137. The answer is B. (*Pediatrics*)
This case provides clinical evidence of coarctation of the aorta. In this condition, there is a narrowing of the aortic lumen usually located just distal to the subclavian artery (at the junction of the ductus arteriosus with the aortic arch). This narrowing leads to left ventricular hypertrophy secondary to increased afterload; hypertension secondary to decreased renal blood flow; and decreased blood flow, growth, and mottling in the lower extremities. Coarctation of the aorta is associated with an increased incidence of a bicuspid aortic valve in approximately 70% of patients. Rib notching, evident on chest radiographs, is an interesting radiographic finding in long-standing coarctation of the aorta secondary to increased collateral flow through the intercostal arteries to the lower extremities. Cyanosis is secondary to deoxygenated hemoglobin and does not typically occur in this condition unless patients are markedly anemic.

138. The answer is D. (*Pediatrics*)
Tetralogy of Fallot accounts for approximately 10% of congenital heart lesions and is the most common cyanotic, congenital, cardiac abnormality. It is characterized by variable obstruction to right ventricular outflow (pulmonic stenosis), dextroposition of the aorta or overriding of the ventricular septum, ventricular septal defect, and right ventricular hypertrophy. Of these abnormalities, ventricular septal defect and right ventricular outflow obstruction are the most important. There is equalization of the right and left ventricular pressures, and shunting of blood to either the right or left side of the heart is critically dependent on the degree of right ventricular outflow obstruction. The greater the degree of left-to-right shunting, the greater the degree of cyanosis. Signs of tetralogy of Fallot include variable degrees of cyanosis, digital clubbing, hyperpnea, a right ventricular heave, and a harsh systolic murmur along the sternal border.

Interestingly, children learn that squatting decreases the hypoxemia and cyanosis; the maneuver increases left ventricular afterload and decreases the left-to-right shunt. For this reason, hypoxemia spells are treated by placing the child in a knee–chest position to increase systemic vascular resistance. Surgical correction is recommended for children with a hypoxemic spell. The other maneuvers (raising or lowering the lower extremities, placing in the Trendelenburg position) do not affect the degree of left-to-right shunting and would have no effect on hypoxemia and cyanosis.

139–141. The answers are: 139-D, 140-E, 141-A. (*Internal medicine*)
It is not uncommon for individuals with type 2 diabetes to display a constellation of factors that put them at high risk for subsequent cardiovascular disease and morbidity and mortality. This patient exhibits many of these risks: obesity, hypertension, proteinuria and nephropathy, a low serum high-density lipoprotein (HDL) level, and left ventricular hypertrophy. Based on these risks, the American Diabetes Association recommends careful attention to glycemic control (fasting blood sugar of 80 to 120 mg/dL, hemoglobin$_{A1C}$ <7%); lipid parameters (total cholesterol, <200 mg/dL; low-density lipoprotein-C [LDL-C], <100 mg/dL; HDL, >45 mg/dL; triglycerides, <200 mg/dL); and blood pressure (<130/85 mm Hg).

In this patient, the major issues are hypertension and progressive nephropathy with proteinuria. Ramipril is the most efficacious drug compared to the other agents listed as answer choices in question 139. Angiotensin-converting enzyme (ACE) inhibitors have been shown to slow the progression of nephropathy (independent of their blood pressure–lowering characteristics) and also to lead to regression in left ventricular hypertrophy. The addition of insulin would not be necessary because the patient's glycemic control is nearly adequate (but not ideal), and he is suffering from hypoglycemic episodes. Metoprolol would be relatively contraindicated in the setting of these hypoglycemic episodes. Amlodipine, a dihydropyridine calcium channel blocker with little antiproteinuric effect, is a poor choice of antihypertensive medication.

Raising the patient's HDL level significantly affects his risk profile. Of the agents listed as answer choices in question 140, only vitamin E does not increase HDL levels. Of the agents listed as answer choices in question 141, niacin appears to worsen glycemic control, and diabetes mellitus is a relative contraindication to its use.

142–145. The answers are: 142-D, 143-E, 144-D, 145-C. (*Pediatrics, statistics*)
In this instance, the approach to diarrhea first involves assessing the patient's hydration and hemodynamic status. Next, it is often possible to predict the causative pathogen by determining the time from ingestion to the development of symptoms. The two bacteria that cause nausea, vomiting, and diarrhea within 1 to 6 hours are *Staphylococcus aureus* and *Bacillus cereus,* which both carry a preformed toxin that causes symptoms. *S. aureus* is frequently found in mayonnaise-containing salads, and *B. cereus* is classically found in fried rice. *Campylobacter jejuni* is the most common cause of food poisoning by poultry, but the incubation period is generally longer than 16 hours. *Entamoeba histolytica* is a parasitic infection that causes colitis with scant, bloody stools, fever, and abdominal pain. Without fever or blood in the stool, the suspicion for an inflammatory diarrhea is low. The incubation period of *Salmonella* is also greater than 16 hours. *Clostridium difficile* is classically seen after a course of antibiotics. Although this patient recently took antibiotics, the association with the sick families present at the picnic makes infection with *S. aureus* from the potato salad more likely. Stool cultures, *C. difficile* enzyme-linked immunosorbent assay (ELISA), and ova and parasite testing are unnecessary. Supportive therapy with oral hydration therapy is the treatment of choice.

The presence of leukocytes by methylene blue stool study indicates inflammatory diarrhea. Pathogens include *Shigella, Salmonella, Campylobacter,* enterohemorrhagic *E. coli, Yersinia, C. difficile,* enteroinvasive *E. coli,* and *E. histolytica. Vibrio cholerae* causes a secretory diarrhea that is not inflammatory.

To determine the posttest probability from the pretest probability, the sensitivity and specificity characteristics of the ELISA test are necessary. The posttest probability = pretest probability × likelihood ratio, and the likelihood ratio = sensitivity/(1 – specificity). The odds ratio, as reported in retrospective studies, is the probability that patients with the disease have a given risk factor. The sensitivity is the probability of having a positive test in patients with the disease. The positive predictive value is the probability of disease occurrence in patients with a positive test.

146. The answer is D. (*Internal medicine, critical care medicine*)
Acute pancreatitis can be a life-threatening disease. Rapid recognition of those patients at risk for complications is important so that proper therapy can be initiated. Several different clinical scoring systems exist to aid in the identification of patients with poor prognosis. The Ranson criteria are the most commonly used measure of the severity of acute pancreatitis:

Ranson Criteria	
At Diagnosis or Admission	During Initial 48 Hours
Age >55 years	Fall in hematocrit by 10%
Leukocytosis >16,000/mm³	Fluid deficit >6 L
Hyperglycemia >200 mg/dL	Hypocalcemia (<8.0 mg/dL)
Serum lactate dehydrogenase (LDH) >300 U/L	Hypoxemia (PO_2 <60 mm Hg)
Serum aspartate aminotransferase (AST) >250 U/L	Increase in blood urea nitrogen (BUN) to >5 mg/dL after intravenous fluid administration
	Hypoalbuminemia (albumin <3.2 g/dL)

Pulmonary complications of pancreatitis include pleural effusions, atelectasis, mediastinal abscess, and acute respiratory distress syndrome (ARDS). This patient has ARDS, which involves bilateral pulmonary infiltrates, severe hypoxemia (arterial oxygen tension/fraction of inspired oxygen ratio [PaO_2/FIO_2] <200), and the absence of left atrial or pulmonary capillary hypertension.

147. The answer is A. (*Internal medicine*)
The combination of low forced vital capacity (FVC), low forced expiratory volumes (FEVs), low total lung capacity, and a reduced diffusing capacity is characteristic of a restrictive process. The differential diagnosis of a restrictive process includes pleural disease and alveolar diseases (e.g., pulmonary edema, interstitial lung disease, neuromuscular disease, or thoracic cage disease). This patient ultimately receives a diagnosis of interstitial lung disease and idiopathic pulmonary fibrosis. Obstructive lung disease is typically associated with a reduced FEV and a FEV/FVC ratio of less than 75%, with an increased residual volume from air trapping. Extrathoracic lung disease can be diagnosed from a flow–volume loop, which demonstrates the limitation of the inspiratory loop. Neuromuscular disease, which can be diagnosed by decreased inspiratory pressures, may appear similar to restrictive disease with decreased lung volumes; however, the diffusing capacity tends to be preserved.

148–150. The answers are: 148-B, 149-D, 150-D. (*Internal medicine*)
This patient has signs and symptoms of peripheral neuropathy. The differential diagnosis is extensive, including diabetes mellitus, alcohol abuse, nutritional deficiencies (vitamins B_1, B_6, B_{12}, E), toxicity (e.g., lead, arsenic, thallium, vincristine, paclitaxel [Taxol]), hereditary disease (Charcot-Marie-Tooth disease), amyloidosis, Guillain-Barré syndrome, chronic immune demyelinating polyneuropathy, porphyria, infection (HIV), leprosy, Lyme disease, hypothyroidism, myeloma, systemic lupus erythematosus, and paraneoplastic syndromes.

Given this patient's history, he is most likely to have alcoholism. Alcoholic neuropathy is difficult to distinguish from the nutritional deficiency that accompanies it. There is damage to both sensory and motor fibers, and the initial symptoms are plantar pain and paresthesia often described as burning. Distal weakness can occur, and ankle jerks are the first reflexes lost.

Despite the patient's complaint of polyuria, his condition is unlikely to be diabetes. Diabetic polyneuropathy is uncommon at the time of diabetes diagnosis. It usually begins with sensory loss in the feet. Hypothyroidism can cause peripheral neuropathy; however, it is a less common than alcohol abuse and no other symptoms suggest it. Tobacco abuse and potential asbestos exposure are not well-characterized causes of peripheral neuropathy.

In considering the differential diagnosis, the workup might include glycosylated hemoglobin and thyroid function studies. Liver function studies and a complete blood count (CBC) may help support the theory of alcohol abuse. Paraproteinemia is unlikely in this patient; therefore, a serum protein electrophoresis is unnecessary.

A macrocytosis is defined as an mean corpuscular volume (MCV) greater than 95–100 fL, depending on the patient population. The most common causes include alcoholism, vitamin B_{12} deficiency, folate deficiency, hypothyroidism, reticulocytosis, drugs (methotrexate, phenytoin, trimethoprim, zidovudine), and liver dysfunction (secondary to abnormal lipid deposition on red blood cell [RBC] membranes).

Anemia of chronic disease is commonly normocytic or microcytic. The general approach to a macrocytosis includes a peripheral smear, vitamin B_{12} and folate levels, thyroid-stimulating hormone (TSH) level, and liver function tests and ruling out a responsible drug.

Test II

QUESTIONS

DIRECTIONS: For each question, select the letter corresponding to the best answer. All questions have only one correct answer.

Setting: Hospital

Questions 1–4

A 32-year-old woman, who is G_1P_1, gives birth to twin boys at 37 weeks. She had no complications during her pregnancy. One infant has Apgar scores of 7 at 1 minute and 9 at 5 minutes, and the other infant has scores of 8 at 1 minute and 9 at 5 minutes. Approximately 30 minutes after delivery, the mother is still bleeding, despite uterine massage, with an estimated blood loss of 600 mL.

1. The most likely cause of this woman's condition is

(A) cervical laceration
(B) retained placenta
(C) uterine inversion
(D) uterine atony
(E) disseminated intravascular coagulation (DIC)

2. The next management step is

(A) ultrasound
(B) gauze packing
(C) curettage
(D) artery ligation
(E) oxytocin

3. Which of the following conditions is NOT associated with DIC?

(A) Abruptio placentae
(B) Placenta previa
(C) Preeclampsia
(D) Amniotic fluid embolism
(E) Retention of dead fetus

4. Which of the following measures is NOT consistent with DIC?

(A) Prolonged prothrombin time (PT)
(B) Prolonged partial thromboplastin time (PTT)
(C) Increased D-dimer
(D) Increased fibrinogen
(E) Increased fibrin degradation products

Setting: Office

Questions 5–7

A 45-year-old woman with a history of rheumatoid arthritis presents with a 1-day history of left knee pain, swelling, and decreased range of motion. She complains that she cannot put weight on the left leg because of severe pain. Ibuprofen (800 mg) provides only minor pain relief. Her other medications include prednisone 10 mg/day, calcium supplements, naproxen 375 mg 2 times a day, and famotidine 20 mg/day. Physical examination reveals a woman in moderate distress with a temperature of 38.9°C and a blood pressure of 130/80 mm Hg. Her left knee appears swollen, and on palpation there is some increased warmth over the knee joint. On both passive and active range of motion, pain is severe, and movement is limited.

5. The first step in this woman's management should be

(A) plain films of the knee
(B) aspiration and analysis of synovial fluid
(C) increasing the dose of prednisone
(D) intravenous antibiotics
(E) oral colchicine

6. Ultimately, a sample of synovial fluid from the knee is obtained. Analysis of this opaque fluid reveals:

White blood cell (WBC) count	60,000/mm^3
Neutrophils	90%
Serum/glucose ratio	<0.5
Gram's stain	Pending

While culture results are pending, which of the following antibiotic regimens would be most appropriate?

(A) Ciprofloxacin
(B) Nafcillin sodium and cefepime hydrochloride
(C) Ampicillin and gentamicin sulfate
(D) Nafcillin, amphotericin B, and ciprofloxacin
(E) Doxycycline and nafcillin

7. Antibiotics are initiated. Culture demonstrates *Streptococcus pyogenes*. Which of the following measures is indicated?

(A) Open surgical drainage
(B) Repeated needle aspiration
(C) Antibiotics for only 2 weeks
(D) Antibiotics and open surgical drainage
(E) Antibiotics and repeated needle aspiration

Setting: Office

8. A 45-year-old man has abduction weakness of the right fifth finger and decreased pinprick sensation on the palmar surface of the right fifth finger. The lesion is at which of the following sites?

(A) Cervical spine
(B) Right precentral gyrus
(C) Right ulnar nerve
(D) Left postcentral gyrus
(E) Right ulnar nerve or left frontoparietal cortex

Setting: Hospital

Questions 9–12

A 54-year-old man is admitted with complaints of severe abdominal pain. For the past 24 hours, he has had nausea and vomiting, and he has not been able to keep down any food. His abdominal pain radiates through to his back. Of note, he was seen in the emergency department (ED) 1 year ago for a fall. Laboratory studies performed at that time revealed:

White blood cell (WBC) count	7,400/mm³
Hemoglobin	11.2 g/dL
Hematocrit	33.8%
Mean corpuscular volume	101/fL
Platelet count	135,000/mm³

9. Which of the following conditions is the most likely cause of this man's presentation?

(A) Trauma
(B) Gallstones
(C) Alcohol abuse
(D) Viral infection
(E) Malignancy

10. Which of the following laboratory tests would NOT be useful at this time for determining the man's prognosis?

(A) Glucose
(B) Aspartate aminotransferase (AST)
(C) White blood cell (WBC) count
(D) Amylase
(E) Lactate dehydrogenase (LDH)

11. A pleural effusion is apparent on chest radiography. Thoracentesis would likely detect all of the following conditions EXCEPT

(A) effusion restricted to the left chest only
(B) decreased amylase
(C) increased total protein
(D) increased LDH
(E) increased specific gravity

12. Three months later, the man returns with epigastric pain and coffee-ground emesis. He is referred urgently to the ED, where he undergoes an esophagogastroduodenoscopy. Gastric varices are seen, with no evidence of esophageal varices. The patient likely has

(A) hepatic vein thrombosis (Budd-Chiari syndrome)
(B) portal hypertension
(C) pseudocyst formation
(D) bile duct obstruction
(E) splenic vein thrombosis

Setting: Hospital

13. A 6-year-old girl is admitted with a 2-day history of bloody diarrhea, which began several hours after a picnic and has progressively worsened. She has become lethargic and has not been able to eat or drink. Physical examination reveals a child who is extremely ill-appearing, lethargic, and difficult to arouse. Vital signs are: temperature, 38.9°C; blood pressure, 80/54 mm Hg; heart rate, 128 beats/minute; and respiratory rate, 22/ minute. The appearance of numerous petechiae on her legs and a diffusely tender abdomen with decreased bowel sounds are notable. Laboratory studies reveal:

Blood urea nitrogen (BUN)	72 mg/dL
Creatinine	8.1 mg/dL
White blood cell (WBC) count	11,000/mm³
Hemoglobin	5 g/dL
Platelet count	<10,000 mm³
Prothrombin time (PT)	Within normal limits
Partial thromboplastin time (PTT)	Within normal limits

Laboratory analysis also includes a peripheral blood smear (*below*).

Which of the following diagnoses is most likely?

(A) Disseminated intravascular coagulation (DIC)
(B) Crohn disease
(C) Ulcerative colitis
(D) Hemolytic uremic syndrome
(E) Immune thrombocytopenic purpura

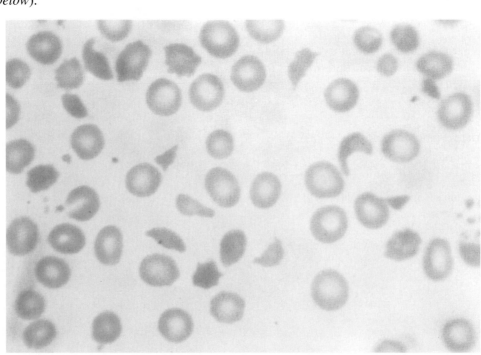

Setting: Office

14. A 2-week-old male infant is brought in by his parents because of persistent vomiting. They state that he forcefully vomits partially digested formula about 1 hour after he is fed. They deny seeing any bile or blood. He is defecating about 3 times a day. Vital signs are: temperature (rectal), 36.8°C; blood pressure, 95/50 mm Hg; heart rate, 130 beats/minute; and respirations, 34/minute. The infant is alert and active and not irritable. Examination is normal except for the presence of a small, nontender, palpable mass in the midepigastrium. Bowel sounds are active and no other masses are palpable. Which of the following procedures is most likely to yield the correct diagnosis in a cost-effective manner?

(A) Computed tomography (CT) of the abdomen
(B) Upper gastrointestinal (GI) series with barium
(C) Ultrasonography
(D) Plain films of the abdomen
(E) Laparoscopy

Setting: Satellite Clinic

Questions 15–18

A 28-year-old woman is brought to the clinic by a friend. She is a corporate attorney but has been missing from work on-and-off for the past 3 months. Her friends believe that she has been agitated and that her personality has changed. Prior to her absence, her performance at the office had been "slipping." On examination, she appears disheveled but is alert and oriented. The rest of the examination is normal.

15. Which of the following conditions likely explains the woman's symptoms?

(A) Major depressive disorder
(B) Drug abuse
(C) Brief psychotic disorder
(D) Schizoaffective disorder
(E) Schizophrenia

16. Which of the following measures is the most important next step?

(A) Assess suicide risk
(B) Screen for drugs of abuse
(C) Obtain a medication list
(D) Order a thyroid-stimulating hormone (TSH) level
(E) Order chemistries

17. Which of the following properties is associated with this disorder?

(A) Affects approximately 5% of the population
(B) More common in women
(C) High levels of TSH
(D) More common in lower socioeconomic groups
(E) Has no "season of birth" correlation

18. Which of the following chemicals is intimately involved with this disease?

(A) Triiodothyronine (T_3)
(B) Serotonin
(C) Norepinephrine
(D) Dopamine hydrochloride
(E) Acetylcholine chloride

Setting: Emergency Department

Questions 19–22

An 18-year-old woman presents with diffuse lower abdominal pain. She complains of fever but has not taken her temperature. She thinks that her last menstrual period was 1 week ago, but she is not sure. Approximately 6 months ago, she had a similar complaint that resolved on its own. She is sexually active; she has had three different sexual partners in the past year; she does not use contraception. Physical examination indicates a temperature of 38.8°C, a blood pressure of 160/90 mm Hg, and a heart rate of 105 beats/minute. Diffuse, lower abdominal tenderness, as well as right upper quadrant tenderness are present.

19. Which of the following procedures is least necessary at this time?

(A) Pelvic examination
(B) Pregnancy test
(C) Ultrasound
(D) Cervical cultures
(E) Complete blood count (CBC)

20. Which of the following conditions is the likely cause of the teenager's right upper quadrant tenderness?

(A) Intrahepatic cholestasis
(B) Perihepatitis
(C) Cholecystitis
(D) Appendicitis
(E) Preeclampsia

21. Which of the following organisms is the least likely to be involved?

(A) *Chlamydia trachomatis*
(B) *Mycoplasma hominis*
(C) *Neisseria gonorrhoeae*
(D) *Ureaplasma urealyticum*
(E) *Staphylococcus aureus*

22. Which of the following antibiotic regimens is likely to be the best treatment?

(A) Ceftriaxone sodium plus doxycycline
(B) Ceftriaxone
(C) Trimethoprim-sulfamethoxazole plus doxycycline
(D) Doxycycline
(E) Doxycycline plus metronidazole

Setting: Office

23. A 23-year-old man has been investigating medically oriented Internet sites. He comes to you, concerned that he may have a precancerous condition. Which of the following conditions is not considered precancerous?

(A) Barrett esophagus
(B) Dysplastic nevus syndrome
(C) Fibroadenoma of the breast
(D) Cervical dysplasia
(E) Squamous metaplasia of the lung

Setting: Office

24. You are reviewing recent papers regarding chest radiography in lung cancer screening. All of the following statements are considered important features of a screening test EXCEPT

(A) the test should detect a disease that is an important health problem
(B) the test should have a low sensitivity but be very specific
(C) an acceptable and effective therapy should be available for patients who have the disease
(D) screening and early treatment should be proved to favorably influence quality of life
(E) the test should be reliable

Setting: Office

25. A 52-year-old man comes in for a "physical" prior to approval for an insurance policy. The patient is asymptomatic, and the physical examination is normal. The physician orders a chest radiograph (*below*). No previous comparison films are available. The patient has smoked 2 packs of cigarettes per day for the past 30 years.

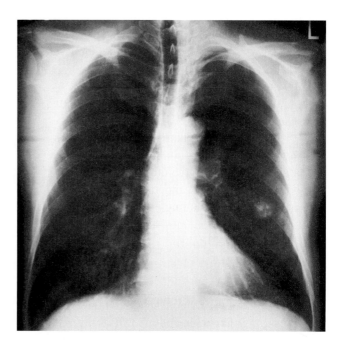

The most appropriate next step in this patient's management would be

(A) Repeat chest radiography in 6 months
(B) Trial regimen of antibiotics for 14 days and repeat chest radiograph in 2 months
(C) Bronchoscopy and needle biopsy
(D) Reassurance and counseling to stop smoking
(E) Resection if there are no contraindications

Setting: Office

Questions 26–29

A 78-year-old man is brought to your office by his daughter for evaluation of his increasing confusion. During the past 6 months, his daughter has noted a progressive deterioration in the man's ability to care for himself. He has become increasingly forgetful and often becomes lost in the neighborhood. Although his memory for remote events has not changed, he easily forgets whatever he is now told. According to his daughter, he occasionally has a beer with dinner.

On being questioned, the man denies any complaints and is not sure why he is in your office. He denies headaches, gait disturbances, visual changes, focal weakness, or sensory loss. His medical history is significant for hypertension and type 2 diabetes mellitus. He takes lisinopril and glyburide. Six months ago, screening laboratory work, including a complete blood count (CBC), liver enzymes, and renal function, were within normal limits.

26. The daughter is concerned that her father may be depressed. Which of the following historic criteria favors a diagnosis of depression over dementia?

(A) Abrupt onset
(B) Abnormal neurologic examination
(C) No patient complaints of memory loss
(D) Progressive deterioration
(E) Few vegetative symptoms

27. Which of the following findings most supports the diagnosis of Alzheimer disease?

(A) CT of the brain, demonstrating marked cortical atrophy
(B) Prominent visuospatial disorientation
(C) Gait instability and incontinence
(D) Myoclonus
(E) Hypersegmented neutrophils

28. On physical examination, you attempt to find causes of the man's progressive deterioration that may be reversible. Which of the following physical findings suggests a reversible cause of the cognitive decline?

(A) Decreased peripheral visual fields
(B) Myoclonus
(C) Delayed relaxation phase of deep tendon reflexes
(D) Labile affect with rapid cycling of emotions from crying to laughter
(E) Choreiform movements of the extremities

29. During the next 6 months, you continue to observe this man, who suffers a progressive decline in his cognitive ability. Especially troublesome to his daughter are periods of extreme agitation in the late evenings. Not uncommonly, the patient awakes at 2:00 AM and begins screaming that people are stealing his clothes and money. The family has attempted reorienting him but, recently, this has become unsuccessful. The daughter does not want to place him in a nursing home, but feels that she is approaching the point at which she is no longer able to care for him. You suggest that pharmacologic therapy may be of benefit. Which of the following agents would you suggest as treatment for the man's behavioral disturbances?

(A) Diphenhydramine
(B) Haloperidol
(C) Diazepam
(D) Vitamin B$_{12}$ injections
(E) Thiamine

Setting: Office

30. A 7-year-old girl is referred by a nurse practitioner about a possible heart murmur. The girl is otherwise healthy, having appropriately reached all developmental milestones. On examination, the precordium is hyperdynamic with a prominent right ventricular heave. A soft murmur is present in the pulmonic position, and the second heart sound has persistent splitting during inspiration and expiration. On electrocardiography (ECG), right axis deviation and rsR′ morphology in the right precordial leads is seen. The most likely diagnosis is

(A) atrial septal defect
(B) ventricular septal defect
(C) patent ductus arteriosus
(D) coarctation of the aorta
(E) pulmonic stenosis

Setting: Office

31. A 6-month-old male infant, who was recently discharged from the hospital after treatment for *Pneumocystis carinii* pneumonia, now has oral thrush. During his hospital stay, he underwent serologic and viral testing for HIV, which was negative. Polymerase chain reaction testing indicates that his parents are HIV-negative, and the infant has never received a blood transfusion. You suspect the presence of a defect in one arm of the immune system. Which of the following tests would confirm your suspicions?

(A) Quantitative serum immunoglobulins
(B) Nitroblue tetrazolium
(C) Delayed hypersensitivity skin testing
(D) Total hemolytic complement
(E) Repeat HIV testing in 3 months

Setting: Office

Questions 32–34

A 49-year-old man presents for a routine checkup with no complaints. He is 5′7″ tall and weighs 240 pounds; this represents an increase of 12 pounds in the past 18 months. During the genitourinary examination, you feel a mass pushing against the lateral aspect of your finger when he bears down. His scrotal examination is within normal limits.

32. Which of the following hernias is the cause of this physical finding?

(A) Hiatal
(B) Direct inguinal
(C) Indirect inguinal
(D) Pantaloon
(E) Femoral

33. The hernia is likely located

(A) medial to the linea semilunaris
(B) inferior to the inguinal ligament
(C) medial to the inferior epigastric vessels
(D) superior to the falciform ligament
(E) lateral to the superior epigastric vessels

34. Which of the following measures is the most appropriate next step?

(A) Elective repair if there is no incarceration
(B) Emergent herniorrhaphy because this type of hernia is at greatest risk for strangulation
(C) Ultrasound
(D) Repair of patent processus vaginalis
(E) Computed tomography (CT) scan

Setting: Office

Questions 35–37

A 38-year-old man has been taking a medication to assist him in alcohol cessation. He later drinks an alcoholic beverage, and flushing, nausea, vomiting, abdominal pain, and headache develop.

35. The patient has an excess of

(A) acetone
(B) free fatty acids
(C) glycerol
(D) β-hydroxybutyrate
(E) acetaldehyde

36. This mode of treatment is an example of

(A) operant conditioning
(B) aversive conditioning
(C) cognitive therapy
(D) systematic desensitization
(E) modeling

37. Which of the following laboratory abnormalities is least consistent with alcohol abuse?

(A) High mean corpuscular volume
(B) Low platelets
(C) Hypoglycemia
(D) Hypermagnesemia
(E) Ketoacidosis

Setting: Satellite Clinic

Questions 38–42

A 21-year-old woman, who is G_1P_0 and 32 weeks' pregnant, complains of bilateral knee pain and hip pain. At 28 weeks, she had contractions that were controlled with terbutaline. On further questioning, she complains of shortness of breath while lying flat. On physical examination, her blood pressure is 150/90 mm Hg, and she is tachycardic. Otherwise, her cardiovascular examination is normal. Her lungs are clear, and her neck examination is normal. Homans sign is negative, and no lower extremity swelling or edema is present. Hyperpigmentation is apparent on her nose and cheeks. Laboratory studies reveal:

Erythrocyte sedimentation rate (ESR)	65 mm/hr
Hematocrit	31%
Hemoglobin	10 g/dL
Platelet count	300,000/mm^3

38. Which of the following measures should be your next step?

(A) Antinuclear antibody
(B) Echocardiogram
(C) Anti-dsDNA
(D) Reassurance
(E) Ventilation-perfusion ($\dot{V}/\dot{Q}$) scan

39. Which of the following conditions best accounts for the tachycardia?

(A) Anemia
(B) Cardiomyopathy
(C) Pulmonary embolism
(D) Rheumatologic disease
(E) Medication side effect

40. The woman mentions that a friend had a clot in her leg while she was pregnant. You tell her that

(A) there is no increased risk of clotting during pregnancy
(B) the risk of clotting is greatest during the third trimester
(C) the risk of clotting is greatest during the second trimester
(D) the risk of clotting is greatest during the puerperium
(E) most pregnancy-related clotting is related to congenital hypercoagulable states

41. The woman asks about her blood pressure. You tell her that

(A) mild hypertension is normally seen at this stage of pregnancy
(B) she has preeclampsia
(C) blood pressure increases early in pregnancy but should normalize by 32 weeks
(D) there is no concern for hypertension after giving birth
(E) blood pressure normally decreases during pregnancy

42. Which of the following statements regarding the woman's anemia is true?

(A) Her hematocrit will likely increase on its own
(B) She will require a transfusion
(C) She has mild hemolysis
(D) Anemia is common secondary to decreased red blood cell (RBC) mass
(E) She will require intravenous iron supplementation

Setting: Hospital

43. A 49-year-old man with a history of asthma undergoes a successful, uncomplicated, laparoscopic, inguinal hernia repair. He remains in the hospital overnight, and he is unable to void on the following morning. The man reports that he was unable to urinate at night, despite drinking a fair amount of liquids. His vital signs are within normal limits. Physical examination reveals a moderately distended bladder and clean, dry, incision sites. He received two tablets of 5 mg of hydrocodone overnight for pain. You administer a 500 mL bolus of normal saline; however, 1 hour later, the patient is still unable to void. After placement of a straight catheter, 900 mL of clear urine is obtained with an unremarkable urinalysis. Which of the following measures would be the next appropriate step?

(A) Administer a diuretic to stimulate urine flow
(B) Discharge with reassurance that he will be able to urinate after the straight catheterization
(C) Order urgent chemistries to determine his serum creatinine level
(D) Order blood cultures and complete blood count (CBC) to examine for occult sepsis
(E) Utilize catheterization and observant management

Setting: Hospital

Questions 44–45

You are the resident on a busy orthopedic service. Yesterday, two previously healthy 59-year-old women were involved in separate motor vehicle accidents. Both women presented with closed comminuted femur fractures (the only injury suffered) and underwent operative fixation with an intramedullary nail. The immediate postoperative course is notable only for pain, which is well controlled with intravenous morphine. However, on postoperative day 2, both patients are febrile (temperature to 39°C). The nurse calls you to evaluate them. Their other vital signs are similar: blood pressure, 120/90 mm Hg; heart rate, 135 beats/minute and regular; and respiratory rate, 30/minute, with oxygen saturation of 85% on room air. You proceed to identify the cause of the decompensation. In both cases, the wounds are clean and dry, without evidence of infection.

44. Patient A is confused and oriented only to name on physical examination, and she has diffuse rales and scattered petechiae on the upper chest and arms. Which of the following tests would be likely to yield the most diagnostic information?

(A) Doppler ultrasound of the lower extremities
(B) Urinalysis and complete blood count (CBC)
(C) CT of the abdomen
(D) Pulmonary angiogram
(E) Radiograph of the femur

45. Patient B is alert and oriented on physical examination, and she complains of dyspnea and chest pain. Examination is notable for a soft, pleural friction rub on the left lower posterior lung field. Which of the following tests would be likely to yield the most diagnostic information?

(A) Radiograph of the femur
(B) CT scan of the chest
(C) Ventilation-perfusion ($\dot{V}/\dot{Q}$) scan of the lungs
(D) CBC and serum chemistries
(E) Chest radiograph

Setting: Clinic

Questions 46–48

You are asked to evaluate the risks of cigarette smoking as a cause of lung cancer based on the following simple risks:

Prevalence of cigarette smoking	56%
Death rate from lung cancer in cigarette smokers	0.96/1,000 per year
Death rate from lung cancer in non-smokers	0.07/1,000 per year
Total death rate from lung cancer	0.56/1,000 per year

46. What is the attributable risk of dying from lung cancer due to cigarette smoking?

(A) 0.40/1,000 per year
(B) 0.56/1,000 per year
(C) 0.89/1,000 per year
(D) 0.96/1,000 per year
(E) 1.05/1,000 per year

47. What is the relative risk of dying from lung cancer due to smoking cigarettes?

(A) 10.0%
(B) 13.7%
(C) 14.5%
(D) 25.0%
(E) 37.5%

48. What is the population attributable risk of dying from lung cancer due to smoking cigarettes?

(A) 0.40/1,000 per year
(B) 0.50/1,000 per year
(C) 0.56/1,000 per year
(D) 0.96/1,000 per year
(E) Cannot be calculated from the information given

Setting: Office

Questions 49–51

A 24-year-old man presents with a small mass on one of his testicles. He initially noticed this mass approximately 1 month ago and thinks that it may have enlarged in the past few weeks. His medical history is unremarkable, and he takes no medications. On physical examination, a firm, nontender mass can be palpated on one of his testicles. The mass does not transilluminate. No abdominal masses and no lymphadenopathy are evident.

49. The factor associated with greatest risk for germ cell tumor of the testis is

(A) family history of testicular cancer
(B) African American race
(C) exogenous estrogen administration to the mother during pregnancy
(D) cryptorchidism
(E) testicular trauma

50. Which of the following measures would be the most appropriate next step in this man's care?

(A) Reassurance and follow-up in 3 months
(B) Inguinal exploration with cross-clamping of the spermatic cord and orchiectomy
(C) Ultrasound-guided biopsy
(D) CT of the abdomen and pelvis
(E) Open testicular biopsy

51. Which of the following statements regarding the spread of testicular tumors is true?

(A) The most common site of metastatic spread is the brain
(B) Inguinal lymphadenopathy is often the first sign of metastatic spread
(C) The retroperitoneum is the most commonly involved site of metastatic spread
(D) Choriocarcinoma only invades locally
(E) The lung is usually spared from metastatic spread

Setting: Hospital

52. You are called to the delivery room after the birth of a full-term infant who has developed respiratory distress. The mother has been in excellent health, and the pregnancy was uncomplicated. An ultrasound at 16 weeks was unremarkable. Physical examination reveals a near total absence of breath sounds bilaterally. No fluid is obtained on suctioning. You immediately intubate the infant and obtain a chest radiograph.

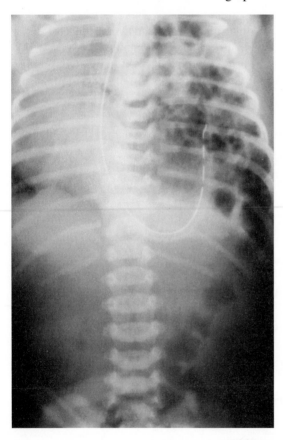

Which of the following conditions is the most likely diagnosis?

(A) Tracheoesophageal fistula

(B) Respiratory distress syndrome (hyaline membrane disease)

(C) Meconium aspiration

(D) Tetralogy of Fallot

(E) Diaphragmatic hernia

Setting: Emergency Department

53. A 2-year-old previously healthy boy is brought to the ED after a brief generalized seizure. For the past day, he has been ill with a cough, rhinorrhea, sore throat, and fever (temperature to 39.5°C). On arrival, he appears lethargic but interactive. Vital signs are: temperature, 39.2°C; blood pressure, 98/50 mm Hg; heart rate, 110 beats/minute; and respiratory rate, 24/minute. Tympanic membranes are normal, oropharynx reveals mild posterior erythema, and chest and neurologic examinations are within normal limits. A complete blood count (CBC) and serum chemistries are within normal limits. Which of the following reports about his prognosis do you give to his parents?

(A) This is probably the first of many such seizures, and referral to a neurologist is warranted

(B) A course of antiseizure medication, for at least 6 months, is warranted

(C) A head CT scan is necessary before determining prognosis

(D) His risk of seizure during another febrile illness may be as high as 30%

(E) Phenytoin can be used for prophylaxis of these seizures, if needed

Setting: Office

54. An 8-year-old boy is brought to see you because his parents are concerned about his lifelong history of bedwetting at night. This behavior occurs an average of five or six nights per week. However, he does not have any daytime wetting or incontinence. His parents have tried several tactics to stop this behavior, including fluid restriction, night awakening, and rewards for dry nights, but the behavior has continued. The boy has had no medical problems and is doing well in school and with his friends. His physical examination is normal. Which of the following diagnostic and therapeutic strategies is most reasonable?

(A) No further studies and a trial of imipramine

(B) Intravenous pyelogram and use of a moisture-sensitive alarm at night

(C) Reassurance that he will grow out of this behavior

(D) Urinalysis and use of a moisture-sensitive alarm at night

(E) Urinalysis and a trial of imipramine

Setting: Satellite Clinic

Questions 55–60

A 24-year-old sexually active woman complains of vaginal itching. She has experienced burning when she urinates but no fever or back pain. She appears well and her abdominal examination is normal, with no costovertebral angle tenderness. Pelvic examination reveals a thin, gray-white, moderately increased, vaginal discharge. Clue cells are present on microscopy of vaginal secretions.

55. Which of the following findings would you also expect?

(A) Hyphae on potassium hydroxide (KOH) examination

(B) Flagellated organisms

(C) Many gram-negative rods

(D) Amine odor on KOH examination

(E) Nits of *Sarcoptes scabiei*

56. Which of the following agents is the most appropriate treatment?

(A) Fluconazole

(B) Metronidazole

(C) Doxycycline

(D) Ciprofloxacin

(E) Ceftriaxone

57. The woman reports that she has had frequent recurrences of this condition. You tell her that

(A) her partner should be treated as well

(B) this disorder is not a sexually transmitted disease

(C) recurrences are common in women because their urethra is short

(D) she should return for treatment immediately if symptoms recur

(E) the parasite is frequently resistant to treatment

58. You discuss the importance of barrier contraception. She consents to an HIV test. The most appropriate screening test for this disease is

(A) p24 polymerase chain reaction
(B) viral load
(C) enzyme-linked immunosorbent assay (ELISA)
(D) Western blot
(E) Southern blot

59. As you are about to leave the room, the woman asks for recommendations regarding contraception. She is currently smoking one-half pack of cigarettes per day but uses no alcohol. Her mother has a history of ovarian cancer. You tell her that

(A) barrier contraceptives are subject to higher failure rates than oral contraceptives
(B) L-norgestrel (Norplant) is injected every 3 months and might be a good choice
(C) her current smoking status is an absolute contraindication to use of oral contraceptives
(D) oral contraceptives can increase the incidence of ovarian cancer
(E) oral contraceptives may increase the incidence of pelvic inflammatory disease (PID)

60. One week later, the results of the woman's HIV test are available. The positive result is confirmed. She does not return your telephone calls. Your next course of action is to

(A) continue calling, because the physician–patient confidentiality relationship may never be suspended
(B) stop calling after several attempts
(C) inform her of the test results at her follow-up appointment
(D) contact the Centers for Disease Control and Prevention (CDC)
(E) seek help in contacting her

Setting: Office

61. A 35-year-old woman is referred to you for evaluation by her family physician, who noted hematuria and hypertension on physical examination. She has no specific complaints and no history of gross hematuria, arthritis or arthralgia, rashes, headaches, and previous illnesses. Her family history is significant for a grandfather who she believes required dialysis. In addition, her parents both died in a motor vehicle accident at 30 years of age. She takes no medications and does not smoke cigarettes. Physical examination reveals a blood pressure of 155/90 mm Hg, and abdominal examination is notable for palpable, nontender masses in both flank regions. Laboratory work indicates microscopic hematuria and proteinuria. Serum creatinine is 5.6 mg/dL, and a 24-hour creatinine clearance is 25 mL/minute. Which of the following tests would most likely yield the correct diagnosis?

(A) Ultrasound of the kidneys
(B) Antinuclear antibody
(C) Anti–glomerular basement membrane antibody
(D) Serum complement levels
(E) Intravenous pyelogram

Setting: Hospital

Questions 62–64

A 32-year-old man undergoes elective colectomy for refractory ulcerative colitis. The patient receives preoperative intravenous cefazolin sodium. The surgery, which involves primary anastomosis, is uncomplicated but, 24 hours postoperatively, the patient has a temperature of 38.2°C. At this time, physical examination is notable only for decreased breath sounds at the left lower lung bases. A chest radiograph is within normal limits. His abdominal wound shows minimal erythema without discharge.

62. Which of the following statements concerning the use of preoperative prophylactic antibiotics is true?

(A) Preoperative antibiotics are useful in prophylaxis of aspiration pneumonia occurring at the time of intubation
(B) Preoperative antibiotics are useful only in those patients with risk factors for bacterial endocarditis
(C) Preoperative antibiotics are effective only if given within 1 hour of the incision and are not effective if given more than 24 hours postoperatively
(D) Antibiotic prophylaxis has been shown to be more important than meticulous surgical debridement
(E) Preoperative antibiotics should only be given to those patients with contaminated wounds

63. On examination of the man's wound, the attending physician is concerned that there may be a local wound infection. Which of the following organisms would most likely lead to early wound infections (i.e., within the first 48 hours)?

(A) Staphylococci
(B) Gram-negative enteric organisms
(C) *Clostridium* species
(D) *Bacillus* species
(E) *Candida* species

64. The man's hospital course becomes complicated; on hospital day 7, he has a temperature of 39°C. Physical examination is notable for left lower chest rales with overlying egophony and dullness to percussion. A chest radiograph confirms the presence of left lower lobe pneumonia. Which of the following antibiotic regimens is most appropriate?

(A) Ceftriaxone
(B) Azithromycin
(C) Cefuroxime and azithromycin
(D) Piperacillin sodium and tazobactam sodium
(E) Ampicillin and gentamicin

Setting: Emergency Department

Questions 65–67

A 23-year-old female nursing student presents with complaints of worsening palpitations, anxiety, and a 20-pound weight loss during the past 2 months. She states that she had been trying to lose weight, but not to this degree. In addition, she complains that she is irritable and is fighting with her friends and parents constantly. She has no medical history, although she admits to possibly having had an eating disorder in high school. She denies taking any medications. Physical examination reveals:

Vital signs	
Temperature	37.9°C
Blood pressure	130/72 mm Hg
Heart rate	130 beats/minute (regular)
Respiratory rate	22/min
Head, eyes, ears, nose, throat	Upper lid lags behind globe when patient looks down
	Somewhat prominent thyroid, with bruit audible over it
Chest	Clear bilaterally
Cardiac	Tachycardia
	Regular, soft systolic ejection murmur over right upper sternal border
Abdomen	Normal bowel sounds
	Nontender without organomegaly
Extremities	Fine tremor of hands
Skin	Warm and moist

65. Hyperthyroidism is suspected, but the laboratory results will not be available until the next morning. In the meantime, which of the following medications should the woman take?

(A) High-dose iodine therapy
(B) Verapamil hydrochloride (sustained-release form)
(C) Propranolol hydrochloride
(D) Propylthiouracil (PTU)
(E) Methimazole

66. The next morning, the laboratory results become available:

Total serum thyroxine (T_4)	45 µg/dL (5.0–12.5 ng/dL)
Triiodothyronine (T_3) resin uptake	56% (25%–35%)
Thyroid-stimulating hormone (TSH)	Undetectable (0.3–5.0 mIU/L)

A radioactive iodine uptake scan of the thyroid shows a diffusely increased rate of uptake. The most likely diagnosis is

(A) factitious hyperthyroidism
(B) thyroiditis
(C) toxic nodular goiter
(D) Graves disease
(E) euthyroid sick syndrome

67. The patient begins taking a medication to control her symptoms and, initially, does well. However, several months later, she returns to the ED with a severe sore throat of 2 days' duration. She appears toxic and has a fever (temperature, 39.4°C). Her condition suggests that she took which of the following agents?

(A) Propranolol
(B) Dexamethasone
(C) Iodine
(D) Propylthiouracil (PTU)
(E) Nonsteroidal anti-inflammatory drugs (NSAIDs)

Setting: Office

68. A 39-year-old woman is referred to you because of easy bruisability. She reports that beginning 1 week ago, every time she bumped into anything, a large bruise appeared. In addition, she has also noted some small, red, nonblanching "bumps" on her legs. She denies any other symptoms and states that she has been healthy all of her life. She takes no medications, and she does not use tobacco or alcohol. Physical examination is notable for numerous bruises of different ages on all of her extremities and petechiae on her anterior tibial surfaces bilaterally. Laboratory studies indicate:

Complete blood count (CBC)	
Hemoglobin	13.1 g/dL
White blood cell (WBC) count	7,200/mm³ (72% neutrophils, 22% lymphocytes, 2% eosinophils, 3% monocytes)
Platelet counts	22,000/mm³
Prothrombin time (PT)	Within normal limits
Partial thromboplastin time (PTT)	Within normal limits
Chemistries	Within normal limits
Liver function tests	Within normal limits

The most likely diagnosis is
(A) disseminated intravascular coagulation (DIC)
(B) idiopathic thrombocytopenic purpura
(C) thrombotic thrombocytopenic purpura
(D) acute myelogenous leukemia
(E) pseudothrombocytopenia

Setting: Satellite Clinic

69. A 35-year-old male prostitute complains of several days of malaise, fevers, arthralgia, and rash. His medical history is notable for several occurrences of gonorrhea and herpes. Physical examination reveals a rash (*below*).

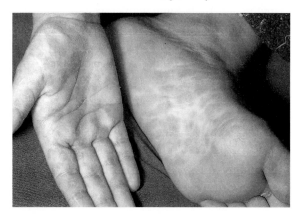

The treatment of choice for this man is
(A) erythromycin
(B) intravenous acyclovir
(C) ceftriaxone
(D) short course of oral corticosteroids
(E) penicillin

Setting: Emergency Department

70. A 6-year-old boy is brought in by his parents. Over the past 3 to 4 hours, he has been complaining of headache, blurry vision, and nausea. In addition, he has had abdominal cramps and diarrhea. The family lives on a farm, and the child has spent the last day helping with crop spraying. The father also reports that the boy has been salivating and sweating quite a bit. Physical examination reveals a lethargic boy with the following findings:

Vital signs	
Temperature	37°C
Blood pressure	90/54 mm Hg
Heart rate	130 beats/min
Respiratory rate	36/min and shallow
Pupils	Miotic
Abdomen	Hyperactive bowel sounds
Skin	Moist and flushed
Neurologic	Fasciculations of the leg muscles, with associated weakness

The next appropriate step would be to

(A) administer succinylcholine chloride and intubate
(B) administer intravenous pralidoxime chloride 25 to 50 mg/kg
(C) administer intravenous glucagon 1 mg
(D) begin intravenous naloxone hydrochloride infusion
(E) administer intravenous atropine sulfate 0.05 mg/kg

Setting: Satellite Clinic

Questions 71–75

A 29-year-old woman, who is G_1P_0 at 10 weeks, presents with concerns about vaginal bleeding. While using the bathroom this morning, she had a "rush" of bleeding. She has had no contractions, abdominal pain, or cramping. She is upset because she has been lifting grocery bags, and her husband is upset because they had sexual intercourse two nights ago.

71. Which of the following is NOT necessary at this time?

(A) Quantitative β-human chorionic gonadotropin (β-hCG)
(B) Speculum examination
(C) Transvaginal ultrasound
(D) Hematocrit
(E) Transabdominal ultrasound

72. On examination, the cervical os is closed and there is no ongoing bleeding or evidence of trophoblastic tissue. Which of the following conditions best characterizes this scenario?

(A) Inevitable abortion
(B) Threatened abortion
(C) Missed abortion
(D) Incompetent cervix
(E) Incomplete abortion

73. Which of the following statements about this situation is NOT true?

(A) There is a risk of low birth weight
(B) There is a greater risk of preterm delivery
(C) There is a higher rate of perinatal mortality
(D) The risk of congenital malformations in the newborn is greater
(E) 50% of pregnant women proceed to spontaneous abortion

74. Which of the following measures is the most appropriate plan?

(A) Admission for close monitoring
(B) Follow-up in 2 weeks
(C) Bed rest
(D) Evacuation of any products of conception
(E) Cerclage

75. Which of the following conditions is the most common cause of spontaneous abortions?

(A) Maternal infection
(B) Luteal phase defect
(C) Alcohol abuse
(D) Asherman syndrome
(E) Chromosomal abnormality

Setting: Office

76. You are asked by the local city council to investigate whether there is any link between a nearby chemical dump and a perceived increased risk of leukemia in the community. You read about various study designs. Which of the following statements about cohort studies is true?

(A) Results are available rapidly
(B) They allow the use of relatively few subjects
(C) They are expensive because of the resources necessary to study a large number of subjects
(D) They cannot establish the absolute risk of an exposure
(E) They only allow for the assessment of one exposure and one outcome

Setting: Emergency Department

77. An 18-year-old adolescent immigrant from Thailand, presents with a 7-cm laceration to his upper thigh, which occurred while he was working with a backhoe at a construction site. After cleansing the wound of debris, you suture it easily. When asked, the young man states that he does not know if he ever received a tetanus vaccination. The most appropriate course of action would be to

(A) initiate tetanus immunization with a full dose of toxoid
(B) administer a booster dose of tetanus toxoid
(C) administer tetanus toxoid and antitetanus immune globulin in the gluteal region
(D) administer antitetanus immune globulin in the nondominant arm and tetanus toxoid in the gluteal region
(E) administer a single dose of ampicillin-sulbactam intravenously followed by a course of oral amoxicillin

Setting: Hospital

Questions 78–81

A 45-year-old man is admitted to the surgical ICU after being rescued from a house fire. At the scene, he was intubated and fluid resuscitation was begun. On arrival at the ICU, examination reveals a sedated man with bilateral rales on chest examination and partial-thickness burns that involve the anterior chest and back and both arms.

78. What is the approximate fluid deficit, in liters, in this 70-kg man?

(A) 2
(B) 5
(C) 10
(D) 15
(E) 20

79. Which of the following physical findings is NOT indicative of secondary infection of the man's wounds?

(A) Blistering
(B) Green pigmentation
(C) Discoloration of burned areas
(D) Fever
(E) Conversion of partial-thickness burns to full-thickness burns

80. The man becomes hypoxemic on hospital day 2 despite ventilatory support. A chest radiograph shows bilateral pulmonary infiltrates. The ventilator settings are synchronized intermittent mandatory ventilation at a rate of 16/minute with fractional oxygen concentration in inspired gas (FIO_2) of 60%, tidal volume of 650 mL, and positive end-expiratory pressure (PEEP) of 4 cm H_2O. An arterial blood gas demonstrates a pH of 7.39, a PO_2 of 50 mm Hg, and a PCO_2 of 35 mm Hg. A pulmonary artery catheter is placed, and the pulmonary capillary wedge pressure is 6 mm Hg. To improve oxygenation in this patient, which of the following measures should be attempted first?

(A) Increase the respiratory rate to 18/minute
(B) Increase the FIO_2 to 100%
(C) Increase the tidal volume to 800 mL
(D) Increase the pulmonary capillary wedge pressure to 13 to 15 mm Hg
(E) Increase PEEP to 8 to 10 cm H_2O

81. After you have changed the ventilator settings, the oxygenation initially improves; however, several hours later, you are called because the man has become hypotensive. The patient's blood pressure is now 60/30 mm Hg, and his oxygenation saturation is 75% with an FIO_2 of 100%. Which of the following diagnoses is most likely?

(A) Sepsis
(B) Tension pneumothorax
(C) Hypovolemia
(D) Pneumonia
(E) Cardiogenic shock

Setting: Emergency Department

82. A previously healthy 25-year-old man presents with acute onset of left scrotal and testicular pain. The pain began approximately 1 hour ago when he was moving heavy boxes. He denies any urethral discharge, high-risk sexual activity, fevers, or chills. His testicle is too painful to allow close examination, but there are no gross abnormalities and no obvious inguinal hernias. Which of the following measures should be taken next?

(A) Urinalysis
(B) Complete blood count (CBC)
(C) Doppler scan of the testis
(D) Blood cultures
(E) Antibiotic coverage

Setting: Hospital

Questions 83–85

A 54-year-old woman with a history of poorly controlled diabetes mellitus, obesity, and hypertension presents with a 6-hour history of worsening abdominal pain. The pain, which is located in the midepigastric region and radiates to the back, is associated with nausea; she has vomited some bilious material. Discussion with the patient indicates that she has recently been binge drinking up to a quart of liquor per day. In addition, 2 weeks ago, she began taking a new antihypertensive medication on the advice of her primary physician. On physical examination, her vital signs are temperature, 38.6°C; blood pressure, 190/100 mm Hg; heart rate, 120 beats/minute; and respiratory rate, 16/minute. Her examination is significant for severe epigastric tenderness, absent bowel sounds, and moderate abdominal distension, with no rebound tenderness.

83. Which of the following tests would most likely yield the diagnosis?

(A) Serum amylase
(B) Abdominal ultrasound
(C) CT of the abdomen
(D) Serum alkaline phosphatase
(E) Serum transaminases

84. Which of the following conditions is least likely to be the cause of the woman's abdominal pain?

(A) Alcohol use
(B) Hydrochlorothiazide use
(C) Gallstones
(D) Hyperlipidemia
(E) Atherosclerosis

85. In the first 48 hours, which of the following abnormalities is NOT associated with a poor prognosis in this condition?

(A) Hematocrit fall of more than 10 percentage points
(B) Blood urea nitrogen (BUN) elevation >5 mg/dL
(C) Serum calcium fall to <8 mg/dL
(D) Arterial P_{O_2} <60 mm Hg
(E) White blood cell (WBC) count <8,000 cells/mm^3

Setting: Hospital

Questions 86–88

A 77-year-old woman is admitted to the medical ICU for respiratory failure. She requires 100% fractional concentration of oxygen in inspired gas (FIO_2) and has a PaO_2 of 56 mm Hg. A central venous catheter indicates a pulmonary capillary wedge pressure of 8 mm Hg. Her chest radiograph is notable for a bilateral alveolar filling process.

86. What is the most likely cause of the woman's respiratory failure?

(A) Aspiration
(B) Sepsis
(C) Trauma
(D) Multiple transfusions
(E) Pneumonia

87. Which of the following would be found on bronchoalveolar lavage?

(A) Lymphocytes
(B) Protein
(C) Blood
(D) Neutrophils
(E) Eosinophils

88. After approximately 10 days on a ventilator, the woman's oxygenation improves, but fever and right upper quadrant pain develop. On examination, her vital signs are within normal limits, and her lung sounds are improving. It is noted that she has lost 12 pounds. Ultrasound finds pericholecystic fluid and a thickened gallbladder wall with no visible stones. The next step is

(A) cholecystostomy
(B) antibiotics and observation
(C) endoscopic retrograde cholangiopancreatography with sphincterotomy
(D) cholecystectomy
(E) CT scan

Setting: Emergency Department

89. A 22-year-old woman presents with severe left lower quadrant abdominal pain of 6 hours' duration that is associated with some moderate vaginal bleeding. She is sexually active. In addition, although she does not use contraception, she denies pregnancy. Her medical history is significant for one previous uncomplicated pregnancy with delivery of a full-term infant and "an episode of something I caught from an old boyfriend." Her last period was 6½ weeks ago. Which of the following modalities provides the least help in confirming your clinical diagnosis?

(A) Quantitative β-human chorionic gonadotropin (β-hCG)
(B) Vaginal ultrasound
(C) Abdominal ultrasound
(D) Culdocentesis
(E) Laparoscopy

Setting: Satellite Clinic

Questions 90–92

A 21-year-old woman presents in extreme emotional distress, stating that she had been raped earlier in the day. She did not know her attacker, who forcibly penetrated her. She is extremely afraid but keeps on insisting that no one else be informed. In addition, she has never been sexually active and does not know what to do.

90. Your obligations at this point include all of the following EXCEPT

(A) informing the police despite her protestations
(B) providing emotional support
(C) providing counseling about the risks of sexually transmitted diseases and pregnancy
(D) offering psychologic counseling
(E) documenting all features of the history and physical examination carefully

91. The woman agrees to a physical examination but still insists that no one be notified. Accordingly, you perform a detailed examination and follow the protocol for obtaining any possible evidence. You advise her that you would recommend presumptive treatment for sexually transmitted diseases. Which of the following regimens would provide the necessary coverage?

(A) Ofloxacin
(B) Penicillin and doxycycline
(C) Clindamycin and ceftriaxone
(D) Ceftriaxone and azithromycin
(E) Metronidazole and ofloxacin

92. You also offer HIV testing. Which of the following statements should you make about the enzyme-linked immunosorbent assay (ELISA)?

(A) If the ELISA is negative, the likelihood of infection is low
(B) ELISA is a baseline test and needs to be repeated in 3 to 6 months to ensure continued absence of serologic signs of infection
(C) ELISA is not very sensitive but is very specific
(D) A polymerase chain reaction test will be used to confirm the ELISA and identify any virus
(E) False-positive results occur in patients with autoimmune disorders

Setting: Emergency Department

Questions 93–94

An 11-month-old girl is brought in by her panic-stricken mother. Her daughter has had a fever of 39°C to 40°C for 3 days, while staying at her father's house. The mother also noticed that the infant had a rash when she picked up her daughter. Her father has not been concerned because the girl has "been herself" and had no complaints.

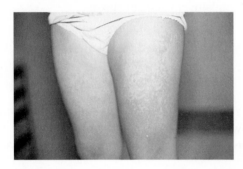

93. The most likely cause of these symptoms is

(A) measles
(B) group A streptococcus
(C) parvovirus B19
(D) human herpesvirus 6
(E) varicella

94. The most appropriate treatment is

(A) observation
(B) acyclovir
(C) immunoglobulin therapy
(D) ribavirin
(E) penicillin

Setting: Satellite Clinic

Questions 95–96

A newborn girl is evaluated for jaundice. At the age of 4 days, her bilirubin is 8 mg/dL and nearly all unconjugated.

95. Which of the following tests is most appropriate?

(A) Complete blood count (CBC)
(B) Blood cultures
(C) Thyroid-stimulating hormone (TSH)
(D) Alanine aminotransferase (ALT) and aspartate aminotransferase (AST)
(E) Blood smear

96. Basic testing suggests no cause for the bilirubin level. Which of the following diagnoses is most likely?

(A) Red blood cell (RBC) enzyme defect
(B) Rubella
(C) Physiologic jaundice
(D) Gilbert syndrome
(E) Crigler-Najjar syndrome

Setting: Emergency Department

97. A 72-year-old man with diabetes mellitus, hypertension, congestive heart failure, and chronic renal insufficiency presents with 1 week of fatigue, nausea, worsening shortness of breath, and worsening lower extremity edema. Physical examination reveals a cachetic man in mild respiratory distress and the following findings:

Vital signs	
Temperature	37°C
Blood pressure	170/98 mm Hg
Heart rate	78 beats/min
Respiratory rate	28/min
Cardiovascular	Jugular venous distension, 10 cm
Cardiac	Prominent S_3 cardiac sound with three-component, pericardial friction rub
Pulmonary	Bilateral pulmonary rales
Extremities	Bilateral lower extremity edema

Laboratory studies reveal:

Na$^+$	130 mEq/L
K$^+$	6.1 mEq/L
HCO$_3$$^-$	18 mEq/L
Blood urea nitrogen (BUN)	105 mg/dL
Creatinine	6.9 mg/dL
Electrocardiogram (ECG)	Normal sinus rhythm Normal intervals and Q waves in leads V_4–V_6 (no change from baseline)

The most appropriate treatment includes all of the following measures EXCEPT

(A) urgent hemodialysis

(B) insulin and glucose infusion

(C) furosemide and nitroglycerin

(D) fluid restriction

(E) potassium-binding resin (sodium polystyrene)

Setting: Satellite Clinic

98. A 28-year-old woman with advanced AIDS (CD4 count: 5/mm^3) presents with worsening dysphagia and odynophagia of 2 weeks' duration. Her dysphagia occurs with solids more than with liquids. She has a history of medication noncompliance, and she admits that the only medication she has been taking is trimethoprim-sulfamethoxazole 3 times a week. Physical examination is notable for marked cachexia and oral thrush; otherwise, physical findings are within normal limits. The next management step is

(A) endoscopy with biopsy

(B) a trial of ganciclovir

(C) a trial of acyclovir

(D) upper gastrointestinal (GI) series with barium

(E) a trial of fluconazole

Setting: Office

Questions 99–100

A 32-year-old woman, who is pregnant for the first time, wishes to initiate obstetric care with your practice. Her medical history is significant for type 2 diabetes mellitus, which she has been able to control with diet and exercise.

99. Which of the following statements regarding her diabetes mellitus and risks during pregnancy is NOT true?

(A) The most common malformations include cardiac and neural tube defects

(B) Ophthalmic evaluation should be performed in each trimester

(C) Optimal glycemic control should include a fasting glucose of 60 to 90 mg/dL

(D) Macrosomia and shoulder dystocia occur with increased frequency

(E) Glipizide should be the initial drug of choice

100. Which of the following statements regarding testing for maternal serum α-fetoprotein (AFP) is true?

(A) Testing should be performed early in the first trimester

(B) The test should be corrected for maternal age, diabetes mellitus, and race

(C) Only 20% of the abnormalities detected by an elevated maternal serum AFP can be seen on ultrasound

(D) Informed consent is not necessary

(E) A low maternal serum AFP value may indicate an increased risk of Down syndrome

Setting: Office

Questions 101–102

A 34-year-old woman presents for evaluation after a diagnosis of cervical cancer. On clinical evaluation, it is apparent that the cancer involves the upper one third of the vagina. There is no parametrial spread. After discussion with the patient, she opts for a combination of external beam irradiation and brachytherapy. In preparing her for this treatment, you want to discuss the possible side effects.

101. Which of the following conditions is NOT a potential side effect of radiotherapy?

(A) Vaginal irritation

(B) Premature menopause

(C) Fibrosis of the colon

(D) Skin irritation

(E) Increased incidence of urinary tract infection

102. The woman returns 2½ years after completing therapy, complaining of flank pain and left leg edema. These symptoms, which began approximately 2 months ago, have progressively worsened. In addition, she has noted some anorexia and a 5-pound weight loss. She denies hematuria, dysuria, or increased urinary frequency. Which of the following diagnostic modalities would provide the most cost-effective approach in determining the correct diagnosis?

(A) Doppler ultrasonography of the lower extremities

(B) Ultrasonography of the kidneys

(C) CT of the abdomen and pelvis

(D) Intravenous pyelogram

(E) Chest radiograph

Setting: Emergency Department

Questions 103–104

A 90-year-old man with Alzheimer disease has had increasing abdominal distension and no stool output for the past 2 days. Although the patient is unable to communicate because of severe dementia, he moans and cries whenever anyone palpates his abdomen. He is bedridden and requires complete assistance for his activities of daily living. His medications include a multivitamin, haloperidol, and verapamil. Physical examination reveals an older, cachectic man in moderate distress, a temperature of 37.5°C, a blood pressure of 160/80 mm Hg, and a heart rate of 150 beats/minute. Abdominal examination reveals moderate distension with few bowel sounds. The abdomen is tender to palpation, but the patient is uncooperative with the examination. You order an abdominal radiograph (*below*).

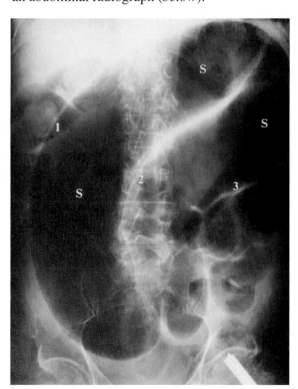

103. Which of the following diagnoses is most likely?

(A) Abdominal perforation
(B) Fecal impaction
(C) Ogilvie syndrome
(D) Sigmoid volvulus
(E) Appendicitis

104. What would be your initial treatment of choice?

(A) Emergent surgical exploration
(B) Enema in the ED and discharge with laxatives
(C) Admission with overnight observation and intravenous hydration
(D) Trial of metoclopramide
(E) Sigmoidoscopy

Setting: Office

105. A 49-year-old man complains of left shoulder pain. He has no associated trauma. On physical examination, he experiences the most pain with crossed arm adduction with applied resistance. Which of the following is the most likely diagnosis?

(A) Acromioclavicular joint inflammation
(B) Subacromial bursitis
(C) Supraspinatus syndrome
(D) Partial rotator cuff tear
(E) Biceps tendinitis

Setting: Office

106. An 8-month-old male infant is seen for a routine checkup. On physical examination, the boy appears normal, except that his right testicle is absent. The left testicle feels normal. His medical history is unremarkable. Which of the following recommendations should you make to the parents?

(A) The testicle is probably absent; this condition is seen in 10% of infants. No further workup is necessary.

(B) The testicle is probably undescended and should be surgically brought down into the scrotum as soon as possible.

(C) The testicle is probably undescended and should be surgically brought down into the scrotum by the time the boy is 6 years of age.

(D) If this condition is repaired, it is not associated with an increased risk of malignancy.

(E) All family members should undergo genetic studies.

Setting: Office

107. A 15-year-old girl is brought in by her mother, who has concerns about her daughter's sexual development. All of the following statements relating to delayed puberty in females are true EXCEPT

(A) The condition is defined as the absence of secondary sexual characteristics by age 13

(B) Bone age is often significantly delayed

(C) There is often a family history of delayed puberty

(D) Autoimmune diseases are the most common cause of this condition

(E) Anorexia nervosa is a common cause

Setting: Office

Questions 108–110

Routine examination shows that a 43-year-old woman has a breast lump. Mammography reveals a density in the left breast. A biopsy finds lobular carcinoma in situ.

108. Which of the following measures is the most appropriate treatment?

(A) Lumpectomy alone
(B) Lumpectomy and radiation therapy
(C) Lumpectomy and lymph node dissection
(D) Screening mammography and, perhaps, tamoxifen
(E) Modified radical mastectomy

109. Which of the following diseases is least associated with increased risk of breast cancer?

(A) Ovarian cancer
(B) Prostate cancer
(C) Endometrial cancer
(D) Melanoma
(E) Lung cancer

110. Which of the following statements is true concerning the role of tamoxifen in the prevention of breast cancer?

(A) The agent has been found to decrease mortality in patients with a history of ductal carcinoma in situ
(B) The agent reduces the risk of invasive breast cancer by 90% in those with lobular carcinoma in situ
(C) Patients with atypical ductal hyperplasia benefit most from therapy with this agent
(D) This agent has the added benefit of decreasing endometrial cancer
(E) Tobacco use is an absolute contraindication to use

Setting: Office

111. A 4-year-old boy is brought in by his parents, who have noted that he has had a fever for the past 4 days (temperature to 39.5°C). Because other family members had suffered from a viral illness, they initially thought that their son had the same condition. However, during the past 24 to 48 hours, he has developed redness on the palms of his hands and the soles of his feet, as well as bilateral redness of the eyes. On physical examination, you also note cracked lips, a bright red tongue, and diffuse cervical lymphadenopathy. All of the following disorders are appropriate considerations in the differential diagnosis EXCEPT

(A) Rocky Mountain spotted fever
(B) juvenile rheumatoid arthritis
(C) toxic shock syndrome
(D) meningococcal sepsis
(E) Kawasaki disease

Setting: Hospital

112. You suspect that a 6-year-old girl who was admitted with bloody diarrhea, renal failure, and thrombocytopenia has hemolytic uremic syndrome. If this is the case, which of the following laboratory patterns would be most likely?

	Platelets	Schistocytes	Prothrombin time (PT)	Partial thromboplastin time (PTT)
(A)	Low	Present	Normal	Normal
(B)	Low	Absent	Normal	Normal
(C)	Low	Present	Increased	Increased
(D)	Low	Present	Increased	Normal
(E)	Low	Present	Normal	Increased

Setting: Office

113. You are seeing a 7-year-old girl with a sore throat and fever. The clinical probability of streptococcal pharyngitis is 25%. A rapid antigen screen is available in your clinic that has a sensitivity of 90% and specificity of 80%. If the test is positive, what is the posttest probability of disease?

(A) 40%
(B) 60%
(C) 80%
(D) 90%
(E) 95%

Setting: Hospital

Questions 114–116

A 28-year-old man who is HIV-positive is admitted with severe headache, nausea, vomiting, and stiff neck. He has a temperature of 39°C.

114. Which of the following tests is most likely to yield a diagnosis?

(A) Computed tomography (CT)
(B) Magnetic resonance imaging (MRI)
(C) Blood cultures
(D) Lumbar puncture
(E) Electroencephalogram (EEG)

115. Which of the following values likely represents this man's CD4 count (cells/mm^3)?

(A) <100
(B) 100 to 150
(C) 150 to 200
(D) 200 to 250
(E) >250

116. Which of the following therapeutic measures is most important at this time?

(A) Lumbar puncture
(B) Ceftriaxone
(C) Vancomycin and ceftriaxone
(D) Amphotericin B
(E) Amphotericin B and flucytosine

Setting: Office

117. A 42-year-old man presents to his primary care physician with complaints of generalized fatigue. He notes that during the past 6 months he can no longer complete his full workout without tiring. He denies cough, shortness of breath, chest pain, edema, bright red blood per rectum, or melena. Physical examination reveals a pale man, with a heart rate of 100 beats/minute and a blood pressure of 110/60 mm Hg. The rest of his examination is within normal limits. Laboratory studies reveal a hematocrit of 26%, a mean corpuscular volume of 72 fL, and a ferritin of 25 ng/mL. The next step in his care should be

(A) initiation of iron therapy
(B) initiation of vitamin B_{12} and folate therapy
(C) referral for colonoscopy
(D) admission for urgent, packed, red blood cell (RBC) transfusion
(E) recommendation to increase the consumption of red meats and follow-up in 2 months

Setting: Hospital

118. A 26-year-old man with AIDS and a CD4 count of $29/mm^3$ presents with a 6-day history of fever and severe headache with associated photophobia. A CT scan of the head, performed in the ED, is within normal limits. The results of a lumbar puncture are glucose, 50 mg/100 mL; white blood cells (WBCs), $100/mm^3$, with 75% lymphocytes; opening pressure, 20 cm H_2O; and protein, 84 mg/100 mL. The most likely diagnosis is

(A) toxoplasmosis
(B) central nervous system (CNS) lymphoma
(C) cryptococcal meningitis
(D) bacterial meningitis
(E) progressive multifocal leukoencephalopathy

Setting: Office

119. A 13-year-old girl comes to the office several hours after injuring her knee during a soccer game. After planting her left foot and turning while running after a ball, she heard a popping noise and then had difficulty on weight-bearing and pain on movement of the knee. Initially, she used ice and ibuprofen to reduce the pain, but she now has noticed swelling and increased pain. On examination, the left knee has a moderate effusion positive anterior drawer and Lachman tests. The most likely diagnosis is

(A) tibial plateau fracture
(B) posterior cruciate ligament tear
(C) anterior cruciate ligament tear
(D) tendonitis
(E) bursitis

Setting: Office

Questions 120–121

A 42-year-old man with no significant medical history has recently returned from Mexico. On arrival home, he experiences severe perianal pain. Several hours later he has a fever (temperature to 39°C). That evening he takes ibuprofen, which relieves his pain and normalizes his temperature. However, the next morning, he has severe pain on defecation. He does not note any bright red blood per rectum or change in stool color. He takes no medications, drinks one beer per week, and has smoked one pack of cigarettes per day for the past 12 years.

On physical examination, the man appears well. His vital signs are notable for a temperature of 39.2°C. The only notable abnormality is a painful, palpable mass at the anal verge. His stool is guaiac-negative.

120. The man is nervous and asks you what you think his problem is. Your answer would be

(A) rectal carcinoma
(B) perirectal abscess
(C) anal fissure
(D) anal fistula
(E) hemorrhoids

121. Your treatment of choice for this condition would be

(A) reassurance and stool softeners
(B) intravenous antibiotics
(C) incision and drainage
(D) sigmoidoscopy
(E) CT of the pelvis

Settings: Emergency Department and Hospital

Questions 122–126

A 49-year-old man with a long history of alcohol abuse and hepatitis C virus infection presents to the emergency department (ED) after several episodes of hematemesis. Although he is somewhat confused on presentation, you are able to determine that he has vomited approximately 2 L of blood during the past 3 hours. He is still actively drinking alcohol. Immediately after entering the ED, he vomits a large amount of bright red blood. His blood pressure is 90/50 mm Hg, and his heart rate is 130 beats/minute. He is somnolent but is oriented to person and place. You secure large-bore intravenous access, order packed red blood cells (RBCs), and initiate resuscitation with intravenous fluids.

122. Which of the following physical findings is indicative of the underlying pathophysiology that is contributing to the man's gastrointestinal (GI) bleeding?

(A) Scleral icterus
(B) Spider angioma
(C) Jaundice
(D) Caput medusae
(E) Hepatomegaly

123. All of the following measures would be appropriate steps in initial management EXCEPT

(A) diazepam prophylaxis for delirium tremens
(B) elective intubation for airway protection
(C) emergent endoscopy with band ligation
(D) intravenous octreotide infusion
(E) placement of a Sengstaken-Blakemore tube

124. The man is stabilized and admitted to the ICU. Two days after a procedure is performed, his hematocrit remains stable, and he is transferred to a medical ward. However, during the next 2 days he becomes increasingly somnolent and confused; he is difficult to arouse and is oriented only to person. His serum ammonia level is elevated. Which of the following conditions would NOT contribute to his worsening encephalopathy?

(A) GI bleeding
(B) Hypokalemia
(C) Metabolic alkalosis
(D) Hypophosphatemia
(E) Alcohol withdrawal

125. The man receives treatment for his encephalopathy, and his condition improves. However, 2 days later, he experiences a fever (temperature to 38.9°C) and some mild abdominal tenderness. Some ascitic fluid is removed from his abdomen; the white blood cell (WBC) count of this fluid is 2,000 cells/mm³, with 90% neutrophils. Which of the following medications is the most appropriate treatment for this condition?

(A) Aldosterone
(B) Intravenous penicillin
(C) Intravenous cefotaxime
(D) Oral ciprofloxacin
(E) Intravenous imipenem

126. The man is discharged home but returns for several other admissions for encephalopathy, esophageal varices, and spontaneous bacterial peritonitis. Because he is still drinking alcohol, he is rejected for consideration as a liver transplant recipient. Ultimately, the patient is discharged to the care of a nursing facility because of his increasing debilitation. You initiate a discussion about resuscitation status, and the patient desires that "everything possible be done." You state (1) that you believe there is no further effective medical therapy to offer, and (2) that the probability of surviving a resuscitation would be extremely low. Despite this discussion, the patient requests that a full resuscitation effort be performed, if needed. He has no living relatives or power of attorney. Two weeks later, you receive a call from the nursing home; staff members have found the patient unarousable, with labored breathing, a blood pressure of 60/30 mm Hg, and an oxygen saturation of 80% on 6 L nasal cannula. They ask you what action is appropriate. The most suitable step would be

(A) urgent ethics team consultation
(B) intravenous morphine
(C) urgent transport to an ED for intubation and admission to an ICU
(D) intravenous naloxone
(E) intravenous normal saline 500-mL bolus

Setting: Office

Questions 127–129

A 22-year-old woman presented as a new patient for general medical care 7 months ago. She had a blood pressure of 180/110 mm Hg. One month after initiation of hydrochlorothiazide, her blood pressure was 175/110 mm Hg. Two other antihypertensive medications were added during the next 6 months with little success. Her social history reveals that she has many sexual partners and does not use contraception; she is G_0P_0. On physical examination, she has short stature as well as cubitus valgus.

127. Which of the following conditions is the most likely cause of the woman's hypertension?

(A) Primary aldosteronism
(B) Primary hyperparathyroidism
(C) Coarctation of the aorta
(D) Pheochromocytoma
(E) Hyperthyroidism

128. Which of the following tests might provide useful information?

(A) Chest radiograph
(B) Thyroid-stimulating hormone (TSH)
(C) Urine metanephrines
(D) Parathyroid hormone
(E) Plasma renin activity

129. According to Sixth Report of the Joint National Committee on Detection, Evaluation and Treatment of High Blood Pressure (JNC VI) guidelines, which of the following agents is a first-line agent for treatment of this woman's hypertension?

(A) Verapamil
(B) Captopril
(C) Amlodipine
(D) Propranolol
(E) Furosemide

Setting: Emergency Department

Questions 130–132

A 25-year-old man with a long history of severe depression presents to the ED after a suicide attempt. He states that he ingested about 60 mL of an alkaline drain cleaner about 20 minutes ago. He is alert but despondent, and his vital signs are stable. Physical examination reveals erythema and ulceration of his posterior pharynx.

130. Which of the following measures would be appropriate in this man's care?

(A) Induction of vomiting
(B) Neutralization of the alkaline solution with acid
(C) Intravenous octreotide
(D) Early endoscopy
(E) Emergency electroconvulsive therapy for his depression

131. The man is appropriately treated and discharged. Six months later he returns complaining that he has difficulty swallowing solid foods, especially meats. In addition to his swallowing difficulty, he also complains of occasional regurgitation. His only medication is paroxetine 20 mg per day. His physical examination is within normal limits. Which of the following diagnoses is the most likely cause of his symptoms?

(A) Esophageal reflux
(B) Zenker diverticulum
(C) Barrett esophagus
(D) Diffuse esophageal spasm
(E) Esophageal stricture

132. Ten years have now passed since the man's initial presentation. During that time, he has suffered from recurrent dysphagia and has required numerous endoscopic procedures. During the past 2 months, he once again reported dysphagia. He now has difficulty swallowing both liquids and solids, and he has lost 10 pounds during the past month. Which of the following findings would be most likely on endoscopy?

(A) Recurrent esophageal ulcerations
(B) Esophageal leiomyoma
(C) Esophageal stricture
(D) Esophageal carcinoma
(E) Gastric carcinoma

Setting: Office

133. A young woman presents with severe itching in the web spaces of her hands of several days' duration. Her husband has similar symptoms but refuses to be seen. On examination, her hands appear as shown in the figure below.

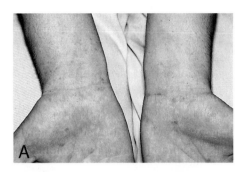
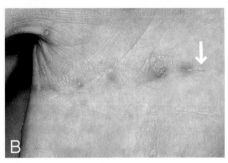

Which of the following measures is the treatment of choice?

(A) Topical steroids
(B) Topical moisturizing lotion
(C) Lindane (lotion)
(D) Reassurance
(E) Ketoconazole (topical lotion)

Setting: Office

134. A 79-year-old man complains of occasional episodes of substernal chest pain associated with exertion. They usually occur in the morning when he walks up a moderately steep incline to collect his mail. The chest pain occasionally radiates to his left inner arm and is associated with some diaphoresis and shortness of breath. On one occasion, he felt as if he might pass out. Rest relieves the condition. On review of symptoms, his only other complaint is worsening fatigue. His only medication is aspirin once a day. His medical history is significant for hospitalization for pneumonia 2 years ago and the removal of a hyperplastic colonic polyp 3 years ago. Physical examination reveals:

Vital signs	
Blood pressure	135/67 mm Hg
Heart rate	65 beats/min
Head, eyes, ears, nose, throat	Delayed carotid pulses with slowly increasing amplitude
Chest	Clear bilaterally
Cardiac	Regular rate and rhythm
	Sustained point of maximal impulse felt in 5th intercostal space, just lateral to midclavicular line
	Loud S_4 and mid-to-late-peaking crescendo–decrescendo murmur along left sternal border
	No change in intensity of murmur with handgrip maneuver
Abdomen	Normal bowel sounds without tenderness or organomegaly
Extremities	Trace lower extremity peripheral edema

The most likely cause of the findings on physical examination is

(A) mitral regurgitation
(B) tricuspid regurgitation
(C) aortic regurgitation
(D) aortic stenosis
(E) pulmonic stenosis

Setting: Satellite Clinic

Questions 135–137

As a medical resident, you have the opportunity to work in a small village in rural Pakistan. A woman who is 31 weeks' pregnant is brought to your clinic by her family with the acute onset of fatigue and jaundice.

135. The most likely cause is

(A) hepatitis A
(B) hepatitis B
(C) hepatitis C
(D) hepatitis E
(E) HIV

136. Serologies are drawn, with the following results:

Hepatitis B surface antigen (HBsAg)	Negative
Hepatitis B surface antibody (HBsAb)	Negative
Hepatitis B core antibody (HBcAb)	Positive
Hepatitis B e antigen (HBeAg)	Negative

The results indicate

(A) infectivity
(B) chronic active hepatitis
(C) immunization
(D) "window" period
(E) acute infection or "old" infection

137. The most common cause of fulminant hepatic failure worldwide is

(A) acetaminophen
(B) hepatitis B
(C) hepatitis C
(D) hepatitis D
(E) *Amanita* ingestion

Setting: Hospital

138. An 80-year-old woman is admitted to the ICU with fever, obtundation, and hypotension. On admission, her blood pressure is 65/30 mm Hg, her oxygen saturation is 80% on 100% oxygen, and her chest radiograph shows bilateral infiltrates. She is emergently intubated and a pulmonary artery flotation catheter is placed. Her right atrial pressure is 3 mm Hg (1 to 6 mm Hg), pulmonary capillary wedge pressure is 8 mm Hg (normal, 6 to 12 mm Hg), cardiac index is 7.0 L/m^2 per minute (normal, 2.4 to 4.0), and the systemic vascular resistance index is 600 dynes m^2/cm^5 per second (normal, 1,600 to 2,400). The cause of her hypotension is most likely

(A) cardiogenic shock
(B) hypovolemia
(C) sepsis
(D) papillary muscle rupture from a myocardial infarction (MI)
(E) cardiac tamponade

Setting: Office

139. A 62-year-old woman with osteoporosis, coronary artery disease, and hypertension presents with vaginal bleeding. She has noted vaginal spotting for the past 3 months but has no other complaints. She has been taking conjugated estrogen, progesterone, simvastatin, and metoprolol. Physical examination is within normal limits. Pelvic examination is also within normal limits. The next appropriate step would be

(A) reassurance that her condition is benign and self-limited
(B) referral to a gynecologist for an endometrial biopsy
(C) stop the hormone replacement therapy and monitor if bleeding recurs
(D) increase the dose of progesterone
(E) increase the dose of estrogen

Setting: Office

140. A 45-year-old man comes in for a "physical" prior to approval for an insurance policy. He has no medical history and takes no medications. His family history is significant for hypertension, diabetes mellitus, and lung cancer in first-degree relatives. He works as a stockbroker, and although he does not smoke, he consumes three or four mixed alcoholic drinks per day. On examination, his blood pressure is 167/90 mm Hg, his weight is 160 pounds, and his height is 5'11". The rest of his physical examination is notable only for an S_4 heart sound. Although the man is concerned about his blood pressure, he does not want to start taking medications. Which of the following measures is likely to have the greatest impact in lowering his blood pressure?

(A) Regular aerobic exercise
(B) Dietary fat reduction
(C) Biofeedback
(D) Discontinuation of alcohol
(E) Dietary potassium reduction

Setting: Satellite Clinic

Questions 141–142

A 53-year-old obese woman with diabetes mellitus presents for routine follow-up. For approximately 6 days, she has been experiencing pain in her right heel. On examination, warmth and swelling over her right heel are evident. There is an ulcer with evidence of a draining tract.

141. Which of the following measures is the most appropriate?

(A) Plain film
(B) Probe for bone
(C) MRI
(D) CT scan
(E) Nuclear bone scan

142. Which of the following statements regarding this woman's disease is true?

(A) Blood cultures are rarely positive in acute disease
(B) Erythrocyte sedimentation rate (ESR) can be used to follow course of disease
(C) Children are most commonly afflicted with vertebral disease
(D) The specificity of an MRI is nearly 100%
(E) Gram-negative rods are the most common pathogen in hematogenous disease

Setting: Emergency Department

Questions 143–145

A 52-year-old man presents with a 1-day history of palpitations, diaphoresis, and shortness of breath. Initial evaluation involves obtaining an ECG (*below*).

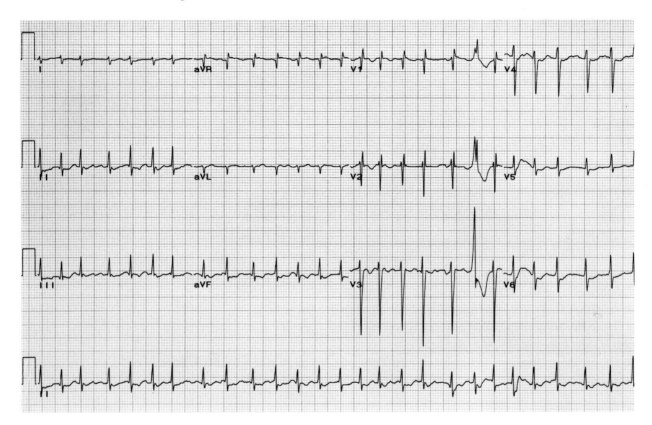

143. All of the following measures are potential therapies EXCEPT

(A) intravenous metoprolol
(B) intravenous verapamil
(C) defibrillation with 300 joules
(D) intravenous procainamide
(E) intravenous digoxin

144. The man does well following this intervention, and his ECG returns to normal. He asks what caused his condition and what further workup he should have. All of the following factors are potential causes of his condition EXCEPT

(A) alcohol
(B) pericarditis
(C) mitral stenosis
(D) pulmonary embolism
(E) anemia

145. The man returns to the ED in 3 days with similar complaints and a return of the cardiac rhythm apparent in the original ECG. This time, metoprolol slows the ventricular rate but the rhythm does not convert to sinus. Long-term management of this rhythm may involve all of the following measures EXCEPT

(A) digoxin
(B) amiodarone
(C) warfarin
(D) diltiazem
(E) attempt at cardioversion in 5 to 7 days

Setting: Office

146. A 20-year-old female college student complains of a cough productive of scant sputum of 3 days' duration. She denies fever, chills, shortness of breath, or other constitutional symptoms. She is concerned that she will become sicker prior to her wedding in 3 days. She has no medical history, and her only medication is an oral contraceptive. She does not smoke cigarettes. Which of the following methods of treatment is most appropriate?

(A) Reassurance
(B) Amoxicillin 500 mg 3 times a day
(C) Azithromycin 500 mg, followed by 250 mg every day for 4 days
(D) Amoxicillin 500 mg 3 times a day and guaifenesin
(E) Trimethoprim 160 mg–sulfamethoxazole 800 mg 2 times a day

Setting: Office

147. A 46-year-old man has a lesion on his arm that initially began as a "freckle" but has enlarged and darkened during the past year (*below*). Occasionally, it bleeds when he scratches it. Which of the following features of the lesion correlates best with prognosis?

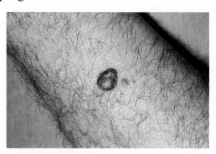

(A) Depth of invasion
(B) Diameter
(C) Pedunculated appearance
(D) Darker pigmentation
(E) Easy bleeding tendency

Setting: Satellite Clinic

Questions 148–149

A 19-year-old Caucasian teenager has a routine sports "physical." He is a runner on the track team at college. Urinalysis shows five red blood cells (RBCs) per high-power field. The adolescent has no known trauma and has no history of previous hematuria.

148. Which of the following measures is the most appropriate next step?

(A) Intravenous pyelogram

(B) Cystoscopy

(C) Radiographic examination of the kidneys, ureters, and bladder

(D) Observation

(E) CT scan

149. While discussing health maintenance issues with the teenager, you inform him that the leading cause of mortality in his age group is

(A) testicular cancer

(B) homicide

(C) AIDS

(D) suicide

(E) motor vehicle accidents

Setting: Satellite Clinic

150. A 40-year-old woman comes to the clinic with many questions regarding the initiation of oral contraceptives. She was told to "ask her doctor" about precautions. Which of the following conditions is considered an absolute contraindication to the use of oral contraceptives?

(A) Epilepsy

(B) Diabetes mellitus

(C) History of pulmonary embolus

(D) Hypertension

(E) HIV infection

ANSWER KEY

1-D	31-C	61-A	91-D	121-C
2-E	32-B	62-C	92-B	122-D
3-B	33-C	63-C	93-D	123-A
4-D	34-A	64-D	94-A	124-D
5-B	35-E	65-C	95-E	125-C
6-B	36-B	66-D	96-C	126-C
7-E	37-D	67-D	97-A	127-C
8-E	38-D	68-B	98-E	128-A
9-C	39-E	69-E	99-E	129-D
10-D	40-D	70-B	100-B	130-D
11-B	41-E	71-C	101-E	131-E
12-E	42-A	72-B	102-C	132-D
13-D	43-E	73-D	103-D	133-C
14-C	44-B	74-B	104-E	134-D
15-E	45-C	75-E	105-A	135-D
16-A	46-D	76-C	106-B	136-E
17-D	47-B	77-D	107-D	137-B
18-D	48-B	78-D	108-D	138-C
19-C	49-D	79-A	109-E	139-B
20-B	50-B	80-E	110-C	140-D
21-E	51-C	81-B	111-D	141-B
22-A	52-E	82-C	112-A	142-B
23-C	53-D	83-C	113-B	143-C
24-B	54-D	84-E	114-D	144-E
25-E	55-D	85-E	115-A	145-E
26-A	56-B	86-B	116-A	146-A
27-B	57-A	87-B	117-C	147-A
28-C	58-C	88-A	118-C	148-C
29-B	59-A	89-C	119-C	149-E
30-A	60-E	90-A	120-B	150-C

ANSWERS AND EXPLANATIONS

1–4. The answers are: 1-D, 2-E, 3-B, 4-D. (*Obstetrics/gynecology*)

Postpartum hemorrhage is defined as blood loss greater than 500 mL associated with delivery. Uterine atony is by far the most common cause. Ordinarily, the body of the uterus contracts promptly after delivery of the placenta, constricting the spiral arteries and preventing excessive bleeding. This muscle contraction plays a larger role than coagulation. Factors that predispose to atony include prolonged labor, leiomyomas, general anesthesia, macrosomia, hydramnios, birth of twins, multiparity, amniotic fluid embolism, and a history of postpartum hemorrhage. On examination, the uterus feels softer and "boggy," as opposed to firm and contracted as it should. Other causes include lower genital tract laceration, retained placenta, hematomas, coagulation defects, amniotic fluid embolism, and uterine inversion.

General management of postpartum hemorrhage involves uterine massage and oxytocin infusion. Gauze packing is a temporizing measure that is rarely used today. Methergine, a potent vasoconstrictor, is occasionally used, but it carries the risk of severe hypertension; for this reason, it is given intramuscularly. Prostaglandins $F_{2\alpha}$ and E_2 have also been used. If these measures do not help, surgical management, including uterine artery ligation, selective arterial embolization, and hysterectomy, may be effective.

The common cause of disseminated intravascular coagulation (DIC) in pregnancy is abruptio placentae. Other causes of this condition include amniotic fluid embolism, preeclampsia, retention of a dead fetus, and sepsis. Clinical manifestations of DIC include epistaxis, hematuria, purpura or petechiae, and bleeding from puncture or incision sites. Laboratory studies show decreased fibrinogen, prolonged prothrombin time (PT)/partial thromboplastin time (PTT), increased D-dimers, increased fibrin split products, and schistocytes on blood smear. Thrombocytopenia may be present. Management includes delivery of the infant and supportive therapy.

5–7. The answers are: 5-B, 6-B, 7-E. (*Internal medicine*)

This patient presents with the classic findings of septic arthritis. The combination of fever, joint pain, limited range of motion, and overlying joint warmth combined with the risk factors of corticosteroid treatment and rheumatoid arthritis make septic arthritis the primary consideration. Bacteria may gain access to a joint space through hematogenous spread, direct inoculation, or direct extension from an adjacent focus of infection. Hematogenous infection, the most common form, usually affects patients with an underlying illness or damage to a joint space. The differential diagnoses in this patient include gout, pseudogout, osteoarthritis, and a flare of rheumatoid arthritis, but the primary concern is ruling out infection. Thus, urgent aspiration of synovial fluid is indicated. None of the other answer choices in question 5 are appropriate in this setting.

The characteristics of the synovial fluid from this patient are clearly indicative of a septic effusion. The presence of a high white blood cell (WBC) count, neutrophil predominance, and low glucose level are characteristic. Effusions seen with gout would have lower WBC counts and higher glucose levels. Effusions seen with rheumatoid arthritis are generally symmetrical and have lower WBC counts with more lymphocytic predominance; glucose levels may be lower. With this cell count, empirical antibiotics must be initiated. The most likely organisms that require antibiotic coverage are *Staphylococcus aureus*, *Streptococcus* species, and gram-negative enteric rods. Thus, the best choice of empiric antibiotic coverage would include nafcillin and cefepime. None of the other choices in question 6 provides adequate coverage.

The management of septic arthritis must include systemic antibiotics. However, because the infection involves a closed space with a potential for inflammatory destruction of the joint space, some form of drainage, involving either repeated needle aspiration of purulent exudates or open surgical drainage, is necessary. For most joints (especially the knee), repeated needle aspiration may be recommended. If symptoms do not resolve in 48 to 72 hours, open drainage may be required. Many experts also advocate open drainage for infections with *S. aureus* and gram-negative enteric bacteria, as well as infections in the hip joint. In all cases, antibiotic therapy should be continued for 4 to 6 weeks.

8. The answer is E. (*Neurology*)

The localization of neurologic complaints requires detailed knowledge of the anatomy of the nervous system. It is necessary to form a mental image of where a lesion might be, often at an intersection between two or more pathways. The ability to abduct the right fifth finger originates in the precentral gyrus of the left cerebral cortex. The signal passes through the left corona radiata and internal capsule, through the cerebral peduncle in the midbrain and basis pontis, to the pyramid of the medulla. From there, it decussates to the right side and proceeds downward in the lateral white matter of the spinal cord, which is referred to as the corticospinal tract. The route then leaves the spinal cord at nerve roots C8 and T1, travels through the lower trunk and medial cord of the brachial plexus, and exits in the ulnar nerve, which terminates at the neuromuscular junction of the abductor digiti minimi muscle.

The ability to feel a pinprick of the fifth finger starts at sensory receptors on the right fifth finger that continue in the right ulnar nerve; this sensation proceeds through the medial cord and lower trunk of the brachial plexus and enters the right C8 nerve root. Pinprick is "pain," so it ascends one or two segments in the cord before crossing to the left and ascending in the left spinothalamic tract. The pathway ascends through the medulla, pons, and midbrain before synapsing in the ventroposterolateral nucleus of the thalamus. It then continues upward through the internal capsule and corona radiata, terminating in the postcentral gyrus of the parietal cortex.

This patient has dysfunction of these two pathways, so the lesion must be in a region where the transmission pathways intersect. That could only be in the right ulnar nerve, the left parietal cortex, or in the ascending pathways of the left brainstem. Other clues in the history and physical examination provide the clinical information necessary to determine the site of the lesion accurately.

9–12. The answers are: 9-C, 10-D, 11-B, 12-E. (*Surgery, internal medicine*)

This patient has acute pancreatitis. The classic presentation is that of steady, boring abdominal pain located in the epigastrium and periumbilical regions that radiates directly through to the back. Frequently, the pain is worse when the patient is supine. Nausea, vomiting, and distension are common as well. Low-grade fever, tachycardia, and, occasionally, hypotension may occur secondary to retroperitoneal third-spacing and the systemic effects of enzymes released into the circulation.

Among the numerous causes of acute pancreatitis are alcohol abuse, biliary tract obstruction, medications, hypertriglyceridemia, hypercalcemia, infection (mumps, coxsackievirus), and trauma. In the United States, the most common causes are alcohol abuse and biliary tract obstruction. This patient has macrocytosis, which correlates best with alcohol abuse in retrospective studies; however, this is still not a specific marker.

At admission, the Ranson criteria help determine the severity of pancreatitis (see explanation for questions 83 to 85). Mortality increases with each additional criterion that the patient satisfies. Note that amylase and lipase are not included in these criteria.

Between 10% and 20% of patients with pancreatitis have pulmonary findings, including pleural effusions, which are primarily left-sided. These effusions are usually exudative and have an elevated total protein, elevated lactate dehydrogenase (LDH), and an elevated specific gravity (less valuable). The high amylase level is a distinguishing feature.

Complications of acute pancreatitis include hemorrhagic pancreatitis, necrotizing pancreatitis, pancreatic abscess and pseudocyst formation, acute respiratory distress syndrome (ARDS), disseminated intravascular coagulation (DIC), splenic vein thrombosis, hypocalcemia, and hypotension. Splenic vein thrombosis manifests with gastric varices in the absence of esophageal varices. Budd-Chiari syndrome is acute thrombosis of the hepatic veins. It manifests acutely with ascites, right upper quadrant abdominal pain, and hepatomegaly. Portal hypertension, which is usually secondary to hepatic cirrhosis, is associated in all cases with both esophageal and gastric varices. Pseudocyst formation can result in persistent abdominal pain and a persistently elevated amylase. However, pseudocysts do not lead to the formation of varices. The same applies to bile duct obstruction.

13. The answer is D. (*Pediatrics*)

This patient has hemolytic uremic syndrome, which is often associated with infection by *Escherichia coli* 0157:H7 and begins with bloody diarrhea and abdominal pain. Pallor, fatigue, and oliguria then follow. In fact, hemolytic uremic syndrome is the most common cause of acute renal failure in children. Findings on physical examination are dehydration, edema, petechiae, hepatosplenomegaly, and irritability or listlessness. The history; physical examination; and laboratory studies, which include a microangiopathic hemolytic anemia with schistocytes (as seen on the peripheral smear), thrombocytopenia, normal coagulation profile, elevated serum creatinine, and urinalysis with mild hematuria and proteinuria support the diagnosis. Treatment is largely supportive, and hemodialysis may be necessary.

Disseminated intravascular coagulation (DIC), which is often confused with hemolytic uremic syndrome, is often seen in sepsis. However, in DIC, coagulation studies are abnormal, with an elevated partial thromboplastin time (PTT), low levels of fibrinogen, and evidence of both clotting and bleeding diathesis. Ulcerative colitis and Crohn disease should be part of the differential diagnosis of any condition characterized by bloody diarrhea and abdominal pain. In this case, the peripheral smear and laboratory values do not support either of these diagnoses. Finally, idiopathic thrombocytopenia purpura is an isolated platelet disorder with immune-mediated destruction of platelets and resulting thrombocytopenia. However, no anemia and renal failure are present.

14. The answer is C. (*Pediatrics*)

This child most likely has pyloric stenosis, which affects approximately 1 of 150 male infants and 1 of 750 female infants. The condition is more likely to occur in firstborn males. Onset occurs in the first 2 to 3 weeks of life. Pyloric stenosis is typified by projectile vomiting after feeding. The vomitus consists of gastric contents only. Diffuse hypertrophy and hyperplasia of the smooth muscle in the pyloric canal, which leads to narrowing and obstruction, is present.

Physical examination reveals varying degrees of dehydration and, sometimes, visible peristalsis proceeding from the left upper quadrant toward the pylorus. Ultrasound is the least invasive, and most highly sensitive and specific and cost-effective diagnostic test. However, the diagnosis is easily made with a variety of radiologic tests. Treatment is surgery, with an incision of the hypertrophied muscle.

15–18. The answers are: 15-E, 16-A, 17-D, 18-D. (*Psychiatry*)

Schizophrenia is characterized by alterations in perception, thinking, social activity, and affect. This disorder, which often begins in late adolescence, starts with social withdrawal and perceptual distortions and progresses to a state of delusions and hallucinations. The age of onset is 15 to 25 years for men and 25 to 35 years for women. Presenting symptoms may be positive (delusions, hallucinations) or negative (anhedonia, decreased emotion, impaired concentration, social withdrawal). The more severe the negative symptoms, the poorer the outcome. The four symptom subtypes of schizophrenia are catatonic, paranoid, disorganized, and residual.

The feature of this patient's presentation that points toward schizophrenia is her previous success and the deterioration that has lasted for more than 6 months. Her agitation, personality change, and lack of interest in her appearance is typical as well. Other disorders may present with psychotic symptoms. However, these should be differentiated from schizophrenia. Schizophreniform disorder satisfies the criteria for schizophrenia, but affected patients have had symptoms for less than 6 months. Schizoaffective disorder is characterized by psychosis resembling schizophrenia but with predominant mood disturbances. Brief psychotic disorder involves the experiencing of a full psychotic episode that is short-lived, often temporally related to a stressor (e.g., pregnancy).

Because individuals with schizophrenia are at high risk for suicide, it is important to assess this patient's suicide risk. One third of persons with schizophrenia attempt suicide; 10% are successful. Risk factors for suicide include male gender, age older than 30 years, and recent hospital discharge. All of the other choices in question 16 represent appropriate measures in the evaluation of the patient. However, the most emergent issue and the one that will alter the therapy is determination of the likelihood that this patient will commit suicide.

Schizophrenia affects 1% of the population. There is no significant gender difference in prevalence of disease. It is diagnosed disproportionately among the lower socioeconomic classes. More individuals with schizophrenia are born during cold weather months.

In addition, dopamine appears to be directly associated with schizophrenia. Dopamine receptor blockers are useful in its treatment. As yet, there is no evidence that other neurotransmitters play a therapeutic role.

19–22. The answers are: 19-C, 20-B, 21-E, 22-A. (*Emergency medicine, obstetrics/gynecology*)
This patient has risk factors, signs, and symptoms consistent with pelvic inflammatory disease (PID), which is the acute clinical syndrome associated with an ascending infection from the vagina to the cervix, endometrium, fallopian tubes, ovaries, or peritoneum. In addition, the perihepatic space can be involved. Risk factors for PID include history of PID, multiple sexual partners, history of a sexually transmitted disease, and use of an intrauterine device for birth control. The relative risk of PID in women with multiple sexual partners is 4.6 times higher than in women with a single partner. Although this particular patient had several sexual partners within a year, she did not become pregnant, despite the lack of use of contraception. This suggests infertility, perhaps secondary to a history of PID.

Based on the clinical criteria and the differential diagnosis, the most important initial tests include a pelvic examination, cervical microscopy/Gram's stain with cultures, complete blood count (CBC), and pregnancy test. Ultrasound might be useful if tubo-ovarian abscess is suspected. Laparoscopy is used for equivocal cases. Hospitalization is suggested for ileus, peritonitis, pregnancy, use of an intrauterine device, significant pain or gastrointestinal (GI) symptoms, temperature higher than 39°C, tubo-ovarian abscess, patient noncompliance, or a white blood cell (WBC) count greater than 20,000/mm^3.

PID occurs more commonly in the days following menstruation because the endocervical mucus resists upward spread, especially during the progesterone-predominant stage of the cycle. Oral contraceptive pills, which mimic this effect, might limit PID. Tubal ligation may provide a barrier to spread of infection as well.

As cervicitis ascends to cause endometritis, it usually rapidly spreads to salpingitis. The salpingitis may remain localized or may spread, causing peritonitis, adhesion formation, or abscess formation. Perihepatitis (Fitz-Hugh and Curtis syndrome) consists of inflammation leading to localized fibrosis with scarring of the anterior surface of the liver and adjacent peritoneum. It is more commonly seen with chlamydial infection. It presents as right upper quadrant pain in the setting of other PID signs and symptoms. The other options in question 20 are not complications of PID. Late sequelae of PID include infertility in 15% to 20% of patients (50% to 75% after three episodes), ectopic pregnancy (risk is increased 7 to 10 times), chronic pelvic pain, and dyspareunia.

The clinical diagnosis of PID is incorrect in up to 35% of women. The correct diagnoses in misdiagnosed PID cases include (in descending order): appendicitis, endometriosis, corpus luteal bleeding, ectopic pregnancy, and adhesions. The clinical criteria for diagnosis includes *all three* of the following conditions: direct abdominal tenderness (usually bilateral), adnexal tenderness, and cervical motion tenderness *and one* of the following signs: positive Gram's stain, temperature higher than 38°C, white blood cell (WBC) count greater than 10,000/mm^3, or pus on culdocentesis or laparoscopy.

The predominant organisms in PID are *Chlamydia trachomatis* and *Neisseria gonorrhoeae*. *Chlamydia* more commonly causes a mucopurulent cervicitis than does *N. gonorrhoeae* but is generally associated with a more indolent course and yet an increased incidence of infertility. Other organisms include *Mycoplasma hominis* and *Ureaplasma urealyticum*. Most cases of PID are believed to be polymicrobial, with combinations of these organisms and anaerobes.

The Centers for Disease Control and Prevention (CDC) recommends the following agents for outpatient treatment of PID:

> Either cefoxitin + doxycycline *or*
> Ceftriaxone + doxycycline for approximately 14 days *or*
> Ofloxacin + clindamycin or metronidazole for 14 days

All regimens should include coverage for both *N. gonorrhoeae* and *C. trachomatis*.

23. The answer is C. (*Internal medicine*)
Cancer progresses through stages, and often, high-risk premalignant lesions can be identified. If treated successfully, the risk of malignancy significantly decreases. Fibroadenoma of the breast is the only lesion listed that is not associated with increased risk of malignancy. The possibility that women who have had fibroadenomas removed surgically have an increased risk of malignancy is controversial. However, no metaplastic changes are seen in these fibroadenomas.

Barrett esophagus, which involves replacement of the squamous epithelium of the esophagus by columnar epithelium, has been associated with severe reflux esophagitis. Adenocarcinoma may occur in 2% to 5% of cases and is usually preceded by dysplasia of the columnar epithelium. Thus, treatment for gastroesophageal reflux must be aggressive, and patients should undergo surveillance endoscopy.

Dysplastic nevus syndrome or familial atypical malignant mole syndrome is characterized by large, numerous, pigmented nevi that have irregular borders and show great variation in pigmentation. Because the likelihood of progression to malignant melanoma is high, careful screening and removal of all suspicious lesions is necessary.

Cervical dysplasia occurs in the junction between the squamous epithelium lining the ectocervix and columnar epithelium lining the endocervix, which is termed the transitional zone. During adulthood, the columnar epithelium recedes and is replaced with the more resistant squamous epithelium (squamous metaplasia). Nearly all cervical cancer originates in this transitional area. This forms the basis for the Papanicolaou smear test, which involves sampling this high-risk area and checking for precancerous changes. Gradual changes from mild to severe dysplasia occur, progressing to carcinoma in situ and, finally, to invasive carcinoma. These neoplastic changes are strongly associated with infection from human papilloma virus.

Squamous metaplasia of the lung also represents a progressive change from a normal to malignant state. It is believed that secondary to repeated injury (i.e., from tobacco and environmental stimuli), the normal columnar epithelium of the bronchi undergoes a change to squamous tissue. From this point onward, there is an increased risk of malignancy. Many trials have attempted to determine if screening for this change through sputum cytology has any impact on mortality from lung cancer. Unfortunately, these trials have failed to show a benefit.

24. The answer is B. (*Statistics*)
Screening can be defined as a means of detecting disease early, in an asymptomatic state, with the goal of preventing morbidity and mortality. It is not equivalent to early detection, which may or may not save lives. To be effective, a screening test should fulfill the following requirements:

1. The screening test should detect a fairly prevalent condition with important health implications.
2. The screening test should have a high sensitivity and specificity. Sensitivity is the proportion of people with the disease who test positive, and specificity refers to the proportion of people who do not have the disease who test negative. In most screening tests, a high degree of sensitivity is required to avoid missing disease. Often, this occurs at the expense of specificity, which necessitates a confirmatory diagnostic test. In addition, the number of false-positive and false-negative tests should be low.
3. Obviously, screening makes sense only if an effective and safe therapy is available for the patients who have the disease in question.
4. There should be evidence (ideally, from a randomized controlled trial) that screening and early treatment have a positive effect on the quality of life.

25. The answer is E. (*Internal medicine*)
This patient has a solitary pulmonary nodule. Given his clinical history and age, this lesion represents a high risk for malignancy ($>40\%$). In evaluating a solitary pulmonary nodule, certain characteristics increase the likelihood of the lesion being benign: (1) presence of calcification, and (2) absence of growth during a 2-year surveillance period. Patients with lesions greater than 3 cm are at high risk of their being malignant.

To evaluate such pulmonary nodules, many authorities advocate CT studies, with high-resolution cuts through the lesion to assess the risk pattern further. However, in high-risk patients, it is prudent to proceed to definitive diagnosis. Diagnosis can be potentially obtained via many modalities, including bronchoscopy with needle biopsy, video-assisted thoracoscopy, transthoracic needle biopsy, or open surgical removal. Surgical resection is the definitive procedure and should be pursued if there are no contraindications to removal. In patients at risk for lung cancer, it would not be appropriate to wait before investigating any lung lesion. Therefore, repeat chest radiographs or a trial of antibiotics would be incorrect. Bronchoscopy with needle biopsy has a relatively high false-negative rate.

26–29. The answers are: 26-A, 27-B, 28-C, 29-B. (*Internal medicine, neurology, psychiatry*)
Dementia is the acquired, generalized, progressive deterioration of cognitive function. It reflects an underlying pathology of the cerebral cortex, its subcortical connections, or both. When evaluating a patient with a disorder of cognitive function, it is important to determine whether a patient is suffering from an acute confusional state or delirium with waxing and waning of symptoms and prominent disturbances in the level of consciousness.

Depression is most commonly mistaken for dementia but is treatable. Both dementia and the pseudodementia of depression can be characterized by mental slowness, apathy, self-neglect, withdrawal, irritability, difficulty with memory and concentration, and changes in behavior and personality. Evidence gathered in the history and physical examination may provide useful information that helps distinguish between dementia and depression. For instance, depression tends to have an abrupt onset with a plateau of dysfunction, unlike dementia, which has an insidious onset and progresses. Furthermore, patients with depression often have a history of the condition. In addition, these patients tend to complain more of memory loss, and exhibit apathy, depressed affect, prominent vegetative symptoms, and somatic complaints. In patients with dementia, symptoms also tend to worsen at night. Of the answer choices in question 26, abrupt onset is most consistent with depression.

Alzheimer disease, the most common cause of dementia, can be diagnosed with certainty only by pathologic examination of the brain. Neuropathologic features include neurofibrillary tangles, neuritic plaques, and granulovacuolar degeneration. Impairment of recent memory is typically the first sign of the disease, and disorientation to time and then place eventually occur. Visuospatial disorientation is very common, and patients often become easily lost. Later in the disease, psychosis with paranoia, hallucinations, or delusions may be prominent. Thus, the occurrence of visuospatial confusion supports the diagnosis of Alzheimer disease. The white matter atrophy seen on CT, which occurs commonly with aging, is a nonspecific finding. Gait instability and incontinence suggest normal pressure hydrocephalus as a cause. Myoclonus is a prominent feature of Creutzfeldt-Jakob disease. Hypersegmented neutrophils should suggest vitamin B_{12} deficiency.

Not all dementia is due to Alzheimer disease. Several causes of cognitive decline are potentially reversible, although they are uncommon. These include depression, as well as hypothyroidism, syphilis, subdural hematomas, vitamin B_{12} deficiency, and infection. It is critical to attempt to detect these reversible causes of dementia, and a careful physical examination can aid this process. The finding of a delayed relaxation phase of the deep tendon reflexes should suggest hypothyroidism and prompt testing for this condition. The other physical examination findings listed in question 28 are found in irreversible dementia. Peripheral visual field defects should suggest a pituitary mass encroaching on the optic chiasm. Myoclonus is seen with Creutzfeldt-Jakob disease, a disease caused by prions and not treatable. A labile affect can be seen in pseudobulbar palsy and is secondary to multiple lacunar strokes. Chorea should suggest Huntington disease.

Agitation, especially at night, is a troublesome symptom in patients with Alzheimer disease. It often leads to placement of patients in nursing homes. The best treatment for this patient's nocturnal agitation is a trial of a low-dose neuroleptic, such as haloperidol, which is safe and effective in a large percentage of individuals. Diphenhydramine, which causes sedation, is strongly anticholinergic and can worsen confusional states and lead to other problems, such as urinary retention. Diazepam is strongly sedating and can lead to paradoxical increases in agitation. Vitamin B_{12} therapy is helpful in deficiency states only. Thiamine therapy is indicated for the treatment of Wernicke encephalopathy, which is characterized by confusion, ataxia, and eye motility disorders.

30. The answer is A. (*Pediatrics*)
The constellation of physical findings in this child is pathognomonic for an atrial septal defect, which is a small opening in the atrial septum that normally separates the right and left sides of the heart. The defect can occur in one of three positions in the atrial septum: (1) high in the septum (sinus venosus defect), (2) in the midportion (ostium secundum defect), and (3) low in the septum (ostium primum defect). An ostium primum defect is usually accompanied by mitral valve incompetence. Many affected children are asymptomatic or may experience mild fatigue and an increase in respiratory infections.

Hemodynamically, an atrial septal defect involves a left-to-right shunt from the left side of the heart, at higher pressure, to the right side, at lower pressure. Thus, flow across the tricuspid and pulmonic valves is increased, with dilation of the right ventricle and pulmonary artery. This gives rise to the characteristic findings of a hyperdynamic right precordium with a right ventricular heave and a systolic murmur in the pulmonic area (secondary to increased flow across the valve). The characteristic fixed split S_2 heart sound is secondary to the increased flow across the pulmonic valve. The ECG reveals right ventricular hypertrophy with right axis deviation and the rSR' in the right precordial leads.

Ventricular septal defects generally cause a harsh murmur beginning before S_1 and ending in midsystole as blood is shunted from the left ventricle to the right ventricle. This murmur is most audible at the lower left sternal border. Patent ductus arteriosus connects the pulmonary artery and the descending aorta and leads to a continuous murmur, which is best heard in the back. Coarctation of the aorta involves stenosis of the descending aorta. Patients with this condition present with lower extremity weakness and severe hypertension. An aortic systolic or diastolic murmur may sometimes be audible. Pulmonic stenosis, an uncommon condition, leads to a systolic murmur in the pulmonic position with gradual onset of right ventricular hypertrophy. It can be easily confused with the findings of an atrial septal defect. However, in individuals with this defect, there is generally a mid-diastolic rumble in the lower right sternal area, representing increased flow across the tricuspid valve, and S_2 is widely and fixed split.

31. The answer is C. (*Pediatrics*)
This child has a defect in T-cell–mediated immunity. In general terms, clinical immunodeficiency states can be divided into four groups: (1) complement disorders, (2) phagocyte disorders, (3) B-cell function defects, and (4) T-cell function defects. Each class of immunodeficiency states leaves a patient susceptible to a particular class of pathogens. For example, complement deficiency increases susceptibility to pyogenic organisms, especially *Neisseria* species. Phagocytic disorders increase the susceptibility to organisms of low virulence such as *Staphylococcus aureus,* and patients are plagued with cutaneous and deep-seated abscesses. B-cell disorders make children susceptible to extracellular pathogens, especially pyogenic and enteric organisms, and these patients typically have recurrent sinopulmonary infections. Defects in T-cell–mediated immunity lead to susceptibility to infection with intracellular organisms, especially fungal and viral infections. It important to keep in mind that some syndromes involve impairment of both T-cell– and B-cell–mediated immunity (e.g., severe combined immunodeficiency, Wiskott-Aldrich syndrome).

Specific testing of immune function can be used to identify the defect in any given patient. Because this patient has recurrent fungal infections, a defect in T-cell–mediated immunity should be suspected, and delayed-type hypersensitivity testing is warranted. Patients with T-cell defects have no delayed-type hypersensitivity reactions. Serum immunoglobulins are decreased in B-cell disorders. The nitroblue tetrazolium test, which is an assay for the presence of catalase function, is abnormal in chronic granulomatous disease (a phagocytic disorder). Total hemolytic complement levels are low in patients with complement deficiency.

32–34. The answers are: 32-B, 33-C, 34-A. (*Internal medicine, surgery*)
A hernia is a protrusion of an organ or tissue outside the body cavity in which it is normally found. The lifetime incidence of hernia occurrence is 5% to 10%. Direct inguinal hernias, which protrude directly through the abdominal wall, account for 25% of all hernias. These hernias lie within the floor of the Hesselbach triangle; the borders are the inguinal ligament inferiorly, inferior epigastric vessels laterally, and the lateral aspect of the rectus abdominus (linea semilunaris) medially. Obesity is a risk factor for direct inguinal hernias, because the cause is mechanical "wear and tear" over time. The frequency increases with age. On examination, the clinician feels the hernia on the *lateral aspect* of the finger when invaginated in the external inguinal ring. Emergent herniorrhaphy is indicated if strangulation of bowel is present; otherwise, an elective procedure is indicated to prevent incarceration.

Indirect inguinal hernias, the most common type of hernia in both men and women, involve protrusion through the internal ring of the inguinal canal, traveling down toward the external ring. They occasionally enter the scrotum if the process vaginalis is patent. On examination, when the finger is invaginated into the external ring, the clinician feels the hernia on the *tip* of the finger while the patient forcibly bears down, as in the Valsalva maneuver. Surgery is necessary if there appears to be strangulation of the hernia contents. Pantaloon hernias are hernial sacs that exist as both direct and indirect hernias straddling the inferior epigastric vessels. Femoral hernias, which are more common in women and during pregnancy, travel beneath the inguinal ligament and down the femoral canal medial to the femoral vessels. They commonly incarcerate because of their narrow neck.

35–37. The answers are: 35-E, 36-B, 37-D. (*Psychiatry, internal medicine*)
An accumulation of acetaldehyde causes flushing, headache, anxiety, and sweating. Alcohol dehydrogenase in the liver breaks down ethanol into acetaldehyde, acetaldehyde dehydrogenase then oxidizes the acetaldehyde to form acetate. Disulfiram blocks this second enzyme, leading to the symptoms described in the clinical scenario, which occur within 10 minutes of alcohol use. Controlled studies of disulfiram have not shown unequivocally that it increases duration of sobriety. Disulfiram therapy is an example of aversive conditioning. It is a classic conditioning method that pairs an unwanted behavior with a painful or aversive stimulus.

Operant conditioning is associated with establishing positive and negative reinforcement to extinguish an unwanted behavior or to encourage a desired behavior. Cognitive therapy is a method of short-term psychotherapy used primarily for depression and anxiety. Systematic desensitization is a classical conditioning method that pairs a frightening stimulus with relaxation procedures in an effort to eliminate phobias. Modeling is observational learning in which an individual adopts the behavior of an admired individual.

Alcohol poisons the bone marrow directly, causing cytopenia, but it also leads to direct platelet destruction. In addition, alcoholics with cirrhosis and splenomegaly have thrombocytopenia secondary to sequestration. A high mean corpuscular volume is a classic finding in alcohol abuse secondary to direct toxic effects on red blood cells (RBCs) as well as nutritional deficiency. Hypoglycemia is common in patients with liver disease; it also occurs secondary to poor nutrition. The deficiency of nicotinamide adenine dinucleotide (NAD) secondary to alcohol metabolism inhibits gluconeogenesis and causes free fatty acid breakdown into ketoacids. Many patients have hypomagnesemia.

38–42. The answers are: 38-D, 39-E, 40-D, 41-E, 42-A. (*Obstetrics/gynecology, internal medicine*)
This woman's joint complaints, facial hyperpigmentation, elevated erythrocyte sedimentation rate (ESR), and shortness of breath are all due to pregnancy. Reassurance is warranted. Knee and hip complaints are common as pregnancy proceeds, and the examination is normal, making a rheumatologic disease unlikely. The facial hyperpigmentation is consistent with melasma and is thought to be secondary to elevated estrogen and melanocyte-stimulating hormone levels. In addition, the ESR is elevated in normal pregnancies and, at one time, was even used as a pregnancy test. Systemic lupus erythematosus is unlikely, and measurement of antinuclear or dsDNA antibodies is unnecessary. Finally, shortness of breath in pregnancy is a common complaint

secondary to diaphragmatic displacement. However, it should raise suspicion of peripartum cardiomyopathy or venous thromboembolism in the correct setting. The cardiovascular examination is normal, which does not indicate cardiomyopathy. (Note that heart murmurs and even extra heart sounds are common in pregnancy.) Peripartum cardiomyopathy occurs later in pregnancy or during the puerperium, making an echocardiogram unnecessary.

Terbutaline sulfate, a β-agonist, is effective in the control of preterm labor. However, secondary to the catecholamine-like effect of the drug, dose-limiting tachycardia is common.

Because blood clot formation is more common in pregnancy, a pregnant woman who presents with complaints of shortness of breath should prompt consideration of thromboembolism. One study found a twofold increased risk during pregnancy and a greater than fivefold increased risk in the puerperium. Some episodes may be secondary to factor V Leiden or other hypercoagulable states but, at this time, it is thought that these situations make up the minority of cases.

It is also believed that blood pressure may decrease for the first 24 to 26 weeks of pregnancy as the result of a reduction in systemic vascular resistance by progesterone. There is a gradual rise to prepregnancy values by term. However, hypertension may manifest during pregnancy and remain elevated thereafter. The American College of Obstetrics and Gynecology classifies this phenomenon as "chronic hypertension during pregnancy."

During pregnancy, a physiologic anemia develops. Maternal plasma volume increases at 6 weeks and peaks at approximately 34 weeks. Red blood cell (RBC) mass increases as well but not as significantly as plasma volume. Hematocrit generally drops until 34 weeks, at which time RBC mass continues to increase while plasma volume stabilizes, causing a small increase in hematocrit. A patient does not require transfusions or intravenous iron for this degree of anemia, but oral iron might be recommended. There is no reason to suspect hemolysis.

43. The answer is E. (*Surgery, internal medicine*)

Postoperative urinary retention, a common problem after laparoscopic hernia surgery, is likely related to anesthetic interference with the autonomic pathways leading to normal bladder emptying. Other possible mechanisms include surgical complications with injury to the autonomic nerve plexus and bladder overdistension that leads to inhibition of smooth muscle contractility. For these reasons, pelvic and perineal procedures are associated with a higher incidence of this complication.

Management includes a careful history with attention to medications that may inhibit normal micturition (e.g., agents with prominent anticholinergic side effects). These side effects may be especially prominent in older men with prostatic hypertrophy. A fluid bolus, which ensures that hypovolemia is not a contributing factor, is a reasonable and safe procedure. Following this, straight catheterization with bladder decompression should be attempted. Often, bladder decompression alone may be enough to allow micturition. However, the catheter should remain in place if the residual volume is greater than 1,000 mL. A trial of clamping the catheter until the patient senses the urge to void can then be attempted; the majority of patients will be able to void in the next 6 to 8 hours. In those few still unable to void, more prolonged catheterization and urologic evaluation may be required.

The use of a diuretic is relatively contraindicated in the setting of urinary retention; the drug will only lead to increased bladder distension and pain. The patient should be discharged only after documentation of adequate urinary bladder emptying or with a Foley catheter to ensure urinary drainage. In the setting of acute urinary retention, chemistries are usually normal; they have no role in management.

44–45. The answers are: 44-B, 45-C. (*Surgery, internal medicine*)

Postoperative fever, a common problem, may be the result of both benign and life-threatening causes. Thus, the occurrence of a fever after surgery always deserves a careful evaluation. Some of the common causes for postoperative fevers include atelectasis, infections (urinary tract, pneumonia, wounds, sepsis), drugs (especially antibiotics), deep venous thrombosis, and pulmonary embolus. A careful history and physical examination, followed by focused laboratory and diagnostic testing, is necessary.

In the first patient, the combination of confusion and petechiae following an operation on a fractured long bone should lead to the consideration of fat embolism. In this condition, bone marrow fat is embolized and leads to occlusion of small vessels throughout the body, especially in the brain, skin, kidney, and lung. Presenting features include shortness of breath, hypoxemia, petechiae (seemingly most prominent on the upper chest), and confusion. Laboratory investigation may reveal serum and urine eosinophilia, as well as fat droplets, in the urine and blood. Thrombocytopenia is also common. Generally, fat embolization is seen up to 72 hours after long-bone trauma. Care is supportive and may involve mechanical ventilation and hemodialysis in severe cases. The other diagnostic tests in question 44 would not be appropriate in this case.

In the second patient, deep venous thrombosis with subsequent pulmonary embolism is the most likely cause of her decompensation. The combination of hypoxemia and a pleural friction rub is highly suspicious for pulmonary embolism and should prompt anticoagulation and a ventilation-perfusion ($\dot{V}/\dot{Q}$) scan. In the case of such high clinical probability, the sensitivity and specificity of a high-probability scan is diagnostic. If the results of the scan are equivocal (intermediate- or low-probability), then lower extremity Doppler ultrasound is warranted. If this is not diagnostic and the clinical suspicion remains high, a pulmonary angiogram is necessary. Neither a chest radiograph nor a CT scan is helpful when the primary consideration is a pulmonary embolus. The only exception to this would be the use of a CT angiogram, which is more invasive and costly than a simple $\dot{V}/\dot{Q}$ scan.

46–48. The answers are: 46-D, 47-B, 48-B. (*Statistics*)
In evaluating whether an exposure may lead to an illness, epidemiologists use several expressions of risk. Incidence, the most basic expression of risk, is defined as the number of new cases of a disease arising in a given population during a given period of observation. However, this yields limited data. In this case, the clinician actually wants to compare two different cohorts of subjects that have different exposures (e.g., the occurrence of death from lung cancer in subjects who smoke cigarettes versus those who do not smoke). Such comparisons are termed measures of effect.

The first measure of effect involves determination of the attributable risk, which estimates the additional risk of exposure over and above that experienced by people who are not exposed. Attributable risk takes into account the background incidence of disease, presumably from other causes, that would have occurred despite the exposure. It is determined by subtracting the incidence of disease in nonexposed persons from the incidence of disease in exposed persons. In this case, the death rate from lung cancer in smokers minus the death rate from lung cancer in nonsmokers is 0.96 to 0.07, or 0.89/1,000 per year.

Relative risk is another useful measure. This expresses how many more times disease is likely to develop in exposed persons versus nonexposed persons. In this question, that would be 0.96 ÷ 0.07, or 13.7. It is important to note that relative risk reveals the strength of association between an exposure and an outcome. In some cases, the relative risk may be very large, although the absolute risk is small. Clinically, attributable risk is a more useful concept because it is a direct expression of the absolute risk.

Population attributable risk is a measure of the excess incidence of disease in a community that is associated with the occurrence of a risk factor. To estimate population risk, it is necessary to take into account the frequency with which members of a community are exposed to a risk factor. In this way, a very prevalent risk factor that may have a weak role may prove to be a valuable intervention point. To determine the population attributable risk, the attributable risk is multiplied by the prevalence of the risk. In our example: 0.89 × 0.56, or 0.50/1,000 per year. It is useful to have estimates of which exposures lead to the greatest risk. For example, a public health department may use population attributable risk to determine the focus of its programs. Population risk deals with the same questions as incidence and relative risk but considers a group of people (population) rather than individuals.

49–51. The answers are: 49-D, 50-B, 51-C. (*Internal medicine, surgery*)

Malignant tumors of the testis are relatively rare in the United States, with an incidence of two to three cases per 100,000 men. Of these tumors, 90% to 95% are germ cell tumors. The major risk factor for the development of testicular cancer is cryptorchidism; approximately 7% to 10% of testicular tumors develop in patients with a history of cryptorchidism. Of these tumors, seminomas are the most common. The relative risk of malignancy is greatest in an intra-abdominal testis (1 of 20). It is important to note that there is an associated increased risk (1 of 80) in the contralateral testis. Surgical placement of the intra-abdominal testis into the scrotum does not remove the risk, but it does facilitate examination. Race is a risk factor; testicular tumors are most common in Caucasians. Several other controversial and less important risk factors include maternal use of estrogens during pregnancy, trauma, family history, and infection.

If cancer cannot be excluded from the physical examination, the next appropriate step is inguinal exploration with cross-clamping of the spermatic cord and orchiectomy. Obviously, reassurance and waiting would not be appropriate whenever cancer is a real concern. Biopsy should not be performed secondary to the high risk of metastatic seeding in the presence of cancer. If cancer is diagnosed, then CT of the abdomen, the pelvis, and, according to some experts, the chest is warranted for staging purposes.

Testicular cancer (with the exception of choriocarcinoma) spreads in a stepwise fashion to the retroperitoneal lymph nodes first (e.g., the iliac, preaortic, para-aortic, paracaval, and renal hilum lymph nodes). Interestingly, inguinal lymph nodes are rarely involved unless scrotal invasion is present. Following retroperitoneal spread, the next most common site of metastatic disease is the lung, followed by the liver, brain, bone, kidney, and adrenal glands. Choriocarcinoma is characterized by early hematogenous spread and often first metastasizes to the lung and unusual sites.

52. The answer is E. (*Pediatrics*)

Inspection of the radiograph reveals a cystic mass in the right chest that looks similar to bowel loops, which is consistent with the diagnosis of diaphragmatic hernia. Herniation most often occurs in the posterolateral segment of the diaphragm; the left side is involved more often. The defect represents a failure of the pleuroperitoneal canal to close completely, with resultant herniation of bowel structures into the pleural cavity. The lung on the affected side is compressed and often hypoplastic. Suspicion of diaphragmatic hernia is warranted in any newborn with respiratory distress, and radiographs confirm the presence of the condition. Initial management centers on stabilizing the infant with respiratory support and, in some cases, extracorporeal support. Surgical treatment is indicated only in those patients who can be initially stabilized.

All of the answer choices, with the exception of tracheoesophageal fistula, are potential causes of acute respiratory distress in a newborn. A tracheoesophageal fistula usually becomes evident on feeding when the esophageal contents are aspirated into the lungs. Respiratory distress syndrome is seen in premature infants who have yet to develop surfactant in their lungs. Meconium aspiration occurs near the time of delivery, and the aspirated contents are usually evident on suctioning. Radiographs generally show bilateral opacities. Tetralogy of Fallot may be a cause of cyanosis in the newborn; however, chest radiographs are usually normal at birth.

53. The answer is D. (*Emergency medicine, pediatrics*)

Febrile seizures occur most often in infants aged 6 months to 3 years. However, it is not uncommon to witness febrile seizures in children up to the age of 6 years. In general, high fevers provoke these events, and they are not considered epileptic seizures. The illnesses most associated with these febrile seizures are upper respiratory infections and ear infections. Typically, temperatures are quite high (>39°C) and are accompanied by a brief (<5 minutes), generalized seizure with postictal lethargy. A careful history, physical examination, and judicial laboratory testing is warranted to exclude metabolic disturbances, intoxications, head injury, central nervous system (CNS) infections, or vascular accidents. The prognosis is excellent in the majority of children; however, up to 30% may experience a recurrent febrile seizure. Epilepsy may develop in a small percentage of children, generally those children with atypical seizure features, such as focal activity, abnormal neurologic examinations, and prolonged seizure activity. Routine CT scanning is controversial in the setting of a normal neurologic examination. Fever control is the only appropriate therapy. In the rare case of recurrent febrile seizures, intrarectal diazepam can be used to terminate the seizures. Antiseizure medications have no demonstrated effect in the prophylaxis or treatment of febrile seizures, and they may result in serious side effects.

54. The answer is D. (*Pediatrics*)

Enuresis is the involuntary loss of urine after an age of continence has been achieved in the majority of children, which typically occurs at 5 years of age in girls and 6 years of age in boys. In school-age children, the incidence of enuresis is 5% to 8%, and it generally decreases with age. The etiology of enuresis is multifactorial and likely involves physical immaturity, sleep disturbances, psychologic factors, and, possibly, genetic factors. It is critical that organic factors be sought and excluded. These include urinary tract infections, urinary tract obstructions, meningomyelocele, diabetes mellitus, diabetes insipidus, chronic stool retention, and sickle cell disease (secondary to defects in urinary concentrating mechanism). However, these organic causes are secondary and account for no more than 5% of all cases.

Evaluation necessitates a careful history, which should involve questions about the pattern of enuresis, history of constipation, and psychologic stressors. The physical examination should focus on a careful neurologic and genital examination. Laboratory studies may be limited to urinalysis to check for specific gravity, glucose, and the possibility of a urinary tract infection. If any abnormalities are evident on physical examination or urinalysis, more detailed studies are appropriate.

Treatment for enuresis centers on behavioral approaches, such as charting, night awakening by parents, and bladder stretching exercises. The use of a moisture-sensitive alarm is one of the most successful treatment modalities and eliminates the condition in 70% of children within the first several months of use. Pharmacologic agents are useful in decreasing the number of episodes of bedwetting but have a high relapse rate. They should be used only when the temporary, rapid elimination of bedwetting is required. Both tricyclic antidepressants and desmopressin acetate are effective. An intravenous pyelogram would be indicated, if the boy had a history of recurrent urinary tract infections, to investigate any possible structural abnormalities of the genitourinary tract. Enuresis is a stigmatizing condition; most families desire a solution and are not satisfied with reassurance.

55–60. The answers are: 55-D, 56-B, 57-A, 58-C, 59-A, 60-E. (*Obstetrics/gynecology*)

Not all vaginal discharge is pathologic and indicates infection. Discharge is often physiologic; it is comprised of cervical mucus, endometrial fluid, exudates from the Skene and Bartholin glands, and vaginal transudate. Exfoliation of squamous cells from the vaginal wall gives the secretions a white color and their characteristic inconsistency. Many factors, including hormonal and fluid status, pregnancy, immunosuppression, and inflammation, influence the amount and character of the vaginal fluid. Normal secretions have no odor. After puberty, increased glycogen favors the growth of lactobacilli in the genital tract. These bacteria break down glycogen to lactic acid, which lowers the pH to 3.5 to 4.5.

Most infectious vaginitis is due to three agents: synergistic bacteria (vaginosis), fungi (*Candida*), and protozoa (*Trichomonas*). Bacteria account for 50% of infectious vaginitis cases, and fungi and protozoa each account for approximately 25%. Bacterial vaginosis is a symbiotic infection of anaerobes (*Bacteroides, Peptococcus, Mobiluncus*, and *Gardnerella*); the normal anaerobe/aerobe ratio of 5:1 shifts to 1,000:1, with an increase in thin, gray-white to yellow discharge. Microscopic examination illustrates the presence of "clue cells," which are epithelial cells studded with bacilli, giving them a ground-glass appearance. Mixing the secretions with 10% potassium hydroxide (KOH) liberates amines with a fishy odor (whiff test). Vulvar irritation is present in 20% of cases. Hyphae on KOH examination are seen in yeast infections. Flagellated organisms indicate infection with *Trichomonas*. Gram-negative rods, which are often seen normally on vaginal smears, represent colonization with normal flora, such as lactobacillus. Scabies does not lead to a vaginal discharge.

The treatment of choice is metronidazole 500 mg 2 times a day for 7 days. The other antibiotic choices in question 56 do not treat anaerobic infections adequately and are inappropriate. Sexual partners should receive treatment, particularly in the presence of frequent recurrences.

In monilial vaginitis, *Candida albicans* causes 90% of cases. Hyphae are apparent. *Candida* vaginitis, which is not considered a sexually transmitted disease, is more common in diabetes, obesity, pregnancy, immunosuppression, and with contraceptive or antibiotic use. Itching is the most common complaint. A thick, odor-free, "cottage cheese" discharge with a 4.0 to 5.0 pH is found. Treatment includes single-dose fluconazole, topical clotrimazole, or topical miconazole nitrate. More than 90% of patients respond initially, but 20% to 30% have recurrent infections after 1 month.

Trichomonas vaginalis, a flagellate protozoan that lives in the vagina, is transmitted by sexual intercourse. Symptoms include itching; burning; dysuria; and copious, frothy discharge with a rancid odor. Microscopic examination reveals the presence of *Trichomonas.* Treatment is metronidazole 1 to 2 g in one or two doses.

In this case, the enzyme-linked immunosorbent assay (ELISA) is most appropriate for screening for HIV. A p24 polymerase chain reaction was once used to test for presence of the virus before seroconversion. Today, most laboratories perform a viral load study to detect virus directly. Neither is appropriate in this setting. If the ELISA is positive, the Western blot is a confirmatory test; it is more specific (there are fewer false-positive results).

All forms of contraception have positive and negative features. Barrier contraceptives are associated with a 5% to 20% failure rate due to improper use. Oral contraceptives have a 1% to 2% first-year failure rate, and cigarette smoking is not an absolute contraindication to their use. Absolute contraindications are pulmonary embolism, deep venous thrombosis, current breast cancer, current endometrial cancer, hepatic disease, severe atherosclerotic disease, and a history of stroke. Oral contraceptives may decrease the incidence of pelvic inflammatory disease (PID), and they also protect from ovarian cancer by inhibiting ovulation.

The physician should immediately seek help in finding this patient, even if it means breaking physician–patient confidentiality. The 1974 Tarasoff decision stated that a clinician may suspend physician–patient confidentiality to warn potential victims and notify law enforcement officials of threats by their patients toward others. The patient with HIV who is unaware of their disease and is sexually active is placing others in harm's way.

61. The answer is A. (*Internal medicine*)

This patient suffers from adult polycystic kidney disease. This autosomal dominant condition leads to renal cyst formation and progressive renal failure, ultimately requiring renal transplantation or dialysis. Presenting features often include microscopic hematuria and hypertension, and these findings, along with the presence of renal impairment, lead to consideration of a broad differential diagnosis. Some of the possible disorders include systemic lupus erythematosus, Goodpasture syndrome, nephrolithiasis, and other vasculitides. However, the presence of bilateral palpable abdominal masses should lead to the suspicion of polycystic kidney disease.

Ultrasonography is the most useful and least invasive diagnostic test. Antinuclear antibody screen, anti–glomerular basement membrane screen, and serum complement levels would all be appropriate if the patient had presented with acute glomerulonephritis. This condition would lead to hematuria, hypertension, and rapidly deteriorating renal function with cellular casts on urinalysis. Glomerulonephritis is not associated with flank masses. Intravenous pyelography would certainly demonstrate cysts but would needlessly expose the patient to intravenous contrast and possibly to dye-induced renal failure.

62–64. The answers are: 62-C, 63-C, 64-D. (*Surgery, internal medicine*)

Preoperative antibiotic prophylaxis (usually with a first- or second-generation cephalosporin) is effective in reducing the incidence of wound infections. However, to be effective, the antibiotic must be given in a timely fashion—preferably within 1 hour of the initial incision. It is important to realize that antibiotic prophylaxis does not prevent the occurrence of other infections, such as pneumonia, endocarditis, or urinary tract infections. Thus, the use of preoperative antibiotic prophylaxis should have no bearing on the workup in postoperative fever. In addition, it is necessary to understand that studies showing a clear-cut benefit from such antibiotic use have involved operations that have an appreciable risk of infection (e.g., acute cholecystitis; large bowel resections; vascular reconstructions; procedures implanting a high-risk prosthesis, such as a hip, knee, or aortic valve).

Wound infections that occur in the first 48 hours are uncommon and should prompt consideration of virulent organisms as the cause. Streptococci and clostridial species are most common. Most often, these organisms are introduced into the wound during the surgical procedure, not in the postoperative period. Prompt initiation of antibiotics that cover these organisms is essential, and surgical debridement of any devitalized tissue is mandatory. When evaluating patients for suspected postoperative infections, it is also important to keep in mind the preoperative risk factors for an increased risk of infection. These include increasing age, diabetes mellitus, malnutrition, and immunosuppression.

The nosocomial pneumonia that eventually affects this patient has various definitions, but the disorder is generally said to develop after 48 to 72 hours of hospitalization. Nosocomial pneumonia, which leads to longer hospital stays with increased costs, is associated with a high mortality rate. It is important to realize that the organisms associated with nosocomial pneumonia are more virulent. The pathogens include resistant, enteric, gram-negative bacteria such as *Enterobacter* species, *Klebsiella pneumoniae,* and *Escherichia coli,* as well as other organisms such as *Staphylococcus aureus* and *Pseudomonas aeruginosa.* Antibiotic coverage must include these organisms. Coverage for community-acquired pneumonia may include ceftriaxone, azithromycin, or cefuroxime; these regimens would be inadequate for nosocomial pneumonia. Furthermore, so-called atypical organisms such as *Chlamydia* and *Mycoplasma* are not causes of nosocomial pneumonia. A reasonable initial antibiotic regimen would be a broad-spectrum penicillin (with antipseudomonal properties) with a β-lactamase inhibitor. Ampicillin has no antipseudomonal activity and would provide inadequate coverage.

65–67. The answers are: 65-C, 66-D, 67-D. (*Emergency medicine, internal medicine*)
This patient presents with the classic findings of symptomatic hyperthyroidism (palpitations, irritability, fatigue, weight loss, increased appetite, hypersensitivity to heat). The acute treatment should focus on the control of these symptoms. Propranolol or other antiadrenergic agents significantly reduce some of the symptoms of thyrotoxicosis. High-dose iodine therapy may be used to decrease hormone release in the setting of thyroid storm. Verapamil hydrochloride would have no effect on the symptoms. Antithyroid agents, such as methimazole and propylthiouracil (PTU), inhibit the organification of iodine into thyroid hormone; they should not be used until the diagnosis is confirmed. PTU has the added advantage of inhibiting peripheral conversion of thyroxine (T_4) to triiodothyronine (T_3). It should be noted that several days may pass before both the antithyroid effect of methimazole and PTU is discernible.

This patient's thyroid tests indicate elevated thyroid hormone levels and a suppressed thyroid-stimulating hormone (TSH). Thus, the differential diagnoses includes Graves disease, factitious disorder, toxic nodular goiter, and thyroiditis. The only way to distinguish among these conditions involves the use of a radioactive iodine uptake scan. In Graves disease, autoantibodies are stimulating the thyroid, resulting in increased uptake. In either factitious disorder or thyroiditis, the uptake is low. It is possible to differentiate between these two conditions by checking the thyroglobulin level, which is elevated in thyroid inflammation—and not by exogenous thyroid hormone. Therefore, this patient has Graves disease; this diagnosis is consistent with the physical examination. On radionuclide scan, toxic nodular goiter shows patchy cases of increased activity with surrounding areas with suppressed uptake.

Agranulocytosis, a severe complication of antithyroid medications, has developed in this patient. This condition affects a reported 0.8% of patients who take PTU. It is essential that patients who take this agent be warned about this complication. Thorough evaluation with a complete blood count (CBC) is necessary when they present with a febrile illness.

68. The answer is B. (*Internal medicine*)
This patient presents with idiopathic thrombocytopenic purpura. This autoimmune disease, which more commonly affects women of childbearing age, is a result of the presence of an antibody against platelets. The diagnosis is one of exclusion; it is necessary to rule out drugs, infections, disseminated intravascular coagulation (DIC), thrombotic thrombocytopenic purpura, bone marrow–infiltrating processes, splenomegaly, and pseudothrombocytopenia. Evaluation relies on a careful history and physical examination. Patients with suspected disease should stop taking all potentially causative medications. Detailed analysis of the peripheral blood smear for signs of malignancy and hemolysis is necessary. In idiopathic thrombocytopenic purpura, all other blood cell lines except platelet counts are normal. DIC is excluded in the setting of a normal prothrombin time (PT) or partial thromboplastin time (PTT). Acute myelogenous leukemia is excluded by the normal white blood cell (WBC) count and differential. Pseudothrombocytopenia results from clumping and clotting of the platelets in the tube. Treatment entails the use of high-dose corticosteroids or intravenous immunoglobulin.

69. The answer is E. (*Internal medicine*)
This patient presents with a rash and symptoms characteristic of secondary syphilis. Syphilis, which is caused by a sexually transmitted spirochete (*Treponema pallidum*), progresses through stages of illness. The primary stage usually develops within 2 to 6 weeks of exposure. Typically, a painless chancre appears that heals in 1 to 4 weeks. An early latent stage then ensues, which is only manifested by positive serologic findings. The secondary stage occurs several weeks later, when presenting features such as fever, lymphadenopathy, malaise, arthralgia, and rash develop. The rash may be manifested in several ways, including macular, papular, pustular, eroded, or any combination of these types, and a high index of suspicion is required to make the diagnosis. Frequently the rash may involve the whole body or affect only the palms and soles. A flat, wart-like lesion known as condyloma latum may occasionally occur in regions of skin apposition. A long, latent phase with only positive serology occurs following the secondary stage. Tertiary syphilis develops in some patients 5 to 20 years after the initial infection, with changes in the central nervous system (CNS); the cardiovascular system; and the bones, eyes, and other tissues.

The diagnosis can be established with a nonspecific serologic screen (rapid plasma reagin or Venereal Disease Research Laboratory [VDRL]) and a confirmatory specific antibody test (fluorescent treponemal antibody). Treatment is high-dose penicillin therapy. All other antibiotics provide suboptimal coverage. In fact, some infectious disease experts recommend that penicillin-allergic patients be desensitized so that penicillin can be given to all patients with syphilis.

70. The answer is B. (*Emergency medicine, pediatrics, neurology*)
The organophosphate insecticides used in crop spraying have potent anticholinesterase activity, which results from chemical similarity of the pesticide with acetylcholine and irreversible binding and inhibition of the cholinesterase enzyme. This effect leads to diminished hydrolysis of acetylcholine and increased cholinergic activity at both muscarinic and nicotinic receptors. At high concentrations of acetylcholine, depolarizing blockade occurs at the nicotinic receptor and paralysis of skeletal muscle results. Clinical symptoms of organophosphate poisoning are headache, blurry vision, nausea and vomiting, abdominal cramps, diarrhea, sweating, increased lacrimation and salivation, convulsions, confusion, cardiac arrhythmias, and shock. Additional physical findings include increased glandular secretions, intestinal hypermobility, pupillary miosis, tachyarrhythmias, weakness, fasciculations, and altered sensorium. The most severe complication is respiratory collapse. Pralidoxime chloride is used to reactivate the cholinesterase molecule and terminate the neuromuscular depolarization block. If muscle function does not show a sustained increase in strength, pralidoxime may have to be administered several times. Another vital part of therapy is thorough decontamination of all surfaces exposed to the toxin to prevent further absorption. Medical personnel should take precautions, including wearing protective clothing.

Succinylcholine chloride would obviously be inappropriate because it is a depolarizing neuromuscular blocker. Glucagon can be used to treat life-threatening hypoglycemia and β-blocker overdosage. Naloxone hydrochloride would be appropriate in the setting of opiate overdose. Atropine sulfate is useful in reversing muscarinic side effects (e.g., hypersalivation, arrhythmia) but has no effect in reversing the nicotinic effects of neuromuscular blockade; in addition, it does not reverse the weakness or the possibility of respiratory collapse.

71–75. The answers are: 71-C, 72-B, 73-D, 74-B, 75-E. (*Obstetrics/gynecology*)
Vaginal bleeding during pregnancy, which sometimes occurs, is not all pathologic. It often raises the concern of a spontaneous abortion. Five percent of women report bleeding of some degree during pregnancy. In most cases, antepartum bleeding is mild and often follows sexual intercourse. Small cervical polyps can also cause bleeding. Because this patient is in the first half of her pregnancy, placenta previa and placenta abruptio are unlikely.

Management at the time of bleeding should include a quantitative β-human chorionic gonadotropin (β-hCG), transabdominal ultrasound, speculum examination to evaluate for an open os, and complete blood count (CBC) to help evaluate the extent of bleeding. If the β-hCG is less than 5,000 mIU/mL, transvaginal ultrasound may be helpful.

Bleeding at 10 weeks of pregnancy should prompt concern for spontaneous abortion, which is the termination of pregnancy prior to viability, typically at less than 20 weeks' gestation or with a fetus that weighs less than 500 g. The incidence of spontaneous abortion is thought to be approximately 50%, assuming that many pregnancies terminate without clinical recognition. A large majority of these abortions (80%) occur during the first 12 weeks of pregnancy. Fifty percent of early spontaneous abortions are attributed to chromosomal abnormalities; trisomy accounts for approximately 45%. Second-trimester abortions are less likely to be chromosomal and more likely to be due to maternal systemic disease (diabetes, cancer, hypothyroidism, hyperthyroidism), abnormal placentation, antiphospholipid antibody syndrome, leiomyomas, septate/bicornuate uterus, Asherman syndrome, infection (*Listeria, Mycoplasma hominis, Ureaplasma,* toxoplasmosis, rubella, cytomegalovirus), smoking, alcohol, and luteal phase inadequacy (insufficient progesterone). Risk factors for spontaneous abortion include multiparity, increasing maternal and paternal age, and conception within 3 months of a live birth.

Completed abortion refers to spontaneous abortion of *all* products of conception, and incomplete abortion refers to retention of some tissue. Pain and bleeding usually occur. To avoid infection, suction curettage is usually necessary. Inevitable abortion is defined as rupture of membranes, cervical dilation, or both during the first half of pregnancy. Pregnancy loss is considered unavoidable. Uterine contractions usually follow with expulsion of the products of conception. A missed abortion is the retention of a failed intrauterine pregnancy for more than two menstrual cycles. Disseminated intravascular coagulation (DIC) may occur if retention lasts for more than 6 weeks after fetal death. Recurrent abortion is defined as two consecutive or three spontaneous abortions. Karyotyping is recommended for both parents. Particular causes to consider are septate uterus, incompetent cervix, Asherman syndrome, and antiphospholipid antibody syndrome.

Any vaginal bleeding in the first half of an intrauterine pregnancy is presumptively called a threatened abortion unless another specific diagnosis can be made. Fifty percent of these women proceed to spontaneous abortion. Those who carry a pregnancy complicated by threatened abortion to viability are at greater risk for preterm delivery, low-birth-weight infants, and perinatal mortality. The infants do *not* have a higher incidence of congenital malformations.

Treatment of spontaneous abortion includes reassurance if pregnancy is found to be intact without cervical dilation. Emotional support is important because partners often blame themselves, and the clinician should see patients within 2 weeks of the initial evaluation as a supportive measure. Couples should abstain from intercourse for three or more weeks. Admission is necessary if there is severe bleeding, infection, severe pain, or anemia thought to be due to the bleeding. Bed rest has no documented benefit. Evacuation is necessary if the fetus is not viable or if the pain or bleeding is persistent or severe. Cerclage is only necessary for documented cases of incompetent cervix.

76. The answer is C. (*Statistics*)
In a cohort study, a group of people (the cohort) who do not have a particular disease or outcome are followed-up by researchers. On entry to the study, individuals undergo careful examination, and then researchers classify them according to potential risk factors that may be related to an outcome. For example, suppose a researcher who is interested in the causes of a new form of leukemia believes that several potential exposures may be related to the development of this disease. He assembles a large group of people without the disease, classifies them according to the risks that interest him, and then observes them over time. In this way, it is possible to see how initial characteristics are related to the final outcome. The most famous cohort study, the Framingham Study, observed a large group of citizens in Framingham, Massachusetts, to identify factors that may be related to heart disease.

Cohort studies have two advantages. One, they eliminate possible bias that may occur from knowing the outcome beforehand; and, two, they allow for assessment of the relationship between multiple exposures and multiple diseases. However, cohort studies are also limited. Because they require careful follow-up of large numbers of subjects during a large period of time, they are expensive. Results are not available for a long period of time, and the enrollment of large numbers of subjects is necessary (especially if the disease of interest is rare).

77. The answer is D. (*Emergency medicine, pediatrics*)
In unimmunized patients, it is important to assess the risk of tetanus in a wound. With clean, uncontaminated wounds, it is reasonable to simply begin immunization. However, with a wound that is likely to be contaminated with soil or feces or a wound that has been neglected for more than 24 hours, it is essential to give both tetanus immune globulin and toxoid. To avoid the formation of antigen–antibody complexes at the site of injection, two different sites of administration must be used. In patients with low-risk wounds who have been immunized and have received a booster in the past 10 years, nothing further is necessary. However, with high-risk wounds, a booster is necessary if the last booster was more than 5 years ago. Patients with wounds that have been neglected for more than 24 hours should probably receive antitetanus immune globulin.

78–81. The answers are 78-D, 79-A, 80-E, 81-B. (*Internal medicine, critical care medicine*)
Burns are classified by depth and extent of injury. First-degree burns involve only the epidermis, and the skin is very erythematous and painful. Second-degree burns include superficial partial-thickness burns (intact skin appendages, blistering, very painful) and deep partial-thickness burns (necrosis extending well into the dermis with skin appendages affected and less painful). Third-degree burns involve the entire extent of the dermis, and because nerve endings are destroyed, there is no pain. The extent of burn injury is determined by the "rule of nines;" in adults, the trunk and back each make up 18% of the body surface area, the arms and head each make up 9%, and the legs each make up 18%.

In this case, the patient has burns of the trunk (18%), back (18%), and arms ([9% × 2] = 18%) for a total of 54% of body surface area. To determine the estimated fluid deficit, the Parkland formula is used (for second- and third-degree burns):

$$\text{Volume} = \text{Total body surface area burned (\%)} \times \text{weight (kg)} \times 4 \text{ mL}$$

For this patient, with 54% of his body surface burned, the fluid deficit is 15 L, of which half should be given in the first 8 to 12 hours, with the remainder in the next 12 to 16 hours.

Secondary infections are a common complication in burn patients. The most common infectious agents include *Staphylococcus aureus, Pseudomonas* species, *Streptococcus* species, and *Candida* species. Findings that should prompt suspicion of infection are fever, wound discoloration (especially green discoloration, which often indicates *Pseudomonas* infection), and transformation of a burn from second-degree (partial-thickness) to a full-thickness burn. Blistering is not a sign of infection.

Acute respiratory distress syndrome (ARDS), a complication of massive burns, is likely the end result of massive immune stimulation with release of inflammatory cytokines. The diagnosis is made on the basis of bilateral pulmonary infiltrates, severe hypoxemia despite high fractional oxygen concentration in inspired gas (FIO_2), and the absence of other causes of infiltrates (notably cardiogenic edema, as manifested by a high pulmonary capillary wedge pressure). Treatment of ARDS is supportive, with meticulous attention to the possibility of infection and careful management of ventilatory support. Several studies have shown that both high tidal volumes and high concentrations of inspired oxygen ($>60\%$) are toxic to the lung. To maintain adequate oxygen in the face of ARDS, an increase in mean airway pressure is necessary. This allows alveoli to remain open and recruits closed alveoli for gas exchange. This can be best accomplished by increasing positive end-expiratory pressure (PEEP). The other measures described in question 80 may improve oxygenation but at the expense of increased lung injury.

Increasing PEEP is not without complications. Increased PEEP may lead to decreased venous return and hypotension that is easily treated with intravenous fluids. A more severe complication is pneumothorax secondary to rupture of the alveoli under increased pressure. In this patient, a tension pneumothorax develops, resulting in impaired oxygenation and hypotension. In acute hypotension, sepsis, hypovolemia, and cardiogenic shock are possible but, in the setting of recently increased PEEP, pneumothorax is a strong consideration. If breath sounds are absent on one side of the chest or if there is tracheal deviation or hyperresonance of one side of the chest, urgent chest tube decompression is necessary.

82. The answer is C. (*Internal medicine*)

This patient has acute testicular torsion, a surgical emergency. Torsion of the spermatic cord is the result of a high attachment of the tunica vaginalis around the terminal cord, allowing the testicle to twist freely within the scrotum. When rotation of the testicle on the end of the cord exceeds 90 degrees, vascular compromise may occur, leading to infarction and gangrene of the testicle.

Testicular torsion, which is generally seen in young men, occurs spontaneously. Physical and sexual activity may predispose to torsion. The onset of severe pain, swelling, and often nausea and vomiting is rapid. Fever is rare. Differentiation from acute epididymitis is critical; in torsion, there is no dysuria or pyuria. Rapid diagnosis is critical to save the testicle. Some physicians advocate surgery with a highly suggestive clinical presentation, but the rapid availability of Doppler ultrasound has made the diagnosis more reliable. The other laboratory tests listed as answer choices, which may detect nonspecific abnormalities, are not necessary.

83–85. The answers are: 83-C, 84-E, 85-E. (*Internal medicine*)

This patient presents with severe abdominal pain that is consistent with acute pancreatitis. However, it is important to keep the differential diagnosis of severe epigastric pain in mind to ensure that other life-threatening diagnoses are not overlooked. Other possibilities include gastric or duodenal ulcer, gastric or duodenal ulcer perforation, acute cholecystitis, bowel infarction, diabetic ketoacidosis, and aortic dissection.

To make the diagnosis, the most useful test would be CT of the abdomen. This test would show evidence of pancreatic inflammation (and, if severe, necrosis and hemorrhage) and rule out other causes. Although a serum amylase level would be elevated in acute pancreatitis, this test is nonspecific and would be elevated in diabetic ketoacidosis, bowel infarction, and perforation. Abdominal ultrasound is less sensitive. Alkaline phosphatase levels are nonspecific but would be elevated if the common bile duct was obstructed. Serum transaminases may be abnormal if there is associated hepatitis.

Several conditions may cause acute pancreatitis. In the United States, gallstones and alcohol account for 90% of cases, but other causes warrant consideration. These include trauma, hyperlipidemia, hypercalcemia, and medications (e.g., thiazides, azathioprine), as well as certain procedures (e.g., endoscopic retrograde cholangiopancreatography). Atherosclerosis is not a cause of pancreatitis.

Acute pancreatitis may be a life-threatening disorder. Numerous scoring systems exist to predict which patients may have poor outcomes and may benefit from more intensive therapy. The Ranson scoring system is the most widely used and includes prognostic signs that are scored on admission and at 48 hours after admission.

Ranson Criteria	
At Diagnosis or Admission	During Initial 48 Hours
Age >55 years	Fall in hematocrit by 10%
White blood count (WBC) >16,000/mm³	Estimated fluid deficit >6 L
Blood glucose >200 mg/dL	Serum calcium <8.0 mg/dL
Serum lactate dehydrogenase (LDH) >350 IU/L	Arterial PO_2 <60 mm Hg
Serum aspartate aminotransferase (AST) >250 IU/L	Blood urea nitrogen (BUN) elevation >5 mg/dL
	Base deficit >4 mEq/L

Patients who present with two or fewer of these prognostic signs have essentially no mortality. Patients with three or four prognostic signs generally have a 15% mortality and require intensive care support in nearly 50% of cases. With five or six signs, mortality approaches 50%. A white blood cell (WBC) count less than 8,000/mm³ has no prognostic significance.

86–88. The answers are: 86-B, 87-B, 88-A. (*Internal medicine, critical care medicine*)
Acute respiratory distress syndrome (ARDS) is a condition characterized by acute hypoxemic respiratory failure as a result of pulmonary edema caused by increased permeability of the alveolar-capillary barrier. ARDS is defined by the presence of the following three criteria: bilateral diffuse opacities on chest radiography, pulmonary capillary wedge pressure less than 18 mm Hg, and a PaO_2/FIO_2 ratio of less than 200 mm Hg. This patient fulfills the criteria for ARDS. The most common causes of this condition (in descending order) are sepsis, aspiration, multiple transfusions, pneumonia, near-drowning, pancreatitis, and cardiopulmonary bypass. Statistically, the cause of respiratory failure in this patient is most likely sepsis.

The pathologic changes in ARDS occur in three distinct phases. During the exudative phase, which occurs initially, hyaline membranes comprised of fibrin and other proteins form. At this stage, bronchoscopy with bronchoalveolar lavage would detect protein. During the proliferative phase, which begins after approximately 3 days, the alveolar exudate either resolves or undergoes organization with fibrosis. During this fibrotic phase, which develops after 3 to 4 weeks, the alveolar spaces and ducts undergo fibrosis. The prognosis of patients with ARDS depends largely on the extent of this fibrotic phase.

While this patient is in the medical intensive care unit (ICU), she loses 12 pounds, and her enteral nutrition appears to be inadequate. Her right upper quadrant pain with fever are consistent with acalculous cholecystitis, which occurs most commonly in the setting of trauma, burns, postoperatively, and postpartum, as well as with vasculitis, diabetes mellitus, or parasitic infection of the gallbladder. Ischemia has been implicated as the primary pathologic process secondary to stasis and inflammation. Treatment includes emergent cholecystectomy in low-risk patients or percutaneous cholecystostomy for high-risk patients such as this one. One study found that a percutaneous procedure had a success rate of 99% with 10% mortality.

89. The answer is C. (*Emergency medicine, obstetrics/gynecology*)
This patient presents with a clinical syndrome highly suggestive of ectopic pregnancy. The classic presentation is amenorrhea, abdominal pain, and abnormal vaginal bleeding. Symptoms of pregnancy are unusual. In the United States, 2% of pregnancies are ectopic, but these cases account for 13% of all pregnancy-related deaths. Approximately 95% of cases occur in the fallopian tubes. Risk factors include salpingitis (pelvic inflammatory disease [PID]), previous ectopic pregnancy, tubal ligation, intrauterine device use, and congenital abnormalities of the fallopian tubes. The differential diagnosis of ectopic pregnancy is extensive, includ-

ing appendicitis, PID, abortion, ruptured corpus luteum cyst, adnexal torsion, endometriosis, pancreatitis, gastroenteritis, and dysfunctional uterine bleeding.

Diagnosis is facilitated by the availability of several highly sensitive tests. Virtually any woman of childbearing age with abdominal pain should have a β-human chorionic gonadotropin (β-hCG) measurement. During the first 5 to 6 weeks of pregnancy, the β-hCG titer normally doubles every 2 days. If this expected rise fails to occur, or if a woman is not at the expected level for her estimated dates, this is strong evidence of abnormal gestation. The performance of vaginal ultrasonography greatly aids in the diagnosis because an intrauterine gestational sac is visible at 5 to 6 weeks' gestation. (Generally, the β-hCG level at which the intrauterine sac should be visible is 2,000 to 3,000 mIU/mL.) Culdocentesis and laparoscopy, which are used less frequently, may be helpful in confusing cases. Abdominal ultrasonography does not afford the high degree of sensitivity associated with vaginal ultrasonography; it identifies a tubal gestational sac in only 25% of cases.

90–92. The answers are: 90-A, 91-D, 92-B. (*Obstetrics/gynecology*)
Rape, which is reportedly the fastest growing crime in the United States, is devastating for the victim both physically and emotionally. As a result of the incident, a significant number of victims suffer from posttraumatic stress disorder. All physicians must be sensitive to the difficult issues that present in the rape victim. Provision of a safe setting with emotional support should occur initially. In many cities, specialized counselors are trained to offer the necessary support. Medical concerns include documentation of the history, physical examination, treatment of any injuries, and discussion of the potential risks of sexually transmitted diseases and pregnancy. It is important to realize that informed consent must be obtained in order to notify the police and to gather evidence from the physical examination. Most centers have detailed protocols to ensure that these issues are properly handled.

After any episode of unprotected sexual intercourse, the risk of acquiring gonorrhea may be as high as 6% to 12%, and the risk of acquiring syphilis is up to 3%. Because 40% to 90% of patients are lost to follow-up, it is essential to offer empiric treatment at the time of initial evaluation. Of the answers for question 91, only ceftriaxone and azithromycin provide adequate broad-spectrum coverage for sexually transmittable agents. The clinician should also offer pregnancy counseling. Some women may opt for pregnancy prophylaxis with two, 50-μg, estrogen-containing combination oral contraceptive tablets, taking one tablet immediately and the other in 12 hours.

Testing for HIV is warranted. In most centers, the initial HIV test is a rapid enzyme-linked immunosorbent assay (ELISA) that detects antibodies formed against the virus. It has a sensitivity and specificity of more than 99%. In the acute stage of HIV infection, antibodies have not had time to form, and ELISA is likely be negative. Therefore, retesting in 3 and 6 months is recommended; at which time, the majority of infected patients will have seroconverted. When an ELISA is positive, it is confirmed by a Western blot, which is more specific but less sensitive. Polymerase chain reaction is used to confirm indeterminate Western blot tests. Because an ELISA detects antibodies, any autoimmune condition may yield false-positive results and warrants careful interpretation.

93–94. The answers are: 93-D, 94-A. (*Emergency medicine, pediatrics*)
This rash and scenario are consistent with roseola infantum (exanthema subitum), which is caused by human herpesvirus 6. Classically, roseola presents with 3 to 4 days of high fever (temperature: 39°C to 41°C) without other clinical findings. After the fever, a diffuse exanthem appears over the trunk that then spreads to the arms, neck, face, and legs. This rash lasts approximately 24 hours and leaves no scars. Roseola, which clusters in the spring and fall, most commonly occurs in young children between 6 and 18 months of age.

Measles is uncommon in developed countries where vaccines are used. Fever is accompanied by malaise, cough, coryza, conjunctivitis, and a maculopapular rash that starts on the face. Group A streptococcus infection is associated with pharyngitis and a sandpaper-like rash (scarlet fever) that appears hours to days after the onset of fever. Initially, the rash of parvovirus B19 (erythema infectiosum) is bright red and appears on the cheeks ("slapped cheek"). Then an occasionally pruritic, diffuse, maculopapular rash develops on the trunk and extremities. As the rash fades, it leaves a lacy or reticular pattern. The maculopapular rash, which is not associated with fever, lasts approximately 10 days but can return in 4 to 6 weeks on exposure to sunlight. Varicella presents with fever, malaise, anorexia, and a vesicular rash that crusts over.

Roseola requires no treatment other than antipyretics, which may decrease the risk of febrile seizures.

95–96. The answers are: 95-E, 96-C. (*Pediatrics*)

Before considering this case, it is important to understand bilirubin metabolism in neonates. Bilirubin is the major breakdown product of heme, which is first converted to biliverdin and then reduced to bilirubin. Albumin carries this unconjugated bilirubin to the liver, where it is conjugated with glucuronic acid. The conjugated bilirubin is excreted with bile into the intestine, where it is catabolized to urobilinogen by the bacterial flora. Urobilinogen is converted to stercobilin, which is excreted in the feces. Several aspects of bilirubin metabolism are not fully developed in neonates. The effective half-life of red blood cells (RBCs) and the higher RBC mass account for neonates' increased bilirubin load.

In evaluating jaundice in neonates, it is first necessary to distinguish between conjugated and unconjugated hyperbilirubinemia. This patient has primarily unconjugated bilirubin, and the most important next step is a peripheral smear to evaluate for hemolysis. A complete blood count (CBC) that indicates anemia might suggest hemolysis as well. If hemolysis is present, the most likely causes include a congenital erythrocyte disorder, an erythrocyte enzyme defect, or a blood group incompatibility. If no hemolysis exists and no infection is evident, the probable diagnosis is either physiologic jaundice or breast milk–induced jaundice. After hemolysis is ruled out, a thyroid-stimulating hormone (TSH), alanine aminotransferase (ALT), and aspartate aminotransferase (AST) would be useful to rule out hypothyroidism and liver disease, respectively.

In physiologic jaundice, unconjugated bilirubin may be as high as 8 to 9 mg/dL by 3 to 5 days postnatally and should decrease to approximately 2 mg/dL by the end of the second week. If it remains increased for more than 2 weeks, consideration of hemolysis, impaired conjugation, or breast-feeding jaundice is warranted. For unknown reasons, breast-fed infants commonly have higher levels of unconjugated bilirubin. Peak levels of 10 to 20 mg/dL occur by 2 to 3 weeks after birth and may be secondary to increased intestinal reabsorption of bilirubin. Kernicterus has not been documented in this setting.

Crigler-Najjar syndrome is characterized by absent (type I) or deficient (type II) hepatic glucuronyl transferase activity and unconjugated bilirubin levels of 20 to 40 mg/dL. Kernicterus develops if the hyperbilirubinemia is not treated with phenobarbital and phototherapy. Gilbert syndrome is characterized by mild elevations of unconjugated bilirubin (up to 3 mg/dL), which is believed to be secondary to decreased hepatic bilirubin uptake. An RBC enzyme defect would have caused hemolysis. Rubella is more likely to present with deafness, cataracts, glaucoma, and congenital heart disease.

97. The answer is A. (*Emergency medicine, internal medicine*)

This patient presents in florid congestive heart failure with pulmonary edema and in renal failure with hyperkalemia. Treatment of the pulmonary edema, the most urgent concern, involves furosemide, which reduces preload and volume, and nitroglycerin, which also reduces preload. Fluid restriction is also appropriate, although this is not an acute concern. Treatment of the hyperkalemia should also occur. An ECG is mandatory to assess for any changes that may be a result of serum potassium elevation (tall, peaked T waves; decreased P-wave amplitude; and QRS widening); none of these changes was present in this patient. Insulin and glucose infusion, as well as the use of a β-agonist (albuterol), achieves a rapid shift of extracellular potassium into cells. However, this provides only a temporary solution, and potassium removal from the body through the use of a potassium-binding resin is essential. Because potassium–sodium exchange may occur on these resins, extracellular volume expansion may occur.

Urgent hemodialysis is indicated in several situations: with severe uremic symptoms, pericardial friction rub, severe and nonresponsive hyperkalemia, nonresponsive volume overload, and severe acidemia. Other therapeutic modalities are appropriate initially in this patient. However, hemodialysis may ultimately be necessary.

98. The answer is E. (*Internal medicine*)

Dysphagia and odynophagia are common problems in late-stage HIV disease. Causes include esophageal candidiasis, herpetic ulcers, ulcers secondary to cytomegalovirus, idiopathic ulcerations, and pill esophagitis. The most common cause is candidal infection, and a trial of oral fluconazole is warranted in patients with active oral thrush before diagnostic workup. Ganciclovir would be appropriate treatment for cytomegalovirus and acyclovir for herpes simplex disease.

99–100. The answers are: 99-E, 100-B. (*Obstetrics/gynecology*)

Diabetes mellitus in pregnant women is associated with a higher incidence of congenital malformations and increased perinatal morbidity and mortality. Gestational diabetes, which affects 3% to 12% of pregnant women, is the most common form of diabetes during pregnancy. The key to successful pregnancy is meticulous glycemic control, with fasting blood sugars of 60 to 90 mg/dL and 2-hour postprandial levels less than 120 mg/dL.

The most common birth defects involve the heart and neural tube. Prenatal care is critical for diabetic women; a clinician should typically see them every 1 to 2 weeks. Some of the current recommendations include ophthalmology examinations every trimester, ultrasound surveillance for fetal growth and macrosomia, antepartum fetal surveillance, and α-fetoprotein (AFP) screening. Oral hypoglycemic agents should be avoided, and insulin is the drug of choice.

Maternal serum α-fetoprotein (AFP) testing is available to screen for fetuses with neural tube defects. These conditions, which occur in approximately 1 of 1,000 pregnancies, include a variety of disorders (spina bifida and acephaly). A low maternal serum AFP may be an indication of a missed abortion, hydatiform mole, or fetal trisomy. Testing should be performed between weeks 15 and 17 of gestation. Careful counseling and informed consent should be obtained because the implications of a positive test can be profound and lead to difficult ethical issues for the patient and her family. It is important to realize that any maternal serum AFP level needs to be interpreted in the context of age, race, maternal weight, number of fetuses, history of diabetes mellitus, and past history of neural tube defects.

Patients who have a positive test result should be referred for further workup, which may include ultrasonography, midtrimester amniocentesis, fetal echocardiography, and other tests. Ultrasonography may detect as many as 80% to 90% of neural tube defects at this time. Any workup should be complete by 22 weeks of gestation to allow the patient the option of pregnancy termination, if so desired.

101–102. The answers are: 101-E, 102-C. (*Obstetrics/gynecology*)

This patient has stage IIa cervical cancer. (The "a" means that there is no spread to the parametrium.) Stage I cervical cancer is confined to the cervix, stage II cancer extends into the upper two thirds of the vagina, stage III cancer extends into the lower third of the vagina or results in no cancer-free space between the tumor and pelvic wall, and stage IV cancer extends beyond the true pelvis and involves the bladder or rectum.

For patients with stage IIa cancer, there are two options for therapy: (1) radical hysterectomy and pelvic lymphadenectomy, or (2) radiotherapy with external beam irradiation and brachytherapy (using cesium-137–loaded colpostats in the uterus and vagina). Many younger women prefer surgery to maintain ovarian function and avoid vaginal irradiation. Radiotherapy is preferable for older patients, especially those who are poor surgical candidates. Unfortunately, radiotherapy has both acute and long-term side effects that include ischemic necrosis and scarring of adjacent tissues (vagina, rectum), loss of ovarian function, and skin irritation to name a few. Radiation-induced cystitis, but not infection, is common.

Clearly, when this patient returns 2½ years later, recurrent disease must be a primary concern. In fact, 80% of patients experience recurrence within this time period. It is important to note that long-term side effects from radiation therapy could account for some of these symptoms. For example, the patient's flank pain is likely due to hydronephrosis, which could result either from tumor invasion or radiation-induced fibrosis of the ureter. In this case, a CT scan of the abdomen and pelvis should be able to discern tumor invasion, if present. The other answer choices in question 102 do not produce a specific diagnosis. In equivocal cases, tissue biopsy is warranted. Unfortunately, palliative therapy is usually the only recourse at time of recurrence.

103–104. The answers are: 103-D, 104-E. (*Emergency medicine, surgery*)
As the abdominal radiograph clearly shows, this patient presents with a sigmoid volvulus. This condition occurs when an elongated loop of sigmoid colon rotates around its mesentery, which leads to a high-grade obstruction with abdominal pain, obstipation, and distension. It is more common in the very elderly, especially in bedridden, debilitated patients. On the radiograph, there is a prominent U-shaped loop of dilated bowel in the lower abdomen.

Abdominal perforation is indicated by the presence of free air under the diaphragm on an upright abdominal radiograph. Fecal impaction is evident on physical examination and demonstrates diffuse colonic dilatation. Ogilvie syndrome, or pseudo-obstruction of the large bowel, is often due to electrolyte or metabolic imbalances and leads to diffuse colonic dilatation.

Sigmoidoscopy is the treatment of choice; this procedure is both diagnostic and therapeutic. After decompression by sigmoidoscopy, surgical resection of the redundant sigmoid loops should be considered in patients with no contraindications. Emergent surgery is not necessary unless the sigmoidoscopy fails to reduce the volvulus. Laxatives and observation would be inappropriate. Intravenous hydration would be required. Metoclopramide, a promotility agent, is relatively contraindicated; this drug has little, if any, effect on the distal colon.

105. The answer is A. (*Surgery, internal medicine*)
The most common causes of shoulder pain in adults include rotator cuff tendinitis, rotator cuff tear, subacromial bursitis, adhesive capsulitis (or frozen shoulder biceps tendinitis), and acromioclavicular arthritis. In this case, crossed arm adduction with resistance aggravates an acromioclavicular joint inflammatory condition. Treatment consists of nonsteroidal anti-inflammatory drugs (NSAIDs) and an injection with steroids or lidocaine.

Subacromial bursitis is elicited by palpation over the deltoid. Rotator cuff injuries, which usually involve the supraspinatus tendon, are best elicited with positioning of the greater tubercle of the humerus beneath the acromion (the "empty beer can" sign). Biceps tendinitis is aggravated by flexion or supination of the upper extremity.

106. The answer is B. (*Pediatrics*)
An undescended testis poses several risks: (1) the testis is susceptible to torsion and trauma, (2) it may be associated with infertility, and (3) it has an increased risk for malignancy. Treatment should occur as early as possible. The longer the testis remains undescended, the higher the risk of infertility. It is critical to remember that even after the testis is brought down into the scrotum, there is still a risk of malignancy; careful, lifelong, routine examination of the testicle is necessary.

Cryptorchidism, which is present in approximately 1% of 1-year-old boys, is usually unilateral but may be bilateral (up to 30% of the time). In most cases, the absent testis is undescended, but in 20% of cases it can be absent. An inguinal hernia is often present on the involved side. Genetic studies are rarely necessary.

107. The answer is D. (*Pediatrics*)
Delayed puberty in girls is defined as the absence of secondary sexual characteristics by the age of 13. Constitutional delay of puberty is a term applied to otherwise healthy children who have an isolated delay in the onset of puberty. Bone age is also significantly delayed in girls with delayed puberty. There is often a strong

family history of delayed puberty or menarche. The extensive list of causes of delayed puberty includes hypothyroidism, connective tissue disease, inflammatory bowel disease, and chronic renal failure, as well as causes of primary ovarian failure (e.g., Turner syndrome) and autoimmune ovarian failure. Other conditions that may lead to delayed puberty are those associated with hypogonadotropic hypogonadism such as Kallmann syndrome, pituitary tumors, anorexia nervosa, and hypopituitarism. Autoimmune causes are rare.

108–110. The answers are: 108-D, 109-E, 110-C. (*Obstetrics/gynecology, surgery*)
Lobular carcinoma in situ is not a premalignant lesion. Ductal carcinoma in situ may itself become an infiltrating, invasive ductal carcinoma. Like early menarche, late menopause, positive family history, personal history of breast cancer, and nulliparity, lobular carcinoma in situ is a risk factor for breast cancer. Thus, diligent screening mammography is necessary for the lobular carcinoma in situ lesion, as it would be with any other risk factor.

Lumpectomy is the treatment for ductal carcinoma in situ. Lumpectomy, radiation, and lymph node sampling is appropriate for most invasive carcinomas, and modified radical mastectomy is warranted for carcinomas involving the skin or nipple. Of note, there is no clear evidence that modified radical mastectomy is superior to lumpectomy plus radiation unless the mass cannot be removed with clear margins (e.g., close proximity to the nipple or skin). Whether a sentinel lymph node biopsy is equivalent to complete lymphadenectomy is still questionable.

At this time, breast cancer is thought to be hereditary in 5% to 10% of cases. BRCA1 and BRCA2 genes are associated with breast cancer, ovarian cancer, prostate cancer, and melanoma. The tumor suppressor gene P53 is associated with breast cancer, brain cancer, sarcomas, laryngeal cancers, vascular tumors, and adrenal cortex cancers. Cowden disease is associated with colon cancer, thyroid cancer, and breast cancer. Endometrial cancer, ovarian cancer, and other gastrointestinal (GI) cancers are seen in hereditary nonpolyposis colorectal cancer (Lynch syndrome II). Currently, there is no well-supported genetic association between lung cancer and breast cancer.

In the early years of the 21st century, the issue of tamoxifen is still controversial. The National Surgical Adjuvant Breast and Bowel Project (NSABP) trials support the conclusion that tamoxifen results in a decrease in the incidence of invasive breast cancer by approximately 50% in ductal carcinoma in situ, lobular carcinoma in situ, and high-risk disease (by Gail index). The reduction in risk appears to be even more significant for those with a history of atypical ductal hyperplasia. But no study to date has found a decrease in mortality, only a decrease in the number of breast cancers. Studies have found that tamoxifen increases the incidence of endometrial cancer by approximately 1/1,000 per year. Smoking is not a contraindication to tamoxifen, but it probably increases the already significant risk of deep venous thrombosis.

111. The answer is D. (*Pediatrics*)
This child has Kawasaki disease. This generalized vasculitis with no known cause typically affects children younger than 4 years. Diagnosis is based on a fever of at least 5 days' duration and four of the following five conditions: (1) induration and erythema of the hands and feet, (2) a polymorphous exanthem, (3) bilateral conjunctivitis, (4) erythema of the oropharynx with a strawberry tongue and cracked lips, and (5) cervical lymphadenopathy. The differential diagnosis of Kawasaki disease includes several infectious diseases that may cause exanthem and fever, such as scarlet fever, staphylococcal scalded skin syndrome, toxic shock syndrome, Rocky Mountain spotted fever, and leptospirosis. Other diseases that should be considered include juvenile rheumatoid arthritis (Still disease) and Stevens-Johnson syndrome. However, meningococcal sepsis is distinct. There is a rapid progression to shock during the course of several hours, generally with a petechial rash.

112. The answer is A. (*Pediatrics*)
Hemolytic uremic syndrome, a potentially fatal disease, has been associated with enteric infection by *Escherichia coli* O157:H7. Although the pathophysiology is not clear, the disease process almost certainly in-

volves endothelial injury and platelet activation. Clinical features of the disorder include a microangiopathic hemolytic anemia, acute renal failure, thrombocytopenia, and, in some cases, systemic involvement. Characteristically, the platelet count is low, schistocytes (fragmented red blood cells [RBCs]) are apparent on a peripheral smear, and the prothrombin and partial thromboplastin times (PT and PTT) are normal (answer A). An isolated fall in platelets (answer B) is characteristic of immune-mediated thrombocytopenic purpura. In disseminated intravascular coagulation (DIC), fibrinogen consumption leads to an increase in PT and PTT (answer C). The patterns described in answers D and E are not typically seen clinically.

113. The answer is B. (*Statistics*)
This question demonstrates the importance of the prevalence of a disease (or pretest probability) on the operating characteristics of a test. In this example, the likelihood ratio (or the chance that a patient has a particular disease given a positive result) can be expressed as:

$$\text{Likelihood ratio (positive test)} = \frac{\text{Sensitivity}}{(1 - \text{specificity})}$$

In essence, this is dividing the probability of a positive test result in a patient with a disease (sensitivity) by the probability of a positive test in a patient without the disease.
In this case:

$$\text{Likelihood ratio} = \frac{0.90}{(1 - 0.80)} = 4.5$$

The probability of pharyngitis is 25%, or 1:3. Thus, the posttest probability is simply:

$$4.5 \times 1:3 \text{ or } 4.5:3 \text{ or } 4.5/7.5 = 60\%$$

114–116. The answers are: 114-D, 115-A, 116-A. (*Internal medicine, neurology*)
Fever and headache in patients with AIDS or with risk factors for HIV suggest the possibility of cryptococcosis, toxoplasmosis, or central nervous system (CNS) lymphoma. In individuals with significant meningismus, such as this one, a lumbar puncture is the single most important diagnostic and, potentially, therapeutic test; cryptococcal meningitis is the most likely cause of symptoms. In individuals who do not have AIDS, significant lymphocytic pleocytosis with protein elevation and low glucose levels is seen, but in patients with AIDS, often these changes are less pronounced. In addition, patients with cryptococcomas (mass lesions due to focal accumulation of cryptococci, which are rare in patients with AIDS) often have completely normal protein and glucose levels in the cerebrospinal fluid (CSF). Approximately 90% of patients who have AIDS and cryptococcal meningitis have positive serum cryptococcal antigen by the latex agglutination test. Nearly 100% are positive in the CSF. Fungemia is present in 10% to 30% of patients; at times, prevalence approaches 50% in patients with AIDS.

Most cryptococcal infections occur when the CD4 count falls below 100 cells/mm³. *Pneumocystis carinii* pneumonia occurs when CD4 falls below 200 cells/mm³, whereas toxoplasmosis, cytomegalovirus, and *Mycobacterium avium-intracellulare* complex are most common when the CD4 count is less than 50 cells/mm³.

The most important immediate therapeutic measure is the evaluation of CSF pressure by lumbar puncture. It is believed that the lipopolysaccharide capsule obstructs CSF resorption via the arachnoid granulations. To maintain CSF pressures below 10 cm H_2O, serial lumbar punctures are essential; daily performance is necessary, at least initially. Amphotericin with or without flucytosine is the treatment for cryptococcal meningitis.

117. The answer is C. (*Internal medicine*)
This patient presents with iron deficiency anemia. The most common cause of this condition in men is gastrointestinal (GI) bleeding, and the most worrisome possibility is colonic carcinoma. The next step should

be referral for colonoscopy. Initiation of iron therapy should wait until a diagnosis is more certain because it can obscure endoscopic visualization of suspect lesions. Vitamin B_{12} and folate deficiency both lead to a macrocytic anemia. Because the patient is only mildly symptomatic, urgent transfusion is not necessary and should be avoided. Follow-up in several months would not be appropriate if a diagnosis of cancer is a possibility.

118. The answer is C. (*Internal medicine, neurology*)
Central nervous system (CNS) infections in a patient with AIDS are varied and include bacterial meningitis, viral meningitis, cryptococcal meningitis, tuberculous meningitis, toxoplasmosis, brain abscess, and progressive multifocal leukoencephalopathy. The incidence of CNS lymphomas and dementia is also higher in a patient with AIDS. This patient's presentation of a subacute meningitis with a lymphocytic predominance is characteristic of cryptococcal meningitis. Toxoplasmosis and CNS lymphoma both present with mass lesions, and although headache may be prominent, focal neurologic findings, seizures, and a positive CT scan are characteristic. Bacterial meningitis presents in a more acute fashion and usually with a neutrophilic predominance in the cerebrospinal fluid (CSF). Progressive multifocal leukoencephalopathy is thought to be due to JC virus, and presenting features include focal neurologic findings and cognitive decline. Treatment with amphotericin B initially followed by fluconazole is appropriate.

119. The answer is C. (*Surgery*)
The anterior cruciate ligament acts as the primary stabilizer preventing forward displacement of the tibia on the femur. Tears of the anterior cruciate ligament may occur as the result of contact injuries or simply hyperextension or a twisting injury of the knee. A joint effusion, which is due to bleeding within the joint space, develops rapidly. The diagnosis can be made by finding abnormal anterior displacement of the tibia. The Lachman test, one of several methods used to diagnose tears of the anterior cruciate ligament, is believed to be the most sensitive test for anterior cruciate ligament instability. In active young adults, surgical repair or reconstruction should be considered.

120–121. The answers are: 120-B, 121-C. (*Internal medicine, surgery*)
The primary diagnostic concern in a patient with perirectal pain and fever should be perirectal abscess. With an anorectal abscess, which typically occurs in the perianal and intersphincteric spaces of the rectum, infection usually begins in one of the anal glands and then spreads vertically, horizontally, or circumferentially. A perianal abscess is the result of distal vertical spread of the infection to the anal margin. Affected patients present with a tender, red, swollen, palpable mass. Rectal carcinoma usually manifests as a painless mass lesion and is often found incidentally on digital rectal examination. A fissure may be present, making the diagnosis difficult, but the presence of swelling and fever should strongly suggest an abscess. A thrombosed hemorrhoid may manifest in a similar fashion, but fever is not usual.

Prompt treatment is critical because untreated infections may lead to severe necrotizing infections of the entire perineum. Therapy involves incision and drainage of the abscess. A perianal abscess simply requires incision of the perianal skin, and an intersphincteric abscess necessitates more involved procedures. Antibiotics are not needed. CT of the pelvis is important with a recurrent abscess when an unsuspected source of pus is a concern. Sigmoidoscopy and stool softeners would not be indicated at this point in the management.

122–126. The answers are: 122-D, 123-A, 124-D, 125-C, 126-C. (*Emergency medicine, internal medicine, critical care medicine*)
In this patient, who most likely suffers from cirrhosis, the hematemesis is probably due to a ruptured esophageal varix. Although bleeding esophageal varices cause most episodes of gastrointestinal (GI) bleeding, it is important to recognize that, even in the setting of end-stage liver disease and portal hypertension, not all patients who present with upper GI bleeding have bleeding varices. In a substantial number of patients,

Mallory-Weiss tears or ulcers may be the source of bleeding. Esophageal varices, which develop secondary to portal hypertension, result from shunting of blood around the portal system. The four major consequences of portal hypertension are ascites, portosystemic shunts (esophageal varices, caput medusae, hemorrhoids), congestive splenomegaly, and hepatic encephalopathy. Of the answers listed, the finding of caput medusae clearly supports the presence of portal hypertension, which may suggest esophageal variceal bleeding. Jaundice and scleral icterus may be evident with any cause of hepatic dysfunction or hemolysis; these signs are not specific for portal hypertension. Although the presence of numerous spider angioma suggests that cirrhosis may be present, this feature is not specific for the finding of portal hypertension. Hepatomegaly would be extremely uncommon because most patients with cirrhosis have small, scarred livers.

Emergent management of esophageal variceal bleeding involves resuscitation, airway stabilization, and control of bleeding. Intubation, especially if there are signs of mental status deterioration and concerns over airway protection, is warranted. Endoscopy should be performed as soon as possible. Intravenous octreotide infusion should be initiated in order to decrease the portal pressure. If endoscopy is not readily available, a Sengstaken-Blakemore tube can be used to tamponade the bleeding (patients must be intubated for this procedure). Although diazepam is used to treat alcohol withdrawal, it should be avoided in this patient for several reasons: (1) the half-life of the drug is prolonged, and in the presence of liver disease, active metabolites accumulate; (2) alcohol withdrawal is a consideration, but it would be unusual within the first few hours of admission; and (3) shorter-acting agents would be more desirable for the purposes of sedation.

Hepatic encephalopathy, a common manifestation of end-stage liver disease, develops in this patient. Although the cause of encephalopathy is not clearly understood, several factors clearly exacerbate the condition, including GI bleeding, hypokalemia and metabolic alkalosis (both of which increase renal ammonia production), high-protein meals, infection from any source, sedative drugs, dehydration, and constipation. Hypophosphatemia is not a cause of hepatic encephalopathy.

Soon after receiving treatment for the encephalopathy, the man shows signs of an infectious condition known as spontaneous bacterial peritonitis. This disorder is defined as the presence of more than 500 white blood cells (WBCs)/mm^3, with more than 250 neutrophils/mm^3. The signs of spontaneous bacterial peritonitis can be subtle and include fever, abdominal pain, worsening encephalopathy, and serum leukocytosis. Typically the infection is monomicrobial, with *Escherichia coli* and *Streptococcus pneumoniae* accounting for the majority of cases. Empirical antibiotic coverage should include activity against these organisms, and intravenous cefotaxime would be an excellent choice. Aldosterone would clearly not be indicated. Ciprofloxacin, ampicillin, and penicillin would provide inadequate coverage. Imipenem is too broad and, more importantly, carries a significant risk of seizures in patients with altered mental status.

Patients who suffer from terminal disease such as end-stage liver disease should receive education about the natural course of their condition. Part of this education includes a discussion of end-of-life issues and whether cardiopulmonary resuscitation, if necessary, is desired. If patients are able to make rational decisions and understand the implications of their choices, the physician must respect their decisions. In this particular case, despite what the physician believes to be a futile medical situation, the patient desires that all resuscitation efforts be performed. Thus, the only appropriate decision would be to honor the patient's wishes and proceed with intubation and intensive care support.

127–129. The answers are: 127-C, 128-A, 129-D. (*Internal medicine*)
In the evaluation of a patient with early onset of hypertension, it is essential to consider secondary causes of the condition. The differential diagnosis includes renal parenchymal disease, renovascular disease, primary aldosteronism, hyperparathyroidism, coarctation of the aorta, pheochromocytoma, and Cushing syndrome. This patient may have Turner syndrome; her short stature and cubitus valgus are consistent with this condition. Other features of this 45,X disease are low hairline, shield chest, widely spaced nipples, and a webbed neck. Patients are infertile; despite frequent, unprotected sexual encounters, this patient is G$_0$P$_0$, which might raise the suspicion for infertility. Amenorrhea is also present. Cardiac abnormalities include bicuspid aortic valve

and coarctation of the aorta. None of the conditions named in question 127 are present, so coarctation of the aorta is the cause of this patient's hypertension.

A chest radiograph might show rib notching secondary to erosion by collateral vessels, as well as the "3 sign" in the paramediastinal shadow secondary to aortic indentation with prestenotic and poststenotic dilatation of the vessel. Urine metanephrines are useful in the diagnosis of pheochromocytoma, parathyroid hormone for hyperparathyroidism, and plasma renin activity–aldosterone level for primary aldosteronism.

The Sixth Report of the Joint National Committee on Detection, Evaluation and Treatment of High Blood Pressure (JNC VI) guidelines recommend thiazide diuretics and β-blockers as the first-line agents for hypertension. Thus, propranolol is the best choice of the agents in question 129 for the patient's essential hypertension.

130–132. The answers are: 130-D, 131-E, 132-D. (*Emergency medicine, internal medicine*)
Caustic injuries to the esophagus result in serious morbidity and mortality. The initial management of caustic injuries should include early endoscopy to evaluate the severity and extent of injury. Alkaline ingestion leads to liquefaction necrosis of the esophageal lining and severe injury. Early complications may include esophageal perforation and sepsis. The extent of injury to the oropharynx is not a useful indicator of the magnitude of esophageal injury. Neither induction of vomiting nor acid neutralization are appropriate because both of these measures exacerbate injury.

Several months after the injury, a complication of alkaline injury to the esophagus—esophageal strictures—becomes apparent. Strictures, which develop as fibrotic healing occurs, result in recurrent episodes of dysphagia and require endoscopic dilation procedures. Zenker diverticulum, an outpouching of the esophagus occurring just proximal to the cricopharyngeus muscle, leads to symptoms of dysphagia, regurgitation of food, choking, and halitosis. Barrett esophagus results from the replacement of the normal squamous epithelium with gastric epithelium. This premalignant lesion often occurs in the setting of severe gastroesophageal reflux disease.

Eventually, the patient develops esophageal cancer, another late-term complication of alkaline injury. Esophageal cancer is up to 500 times more common in the setting of a caustic injury. The patient's symptoms of severe, progressive dysphagia, and weight loss are classic of this condition. Esophageal leiomyomas are rare; given this patient's history, they would be unlikely, even though dysphagia is a presenting symptom. Gastric carcinoma would be unlikely to lead to dysphagia.

133. The answer is C. (*Internal medicine*)
Scabies, a highly contagious condition, generally affects persons with poor personal hygiene. The mite *Sarcoptes scabiei,* which causes the lesion, burrows into the skin, creating an inflammatory condition with very pruritic excoriations. Treatment includes investigating other close contacts of the patient, thorough bathing, and the use of permethrin cream or lindane (Kwell) lotion.

134. The answer is D. (*Internal medicine*)
The history and physical examination in this patient are most consistent with aortic stenosis. Affected patients may present with several clinical complaints, including chest pain, shortness of breath, syncope, and heart failure. Chest pain is often due to supply–demand mismatch secondary to increased left ventricular mass and wall tension. In fact, two thirds of patients experience angina, but only 50% have coronary artery disease. On examination, several findings are characteristic: a slow rising, low amplitude carotid pulse (pulsus parvus et tardus); a discrete, but sustained and laterally displaced, point of maximal impulse (secondary to left ventricular hypertrophy); a decreased intensity of A_2 (from valve calcification and reduced leaflet mobility); and a diamond-shaped crescendo–decrescendo murmur loudest at the upper left sternal border with radiation to the carotids. As the stenosis worsens, the murmur peaks later. The intensity of the murmur bears no relation to severity of the stenosis.

It is important to distinguish aortic stenosis from other systolic murmurs such as those from hypertrophic obstructive cardiomyopathy and mitral regurgitation. In the cardiomyopathy, the murmur increases during the strain phase of the Valsalva maneuver, whereas in aortic stenosis, the murmur does not change and changes little with handgripping. In mitral regurgitation, the carotid pulse is normal, the murmur is holosystolic with radiation to the axilla, and the murmur increases with handgripping.

135–137. The answers are: 135-D, 136-E, 137-B. (*Internal medicine*)
This woman likely has fulminant hepatic failure secondary to hepatitis E virus. Fulminant hepatic failure is defined as acute liver disease, occurring in the absence of preexisting liver disease leading to encephalopathy within 8 weeks of the onset of symptoms, *or* liver disease, leading to encephalopathy within 2 weeks of the onset of jaundice. The differential diagnoses include viral illness, toxins, drugs, metabolic diseases, and, occasionally, cardiovascular disease.

Acetaminophen overdose is the most common cause of fulminant hepatic failure in the United Kingdom, but acute viral hepatitis is the leading cause worldwide. The incidence of acetaminophen overdose is rising in the United States as well. Hepatitis E, which is endemic in India, Pakistan, and Mexico, is associated with an unusually high incidence of fulminant hepatic failure in the third trimester of pregnancy, with mortality approaching 40%. Hepatitis A causes fulminant hepatic failure in 0.35% of cases. Hepatitis B, which causes fulminant hepatic failure in 1% of cases, is the most common cause of fulminant hepatic failure worldwide and causes fulminant hepatic failure more often in the setting of coinfection or superinfection with hepatitis D. Hepatitis C is a rare cause of fulminant hepatic failure. Other causes include adenovirus; herpes simplex virus; human herpesvirus 6; cytomegalovirus; Epstein-Barr virus; methylenedioxymethamphetamine (the recreational drug, Ecstasy); *Amanita phalloides;* Wilson disease; Budd-Chiari syndrome; Reye syndrome; autoimmune hepatitis; and hemolysis, elevated liver enzymes, low platelet count (HELLP syndrome).

When evaluating hepatitis B serologies, it is important to recall that a positive hepatitis B surface antigen (HBsAg) for more than 6 months defines chronic infection. The "window" is that brief period (4 to 6 months after infection) when HBsAg has been cleared but hepatitis B surface antibody (HBsAb) is not yet detectable. If hepatitis B core antibody (HBcAb) is present, as in this case, actual virus has been "seen." Because HBcAb is the first antibody seen, it is the only marker of hepatitis B present in the window period. Alternatively, HBcAb is the only marker of hepatitis B in the setting of "old" infection when HBsAb has waned and HBcAb remains detectable. Hepatitis B e antigen (HBeAg) reflects viral replication (other than in a precore mutant that is void of HBeAg despite replication). Immunization is reflected by the presence of HBsAb only. Patients are still immune to hepatitis B as their HBsAb levels return when exposed to the virus.

138. The answer is C. (*Internal medicine, critical care medicine*)
This patient is suffering from septic shock, which is consistent with both her history (fever) and hemodynamic data. Hypotension is present, filling pressures are low (both right atrial and pulmonary capillary wedge pressure), cardiac output is increased, and vascular resistance is low. In cardiogenic shock, filling pressures are high, cardiac index is low, and vascular resistance is high. In hypovolemia, both filling pressures and cardiac index are low and vascular resistance is high. With papillary muscle rupture, pulmonary capillary wedge pressures are high, and cardiac output is low. In cardiac tamponade, there is equalization and elevation of all filling pressures, low cardiac output, and high vascular resistance.

139. The answer is B. (*Internal medicine*)
Postmenopausal bleeding is always abnormal and should prompt concerns of malignancy. Endometrial carcinoma is the most common cancerous cause; cervical cancer may also lead to postmenopausal bleeding; however, uterine fibroids are the most common cause of such bleeding. Other causes include atrophic vaginitis and polyps. The workup should include a detailed history focusing on risk factors for malignancy (e.g., unopposed estrogen use), careful physical examination, and appropriate laboratory testing (complete blood count [CBC],

coagulation profile). A pelvic ultrasound and endometrial biopsy should be performed to assess for endometrial malignancy.

140. The answer is D. (*Internal medicine*)
Lifestyle modifications can significantly decrease blood pressure. These include limiting alcohol intake, maintaining an active lifestyle, remaining at or near ideal body weight, and watching dietary sodium intake. High alcohol intake is strongly associated with hypertension, and up to 10% of all cases of hypertension are attributable to the use of alcohol. Aerobic exercise and limiting the amount of fat in the diet are useful measures, but in this patient, limiting alcohol intake would have a larger overall effect on blood pressure. Decreasing the amount of potassium in the diet might actually lower blood pressure.

141–142. The answers are: 141-B, 142-B. (*Surgery, internal medicine*)
This patient, who has diabetes mellitus, is at particular risk of osteomyelitis secondary to poor vascular flow, neuropathy, and immunodeficiency. In most cases, the diagnosis is missed for two reasons: (1) ulcers do not contain exposed bone, and (2) no evidence of inflammation is present on physical examination. Probing for bone, a simple test that may be performed at the bedside, allows immediate diagnosis with good accuracy in patients with diabetes. In one series, the presence of bone palpation by probe had an 89% positive predictive value; however, the prevalence of osteomyelitis was 61% by bone biopsy. Size is also useful in the diagnosis of ulcers in diabetics. Ulcers that are greater than 2 cm^2 in area are likely to be a sign of osteomyelitis.

Magnetic resonance imaging (MRI) is the imaging study of choice for osteomyelitis in this population, with a sensitivity of approximately 95%. However, MRI can lead to false-positive results in the setting of bone infarct, fracture, or healed osteomyelitis. Thus, specificity of MRI in the diagnosis of osteomyelitis is not nearly 100%. In one series, plain films, bone scan, and indium scan had sensitivities in the 50% to 70% range.

The erythrocyte sedimentation rate (ESR) may be increased in osteomyelitis. If it is high initially, it can be followed to assess treatment and recurrence. Hematogenous osteomyelitis accounts for 20% of cases. *Staphylococcus* species are the most common isolate, while *Pseudomonas* and *Peptostreptococcus* are the most common gram-negative rods and anaerobes, respectively. Blood cultures are positive in 50% of acute osteomyelitis cases. If radiologic studies are positive as well, it obviates the need for a bone biopsy. In children, the long bones of the femur, tibia, and humerus are most commonly involved. Adults more commonly have involvement of the vertebrae, sternum, clavicle, and sacroiliac bones.

143–145. The answers are: 143-C, 144-E, 145-E. (*Emergency department, internal medicine*)
Atrial fibrillation, a common condition affecting more than 1 million patients in the United States, carries an increased risk of stroke and decreased functional capacity (5 to 7 times). Acute treatment of atrial fibrillation may include either rate control or cardioversion. Drugs such as metoprolol, verapamil, digoxin, or diltiazem may result in rate control, with a goal of ventricular response between 60 to 90 beats/minute. If documentation indicates that the atrial fibrillation has been present for less than 2 days, attempts at either electrical or chemical cardioversion are warranted. Cardioversion is initially attempted at 100 joules, then 200 to 360 joules. Class IA, IC, or III agents are preferred for chemical cardioversion.

Many conditions are commonly associated with the development of atrial fibrillation, including mitral valve disease (especially from rheumatic disease), hypertension, ischemic heart disease, thyrotoxicosis, pulmonary embolism, chronic lung disease, heart failure, electrolyte abnormalities, alcohol binging, and pericarditis. At a minimum, it is important to check thyroid function tests and serum electrolytes in all at-risk patients.

Anticoagulation with warfarin is essential in patients with persistent atrial fibrillation to decrease the risk of embolic stroke (international normalized ratio [INR] of 2.0 to 3.0). Cardioversion can be attempted after at least 3 weeks of adequate anticoagulation. Rate control with atrioventricular nodal blocking agents and, for some patients, treatment with an antiarrhythmic agent are other important options.

146. The answer is A. (*Internal medicine*)

In all likelihood, this patient is suffering from a viral infection. She has no worrisome comorbidities, and observation is safe. Antibiotics are not warranted. The overprescribing of antibiotics for nonindicated conditions is one of the primary reasons for the emergence of antibiotic-resistant bacteria. Symptomatic therapy with dextromethorphan for cough suppression is safe.

147. The answer is A. (*Internal medicine*)

This patient presents with malignant melanoma. The incidence of this condition has increased greatly in the past decade and may relate to increases in recreational sun exposure in early life. The most important prognostic factor involves the stage at presentation. Depth of invasion (i.e., thickness) is the single most important prognostic factor in all existing staging systems. For patients with lesions less than 0.7 mm in depth, overall survival is 96%. In contrast, with lesions greater than 4.0 mm in depth, survival is only 47%.

148–149. The answers are: 148-C, 149-E. (*Pediatrics*)

The number of red blood cells (RBCs) in the urine that defines an abnormality is controversial. Most studies support the finding that three or more RBCs per high-power field is significant for microscopic hematuria. Most significant lesions that cause microscopic hematuria, including bladder cancer, renal stones, and renal cell cancer, occur in patients older than 50 years. The likelihood of finding a significant lesion is less than 1% in an asymptomatic patient who is younger than 50 years, who has no known risk factors, and who has a normal physical examination and basic laboratory tests. To rule out a significant stone or a glomerulonephritis, only radiographic examination of the kidneys, ureters, and bladder and measurement of a serum creatinine is necessary. If the radiographic examination is positive, an intravenous pyelogram, which is useful for finding upper genitourinary tract lesions, is appropriate. If the radiographic examination is negative, follow-up is reasonable. Cystoscopy is the gold standard for detecting lesions of the lower urinary tract.

In a Caucasian adolescent (younger than 18), motor vehicle accidents are the leading cause of mortality, followed by homicides and suicides. In an African American individual of the same age, homicide is a more significant cause of mortality. The *Morbidity and Mortality Weekly Report* should be consulted for the most current statistics.

150. The answer is C. (*Obstetrics/gynecology, internal medicine*)

Oral contraception, using a combination of synthetic estrogen and progestin, is a highly effective technique of birth control. The combination pill appears to prevent the cyclic release of follicle-stimulating hormone (FSH) and luteinizing hormone (LH), which are critical for follicle maturation and ovulation. Other effects of oral contraception include alterations of the cervical mucus and endometrial lining. It is important to be familiar with the adverse effects that may accompany the use of oral contraceptives. The major hazards of oral contraception are related to the increased risk of thromboembolism (4 to 11 times higher). This risk is greater for smokers and for women older than 35 years. Any history of thromboembolic disorders is considered an absolute contraindication to the use of oral contraception. Other absolute contraindications include impaired liver function from any cause, known or suspected estrogen-dependent neoplasm (such as breast or endometrial cancer), undiagnosed vaginal bleeding and known or suspected pregnancy. Relative contraindications to the use of oral contraception include migraine headaches, hypertension, hyperlipidemia, epilepsy, uterine fibroids, tobacco use, diabetes mellitus, age older than 35 years, and patient unreliability.

Test III

QUESTIONS

DIRECTIONS: For each question, select the letter corresponding to the best answer. All questions have only one correct answer.

Setting: Hospital

Questions 1–4

A 42-year-old man is referred to you for evaluation of hypertension. He has been previously healthy, but for the past few months he has suffered from severe headaches and facial flushing. On numerous occasions, he has had blood pressures of 190/100 mm Hg. In addition, the patient notes that he has lost 8 pounds in the past month and has experienced palpitations and diaphoresis. Currently, he is not taking medications. His family history is notable for a history of thyroid cancer and death of his father from stroke. Physical examination reveals a flushed-appearing man with a fine tremor of his hands. His blood pressure in both upper extremities is 180/100 mm Hg, and his heart rate is 120 beats/minute. The rest of the examination is within normal limits.

1. The next most appropriate step in the diagnostic workup is

(A) imaging the thyroid
(B) imaging the adrenal glands
(C) urinary catecholamines
(D) serum electrolytes
(E) parathyroid hormone level

2. A diagnosis is made, and the man is referred for surgery. Which of the following preoperative preparations is critical to ensure a safe operation?

(A) Cardiac stress test
(B) Phenoxybenzamine hydrochloride followed by propranolol hydrochloride
(C) Propranolol alone
(D) Diuresis with furosemide
(E) Computed tomography (CT) of the brain

3. The man is concerned that his condition is malignant, and he asks you to estimate the probability. You tell him that the probability of malignancy in his situation is approximately

(A) 5%
(B) 10%
(C) 20%
(D) 30%
(E) 40%

4. The surgery proceeds uneventfully. The man's blood pressure improves, and his symptoms essentially disappear. However, you are concerned about his family history and ask him to continue to see you. Which of the following laboratory studies would you use for follow-up of this patient?

(A) Serum sodium
(B) Serum calcium
(C) Thyroid-stimulating hormone (TSH)
(D) Serum cortisol
(E) Urinary protein

Setting: Office

Questions 5–9

A 47-year-old Caucasian man complains of weight gain. In the past month he has noticed difficulty buttoning his pants. He works as an accountant for an automotive company that manufactures brake systems. His social history is significant for 20 pack-years of tobacco abuse; he does not use alcohol. He is married with two healthy children. His family history is notable for an uncle who died of liver disease and an aunt who had breast cancer at 48 years of age.

5. Which of the following tests is most necessary at this time?

(A) Chest radiograph
(B) Electrocardiogram (ECG)
(C) Complete blood count (CBC)
(D) Liver function tests
(E) Echocardiogram

6. On abdominal examination, the man has shifting dullness. Paracentesis reveals:

Total protein	2.0 mg/dL
Albumin	2.3 mg/dL
Cell count	230/mm^3
Serum albumin	3.8 mg/dL
Peripheral white blood cell (WBC) count	8.1/mm^3

Which of the following diagnoses is least likely?

(A) Hepatitis C
(B) Budd-Chiari syndrome
(C) Veno-occlusive disease
(D) Portal vein thrombosis
(E) Peritoneal carcinomatosis

7. Which of the following studies is most likely to yield the correct diagnosis?

(A) Antimitochondrial antibodies
(B) Hepatic iron index
(C) Ceruloplasmin
(D) HFE (hemochromatosis) gene studies
(E) Anti–smooth muscle antibody

8. Which of the following statements about this man's disease is true?

(A) It is more common in African Americans
(B) For tobacco users, it poses an increased risk of mesothelioma
(C) For tobacco users, it poses an increased risk of squamous cell carcinoma
(D) It is associated with an increased risk for hepatocellular carcinoma
(E) An ophthalmologic examination may often provide a diagnosis

9. A new genetic test is developed to help diagnose this man's disorder. In a given patient population, the disease prevalence is 50%. The test has a sensitivity of 80% and specificity of 90%. Which of the following statements about this test is true?

(A) If the man is free of the disease, the test is negative with 90% certainty
(B) It is more useful as a screening test than as a confirmatory test
(C) If the man has the disease, he will have a positive test 90% of the time
(D) If the man has a negative test, he has a 20% chance of having the disease
(E) The negative predictive value of the test is 90%

Setting: Office

10. An 80-year-old woman presents with a 2-week history of severe temporal headache, bilateral jaw pain with chewing, malaise, low-grade fever, and proximal limb pain. You immediately believe that you know the diagnosis. Which of the following conditions is a complication of this disease?

(A) Paralysis
(B) Myocardial infarction (MI)
(C) Pulmonary embolism
(D) Blindness
(E) Seizures

Setting: Office

Questions 11–12

A 37-year-old woman has missed her past three menstrual cycles. Previously, her menses were regular. She denies being sexually active and has noted no vaginal spotting during this time. Review of symptoms is notable for occasional headaches and a decreased energy level for the past several months. She has no history of visual changes, no weight loss, no abnormal hair growth, and no galactorrhea. She has never been pregnant. She has no medical history and takes no medications. Family history is significant for premature coronary artery disease in her father (myocardial infarction [MI] at 47 years of age). Physical examination, including pelvic examination, is within normal limits. She receives a prescription for medroxyprogesterone acetate 10 mg, with instructions to take one tablet per day for the next 5 days.

11. The onset of withdrawal bleeding after progestin administration indicates which of the following conditions?

(A) High likelihood of ovarian failure
(B) Presence of occult prolactinoma
(C) Problem with luteinizing hormone (LH) release from the pituitary
(D) Presence of uterine disease
(E) High probability of hypothyroidism

12. The woman experiences no menstrual bleeding in response to the medroxyprogesterone. Which of the following laboratory profiles is consistent with primary ovarian failure?

	Follicle-stimulating Hormone (FSH)	Estradiol	Prolactin
(A)	High	High	Normal
(B)	High	Normal	High
(C)	Low	Low	Normal
(D)	High	Low	High
(E)	High	Low	Normal

Setting: Office

Questions 13–15

A 31-year-old woman with HIV complains of fever since her last visit 6 weeks ago. During the same time, she has had persistent diarrhea. Laboratory studies reveal:

Aspartate amino-transferase (AST)	43 U/L
Alanine amino-transferase (ALT)	40 U/L
Albumin	3.1 g/dL
Alkaline phosphatase	228 U/L
Total bilirubin	1.4 g/dL

13. Her CD4 count (cells/mm^3) is likely to be

(A) <50
(B) 50 to 100
(C) 100 to 150
(D) 150 to 200
(E) >200

14. The most likely cause of her symptoms is

(A) *Cryptosporidium*
(B) *Microsporidium*
(C) *Mycobacterium avium-intracellulare* complex (MAC)
(D) *Isospora belli*
(E) *Giardia lamblia*

15. The most appropriate treatment is

(A) ethambutol hydrochloride and clarithromycin
(B) metronidazole
(C) amphotericin B
(D) ganciclovir
(E) isoniazid and rifampin

Setting: Office

16. An 80-year-old woman complains of fatigue and shortness of breath. Workup reveals:

Hematocrit	22%
Mean corpuscular volume	85 fL
White blood cell (WBC) count	5,000/mm^3
Blood urea nitrogen (BUN)	60 mg/dL
Creatinine	4.1 mg/dL

However, urinary dipstick for protein is negative, with a total urine protein of 2.5 g/24 hours. Which of the following conditions is the likely diagnosis?

(A) Hemolysis
(B) Adrenal insufficiency
(C) Anemia of chronic disease
(D) Multiple myeloma
(E) Anemia of chronic renal disease

Setting: Emergency Department

17. A 32-year-old woman presents with general tonic-clonic seizures, and she requires diazepam and intubation before the seizures are controlled. History reveals that the patient has schizophrenia. In addition, she has been drinking water excessively and has been vomiting for the past 2 days. Laboratory work reveals serum sodium of 110 mEq/L. An infusion of 3% saline is initiated. Two hours later, the serum sodium is 130 mEq/L. Four hours later, the serum sodium is 142 mEq/L. The woman is still on a ventilator 3 days later and, despite no sedation, shows no upper or lower extremity movement to noxious stimuli. Attempts at weaning her from the ventilator are unsuccessful. Which of the following conditions is the likely cause of the woman's deterioration?

(A) Hypocalcemia
(B) Hypermagnesemia
(C) Central pontine myelinolysis
(D) Unrecognized drug intoxication
(E) Hypernatremia

Setting: Office

Questions 18–19

A 25-year-old man, employed as a truck driver, presents with a tender right groin mass. The mass, which has been present intermittently for 1 month, is worse after the man completes a day of work. He notes that the mass is usually not present in the morning. He has no significant medical history and takes no medications. On physical examination, a palpable mass is evident on insertion of the index finger into the scrotal region. The mass is tender and soft. When you ask the patient to bear down in a Valsalva maneuver, the mass becomes more prominent.

18. The mass passes through which of the following anatomical regions?

(A) Deep inguinal ring
(B) Obturator canal
(C) Femoral canal
(D) Superficial inguinal ring
(E) Hesselbach triangle

19. The man undergoes repair of the hernia (Lichtenstein procedure with placement of synthetic mesh) and presents 12 days later with severe pain over the incision site. The wound site is erythematous, with purulent drainage, and a soft, easily reducible tissue mass is present. Which of the following measures should be performed next?

(A) Wound exploration, removal of mesh, and repair with new mesh
(B) Admission with intravenous antibiotics
(C) Wound exploration, removal of mesh, and hernia repair with a different technique
(D) Discharge with dressing changes
(E) Insertion of a percutaneous drain, antibiotics, and close follow-up

Setting: Office

20. A 58-year-old woman with diabetes mellitus presents with shoulder pain. On examination, she has decreased range of motion in flexion, extension, and abduction. Which of the following conditions is the most likely cause of her problem?

(A) Rotator cuff tear
(B) Impingement syndrome
(C) Adhesive capsulitis
(D) Glenohumeral arthritis
(E) Subacromial bursitis

Setting: Satellite Clinic

Questions 21–23

A 31-year-old woman presents to your clinic with concerns regarding hair growth. Within the past 6 months she has noticed increased hair on her chin and abdomen that is darker in color. On examination, she is normotensive, has a normal body habitus, and has dark, coarse hair on her chin and abdomen.

21. Which of the following measures is the most appropriate next step?

(A) Luteinizing hormone (LH) and follicle-stimulating hormone (FSH) levels
(B) Bimanual examination of the pelvis
(C) Dehydroepiandrosterone sulfate (DHEAS) levels
(D) Urine free cortisol
(E) Testosterone

22. A battery of tests yields:

LH/FSH	1.9
DHEAS	500 mg/dL (normal, <700 mg/dL)
Testosterone	6.5 ng/mL (normal, <2.0 ng/mL)
Urine free cortisol	75 μg/24 hours (normal, <100 μg/24 hours)

Which of the following procedures is the most appropriate next step?

(A) Computed tomography (CT) of the abdomen
(B) Transvaginal ultrasound
(C) Magnetic resonance imaging (MRI) of the brain
(D) High-dose dexamethasone suppression test
(E) Low-dose dexamethasone suppression test

23. Which of the following substances directly inhibits the conversion of testosterone to dihydrotestosterone?

(A) Leuprolide acetate
(B) Flutamide
(C) Cyproterone
(D) Finasteride
(E) Spironolactone

Setting: Satellite Clinic

24. A 56-year-old woman presents with a 2-month history of intermittent vaginal bleeding. She has been spotting nearly every day for 1 week. Postmenopausal for 7 years, she has been taking estrogen replacement therapy secondary to severe hot flashes. She has no significant medical history and takes no other medications. She has been pregnant twice with normal vaginal deliveries. Review of symptoms is otherwise negative. Family history is significant for a mother who died with colon cancer at 85 years of age. Physical examination is within normal limits. Pelvic examination reveals external genitalia, vagina, and cervix appearing normal, without visible bleeding. Bimanual examination is within normal limits. The next step in the care of this patient should involve which of the following measures?

(A) Trial of progestin
(B) Reassurance
(C) Referral for endometrial biopsy
(D) Pelvic ultrasound
(E) CA-125 level

Setting: Satellite Clinic

25. A 23-year-old woman returns to see you because of recurrent vaginal yeast infections. Her first yeast infection was 6 months ago, and intravaginal treatment with clotrimazole was successful. After a second yeast infection 2 months later, she again received clotrimazole; however, she required a second course of treatment with oral fluconazole to eradicate the infection. She now returns with complaints of vaginal burning, pruritus, and a white, vaginal discharge. Except for the yeast infections, her medical history is significant only for genital herpes. She denies taking any medications. Review of symptoms is only notable for mild, generalized fatigue and dysuria. On examination, a thick, white, vaginal discharge is present, which shows hyphae and budding yeast forms on slide examination with potassium hydroxide. Which of the following conditions could explain her recurrent yeast infections?

(A) Sarcoidosis
(B) Systemic lupus erythematosus (SLE)
(C) Diabetes mellitus
(D) Herpes simplex virus infection
(E) Cervical dysplasia

Setting: Emergency Department

Questions 26–29

A 74-year-old man complains of right-sided knee pain. When he awoke 6 hours ago, he noticed the knee pain, which has since worsened. He has felt warm but has not taken his temperature, and he has had diarrhea all morning. He has a history of diabetes mellitus, hypertension, and osteoarthritis involving his knees bilaterally, and his medications include propranolol and hydrochlorothiazide. On review of symptoms, he has a history of a painful toe on two occasions that resolved in several weeks with ibuprofen. On examination, his temperature is 39°C, and he has a 2/6 systolic murmur loudest at the upper sternal border. His right knee is erythematous and warm; no other joints are involved. He experiences pain to both passive and active motion of the right knee.

26. Which of the following measures is the next most appropriate test?

(A) Complete blood count (CBC)
(B) Echocardiogram
(C) Joint aspiration
(D) Knee radiograph
(E) Magnetic resonance imaging (MRI)

27. Radiographs find evidence of a joint effusion and osteoarthritis. Complete blood count (CBC) and joint aspirate reveal:

CBC

White blood cell (WBC) count	2,900/mm^3
Hemoglobin	10.5 g/dL
Hematocrit	32%
Platelet count	175,000/mm^3

Joint Aspirate

WBC count	65,000/mm^3, with 76% segs
Gram's stain	Pending
Cultures	Pending

Which of the following conditions is the most likely cause of the pain?

(A) Gout
(B) Pseudogout
(C) Bacterial infection
(D) Reiter syndrome
(E) Rheumatoid arthritis

28. Which of the following organisms is the most common pathogen involved in native joint infectious arthritis?

(A) *Escherichia coli*
(B) *Neisseria gonorrhoeae*
(C) *Staphylococcus epidermidis*
(D) *Staphylococcus aureus*
(E) *Mycobacterium tuberculosis*

29. Which of the following agents is the most appropriate treatment?

(A) Colchicine
(B) Allopurinol
(C) Antibiotics
(D) Prednisone
(E) Naproxen

Setting: Emergency Department

30. A 40-year-old woman with severe asthma and depression, who lives alone, is found unresponsive at home. Her neighbors have noticed that she has been increasingly depressed, and they saw her throwing away medications several days ago. One month ago, she received treatment in the medical ICU for a severe asthma exacerbation. No further history is available. The rescue squad finds no evidence of toxic ingestion at the scene. On arrival at the emergency department (ED), the woman is unresponsive, with normal respirations and a blood pressure of 60 mm Hg/palpable. Cardiac, pulmonary, and abdominal examinations are within normal limits. She is emergently intubated; intravenous sodium chloride and dextrose do not improve her blood pressure. Which of the following interventions is indicated next?

(A) Emergent chest radiograph for pneumothorax
(B) Trial of intravenous naloxone
(C) Intravenous dexamethasone
(D) Emergent head CT for intracerebral hemorrhage
(E) Broad-spectrum antibiotic therapy

Setting: Emergency Department

31. A 78-year-old man with long-standing, poorly controlled, hypertension presents with the acute onset of a tearing-like, severe pain in his chest that radiates to his back. His blood pressure is 210/105 mm Hg, and he is writhing in bed. An electrocardiogram (ECG) is notable for sinus tachycardia, left ventricular hypertrophy, and nonspecific ST-segment and T-wave changes. A chest radiograph shows possible mediastinal widening. Which of the following medications is indicated?

(A) Thrombolytics
(B) Heparin
(C) Aspirin
(D) Labetalol hydrochloride
(E) Sodium nitroprusside

Setting: Office

Questions 32–33

A study is performed concerning the relationship of blood transfusions and the risk of developing hepatitis C. A group of patients is studied for 3 years, and the following results are obtained.

	Transfusion	Hepatitis C
YES	595	75
NO	712	16

32. This project represents which of the following types of studies?

(A) Cohort study
(B) Case-control study
(C) Randomized study
(D) Retrospective study
(E) Randomized prospective study

33. What is the relative risk of developing hepatitis C if an individual receives a blood transfusion?

(A) 3.2
(B) 4.0
(C) 5.7
(D) 7.5
(E) 10.5

Setting: Office

Questions 34–35

A 32-year-old man is referred to you as part of an infertility workup. You order a semen analysis.

34. Which of the following findings is consistent with obstruction of the seminal vesicles?

(A) High follicle-stimulating hormone (FSH) levels
(B) Low FSH levels
(C) High fructose levels
(D) Low fructose levels
(E) High prolactin levels

35. Semen analysis reveals significantly decreased sperm numbers with normal motility. Further workup shows low luteinizing hormone (LH), low FSH, and low testosterone levels. Which of the following is most likely to cause this man's oligospermia?

(A) Genetic abnormality
(B) Diabetes mellitus
(C) Alcoholism
(D) Prolactinoma
(E) Hypothyroidism

Setting: Office

Questions 36–39

A 55-year-old man is referred to you for further evaluation of a heart murmur that was discovered on a physical examination for insurance. The patient denies any complaints except for occasional back pain, which has plagued him for 20 years. His medical history is notable for a cholecystectomy and appendectomy. He takes one aspirin a day. He does not smoke tobacco and does not drink alcohol. His family history is significant for diabetes mellitus, hypertension, and colon cancer.

On physical examination, the man's blood pressure is 110/60 mm Hg, and his heart rate is 65 beats/minute. Cardiac examination reveals a normal point of maximal impulse; regular rate and rhythm; and a harsh 3/6 systolic murmur that peaks in early systole, which is best heard over the second right intercostal space. The murmur radiates to the carotid region in the neck. The rest of the physical examination is within normal limits.

36. Which of the following diagnoses is consistent with this heart murmur?

(A) Aortic regurgitation
(B) Mitral regurgitation
(C) Mitral stenosis
(D) Aortic stenosis
(E) Tricuspid regurgitation

37. Which of the following physical examination findings correlates with a severe lesion?

(A) Early peaking of the murmur in systole
(B) Late peaking of the murmur in systole
(C) Rapid carotid upstrokes
(D) Louder murmur
(E) An early systolic ejection click

38. If an ECG is obtained, which of the following findings may be evident?

(A) Supraventricular tachycardia
(B) Inferior Q waves
(C) Anterior Q waves
(D) R or S wave in limb lead >20 mm
(E) Right axis deviation

39. The patient expresses concern about this new diagnosis and is unsure of what to expect in the future. Which of the following responses is appropriate?

(A) Don't worry, be happy—this is an innocent murmur
(B) You need careful, long-term follow-up, and surgery may be a possibility in the future
(C) Your children should be screened for heart disease
(D) You do not require antibiotic prophylaxis for invasive procedures
(E) You need a cardiac catheterization to obtain any prognostic information

Setting: Emergency Department

Questions 40–42

A 10-year-old girl presents with a rash. Her mother reports that she has abdominal pain, joint complaints, and a purpuric, nonblanching rash on her lower extremities. The rash is tender to touch. The girl has not been taking any medications and has not been playing outside in the woods.

40. A skin biopsy is most likely to find

(A) panniculitis
(B) leukocytoclastic vasculitis
(C) eosinophilic infiltration
(D) subepithelial humps
(E) loss of dermal–epidermal junction

41. Which of the following findings might also be expected?

(A) Increased alanine aminotransferase (ALT)

(B) High serum bicarbonate

(C) Increased creatinine

(D) Low hematocrit

(E) Low erythrocyte sedimentation rate (ESR)

42. The most appropriate therapy is likely to be

(A) observation

(B) plasmapheresis

(C) corticosteroids

(D) intravenous immunoglobulin

(E) recombinant anti–tumor necrosis factor-α

Setting: Emergency Department

Questions 43–45

A 5-year-old girl is stung by a hornet while playing outside. Shortly afterward, she complains of severe pain at the site of the insect bite. She then becomes acutely short of breath, and bystanders notice that she is wheezing. The paramedics arrive on the scene within 10 minutes. On their arrival, she is in acute respiratory distress and audibly wheezing. Her blood pressure is 70/40 mm Hg, and her heart rate is 140 beats/minute. Wheezes are bilateral, and the insect bite on her left leg is erythematous and swollen.

43. Which of the following medications is indicated as a first-line therapy?

(A) Diphenhydramine 5 mg/kg for 24 hours

(B) Hydrocortisone 5 mg/kg every 6 hours

(C) Epinephrine 1:1,000 dilution (0.01 mL/kg subcutaneously)

(D) Epinephrine 1:10,000 dilution (1 mg intravenously)

(E) Cimetidine 5 mg/kg every 6 hours

44. After the initial treatment, the girl stabilizes. She is awake, alert, and interactive at the scene. Her parents ask if she needs to be transported to the hospital. Your response should be

(A) she may stay at home as long as her parents are with her

(B) she should be seen at her pediatrician's office the next morning to begin allergen therapy

(C) she may stay at home, but she needs an emergency kit for treatment if this happens again

(D) she should be monitored at an ED

(E) she may resume normal activities

45. All of the following medications may play a role in the treatment of this condition EXCEPT

(A) albuterol nebulizer treatments

(B) histamine (H_2)-receptor antagonists

(C) corticosteroids

(D) intravenous normal saline

(E) antivenin

Setting: Office

Questions 46–48

You are an intern at a "morning report" conference listening to a patient presentation. A 64-year-old woman presented with fever, headache, and jaw claudication. The erythrocyte sedimentation rate (ESR) was 105 mm/hour. A 3-cm temporal artery biopsy was negative for granulomatous changes.

46. Which of the following measures is the most appropriate next step in such a case?

(A) Ibuprofen

(B) Repeat biopsy

(C) Prednisone

(D) Referral to ophthalmology

(E) Observation

47. Which of the following proteins most contributes to an elevated ESR?

(A) Fibrinogen
(B) Ferritin
(C) Ceruloplasmin
(D) Transferrin
(E) Albumin

48. Which of the following conditions does NOT elevate the ESR?

(A) Myeloma
(B) Macrocytosis
(C) Age
(D) Waldenström macroglobulinemia
(E) Hyperalbuminemia

Setting: Emergency Department

Questions 49–51

A 3-year-old boy is brought in by his parents with a 2-day history of abdominal cramps and diarrhea twice a day. His parents state that he is always irritable and "bad." The boy has no previous medical problems, but he does not have a regular pediatrician. On physical examination, the child appears withdrawn, and you notice several bruises on his upper arms. His abdominal examination is benign and reveals normal bowel sounds. You are concerned about the bruises and ask the father how the child obtained them. He reports that his son fell off a swing yesterday when he was playing.

49. Which of the following statements concerning the bruises most likely supports the father's description of how they were obtained?

(A) They are red with some purple discoloration
(B) They are blue to blue-brown
(C) They are green
(D) They are yellow
(E) They are associated with skin lacerations

50. You are concerned about possible child abuse. Which of the following laboratory studies is NOT appropriate?

(A) Prothrombin time (PT) and partial thromboplastin time (PTT)
(B) Complete blood count (CBC)
(C) Bleeding time
(D) Long bone radiographs
(E) Urinalysis

51. After an appropriate workup, your suspicion of abuse still exists. Which of the following measures is the next appropriate step?

(A) Discharge the boy and notify the police
(B) Report your concerns to protective services and a social worker
(C) Admit the boy to the hospital
(D) Ask the wife privately if she believes the husband is harming their son
(E) Ask a visiting nurse to check on the boy in the next few days

Setting: Office

Questions 52–54

A 64-year-old woman returns to the clinic after the finding of an adenoma in the sigmoid colon on screening colonoscopy. Her family history is significant for colon cancer.

52. Which of the following characteristics of an adenoma is least worrisome for malignancy?

(A) Tubular
(B) Villous
(C) Tubulovillous
(D) Sessile
(E) 3-cm diameter

53. Pathology studies find that the mass is a villous adenoma. You recommend

(A) repeat colonoscopy in 3 years
(B) polypectomy
(C) segmental resection
(D) cauterization
(E) annual colonoscopic observation

54. Polyps are NOT premalignant in which of the following syndromes?

(A) Gardner syndrome
(B) Cronkhite-Canada syndrome
(C) Cowden syndrome
(D) Familial polyposis syndrome
(E) Peutz-Jeghers syndrome

Setting: Office

Questions 55–57

A 51-year-old construction worker presents with concerns regarding facial flushing. He has had the condition for years, particularly with the consumption of alcohol. He presents now because of worsening flushing with skin changes on his nose. He has smoked one-half pack of cigarettes per day for the past 30 years. He takes lisinopril 10 mg/day for hypertension. On examination, the man's skin is very tan, secondary to occupational sun exposure. The skin overlying his nose is reddened and papular, with a waxy appearance.

55. Which of the following conditions is the likely cause of his disorder?

(A) Alcohol abuse
(B) Tobacco abuse
(C) Sun exposure
(D) Neoplasia
(E) Unknown factors

56. Which of the following therapies do you recommend?

(A) Oral tetracycline
(B) Skin biopsy
(C) Fluorinated topical steroids
(D) Topical metronidazole
(E) Trimethoprim-sulfamethoxazole

57. Which of the following conditions is NOT associated with this disorder?

(A) Blepharitis
(B) Cataracts
(C) Iritis
(D) Keratitis
(E) Recurrent chalazia

Setting: Satellite Clinic

Questions 58–63

A 21-year-old man who has had no previous medical problems is brought to your office for evaluation of unusual behavior. His family reports that during the past 2 months he has begun to "talk to people that are not there." He also has come to believe that his radio is broadcasting messages to him every night at 8:00 PM. The family has also noted that he has become more reclusive. The man had worked as a clerk in a department store but was recently fired after he argued with a customer. Apparently, he believed the customer was trying to get him to "do bad things." The man is not taking any medications. He lives at home with his parents.

58. Which of the following conditions should NOT be considered in the differential diagnosis of this man's behavioral change?

(A) Schizophrenia
(B) Psychosis associated with phencyclidine use
(C) Bipolar disorder
(D) Anxiety disorders
(E) Psychosis associated with hallucinogen use (lysergic acid diethylamide [LSD])

59. Which of the following historic features most supports the diagnosis of schizophrenia?

(A) Family history of mood disorders
(B) Intermittent nature of delusional symptoms
(C) Memory impairment
(D) Disorientation
(E) Disorganized speech, such as frequent derailment of ideas

60. Which of the following statements regarding the natural history of schizophrenia is true?

(A) Onset generally occurs in the fourth decade
(B) Prodromal symptoms are unusual
(C) Most people with schizophrenia are dangerous to others
(D) Each recurrence of illness leads to increased impairment in functioning
(E) Prognosis is poor in those with sudden onset of symptoms

61. The man receives neuroleptic medication to control his symptoms. Which of the following statements regarding neuroleptics is true?

(A) A trial of at least 8 to 12 weeks is necessary before an agent can be pronounced ineffective
(B) Tardive dyskinesia is reversible after stopping the agent
(C) Elevation of serum prolactin is common in patients being treated with typical neuroleptics
(D) After control of a patient's symptoms, the dosage can be decreased immediately
(E) Anticholinergic drugs improve tardive dyskinesia

62. The man's symptoms are well controlled with haloperidol. One afternoon, his parents find him lying on his bed unable to move and with unintelligible speech. The rescue squad finds that the patient's vital signs are: temperature, 41°C; blood pressure, 160/95 mm Hg; heart rate, 110 beats/minute; and respirations, 40/minute. The patient is unable to provide any history. On physical examination, his extremities show significantly increased tone. He is transported to the hospital. Which of the following laboratory values is most consistent with the diagnosis you are considering?

(A) Serum sodium: 120 mEq/L
(B) Arterial pH: 7.01
(C) Creatinine kinase: 6,000 IU
(D) Serum calcium: 6.0 mg/dL
(E) Thyroid-stimulating hormone (TSH): undetectable

63. Which of the following medications would you use to treat this man's condition?

(A) Intravenous esmolol hydrochloride
(B) Dantrolene sodium
(C) Ibuprofen
(D) Clozapine
(E) Ceftriaxone sodium, pending lumbar puncture results

Setting: Office

Questions 64–66

A 6-month-old boy is brought to the office for a routine examination. You find an undescended testis on the right side. The testis is palpable in the inguinal canal.

64. The recommended therapy is

(A) gonadotropic-releasing hormone administration
(B) testosterone injection
(C) observation
(D) orchiopexy
(E) dihydrotestosterone

65. This disease is associated with all of the following conditions EXCEPT

(A) malignancy
(B) hernias
(C) torsion
(D) infertility
(E) epididymitis

66. Which of the following statements about this disease is NOT true?

(A) Seminoma is the most commonly associated malignancy
(B) Orchiopexy can decrease the risk of cancer if it is performed early
(C) Malignancy is more common in a unilateral undescended testis
(D) The peak age for development of malignancy is 15 to 45 years
(E) The percentage of seminomatous malignancies diminish after orchiopexy

Setting: Office

Questions 67–68

A 26-year-old woman returns to your clinic 12 months after splenectomy for idiopathic thrombocytopenic purpura. Her platelet count after surgery was 270,000/mm³; today, it is 40,000/mm³. A peripheral smear finds normal red blood cell (RBC) morphology with no RBC inclusions.

67. The next step in the management of this case is

(A) plasmapheresis
(B) steroids
(C) intravenous immunoglobulins
(D) radionuclide spleen scan
(E) platelet transfusion

68. Which of the following organisms is NOT associated with increased mortality after splenectomy?

(A) *Pneumococcus*
(B) *Haemophilus influenzae*
(C) *Babesia*
(D) *Moraxella catarrhalis*
(E) *Capnocytophaga canimorsus*

Setting: Office

Questions 69–72

A 45-year-old construction worker presents with concerns about a pigmented skin lesion on his right forearm. He noticed this lesion approximately 1 year ago but did not seek medical attention. He is now concerned because it seems to have grown and become darker in color during the past month. His work requires that he be exposed to the sun most of the day. The man has no medical history and no family history of cancer. Review of symptoms is negative.

69. On examination of this skin lesion, which of the following characteristics most prompts concern about malignancy?

(A) Smooth border
(B) Dark color throughout the lesion
(C) Light color throughout the lesion
(D) Uniformly smooth elevation
(E) Small region of bleeding in the center of the lesion

70. Which of the following findings does NOT contribute to a poor prognosis in malignant melanoma?

(A) Ulceration of the lesion
(B) Tumor depth >0.75 mm
(C) Tumor location on the arm
(D) Invasion of the reticular dermis
(E) Male sex

71. The skin biopsy reveals a diagnosis of squamous cell cancer. Which of the following statements regarding this form of skin cancer is NOT true?

(A) Immunosuppression is a risk factor
(B) Marjolin ulcers are squamous cell carcinomas that form at the site of old scars
(C) Actinic keratosis is a premalignant, precursor lesion
(D) Metastasis is more frequent in basal cell cancers
(E) Depth of penetration is an important prognostic feature

72. Several years later, the man returns with a new skin lesion on his forehead. The nontender and nonpruritic lesion, which has been present for several months, has increased only minimally in size. On examination, an 8-mm pearly, translucent lesion with smooth margins is evident on the left side of the forehead. There is no associated lymphadenopathy. This lesion is most consistent with which of the following diagnoses?

(A) Nonmelanotic melanoma
(B) A simple skin tag
(C) Acne
(D) An infectious pustule
(E) Basal cell carcinoma

Setting: Satellite Clinic

Questions 73–76

A 28-year-old woman complains of erythematous, raised skin lesions on her shins. The tender lesions have developed during the past 48 hours. She has no significant medical history. She does not smoke or use alcohol and is currently on vacation from college in Arizona. On review of symptoms, she notes having had fever and a sore throat recently, but no cough. On examination, her temperature is 39°C, and her rash is tender. Her oropharynx is erythematous, and tender anterior cervical lymphadenopathy is present.

73. Which of the following conditions is the most likely cause of the skin findings?

(A) Coccidioidomycosis
(B) Blastomycosis
(C) Streptococcal infection
(D) Systemic lupus erythematosus
(E) Sarcoidosis

74. Which of the following tests is least necessary?

(A) Chest radiography
(B) Skin biopsy
(C) Antinuclear antibody (ANA)
(D) Erythrocyte sedimentation rate (ESR)
(E) Antistreptolysin O (ASO)

75. Which of the following measures is the most appropriate treatment?

(A) Observation
(B) Amphotericin B
(C) Hydroxychloroquine sulfate
(D) Prednisone
(E) Penicillin

76. Which of the following markers is the most sensitive study for the diagnosis of systemic lupus erythematosus?

(A) ANA
(B) Anti-ssDNA antibody
(C) Anti-dsDNA antibody
(D) Anti-Smith antibody
(E) Anti-Ro antibody

Setting: Hospital

Questions 77–79

A 49-year-old man is admitted to the ICU with severe pneumonia of unknown cause. Intubation and ventilatory support are necessary. Treatment involves ceftriaxone, azithromycin, and gentamicin, along with blood pressure support with intravenous norepinephrine. On hospital day 1, he undergoes CT with contrast of the chest, which shows bilateral pneumonia and no evidence of pulmonary thromboembolism. On hospital day 3, his urine output decreases to 400 mL per 24 hours and his serum creatinine rises to 2.0 mg/dL (admission creatinine: 1.2 mg/dL). His serum blood urea nitrogen (BUN) is 65 mg/dL. The intravenous boluses of furosemide administered to increase his urine output have not been effective. You have been called to see this patient regarding his deteriorating renal function.

77. In assessing this man's volume status, which of the following measurements is most helpful?

(A) Urine sodium
(B) Urine urea
(C) Blood pressure
(D) Pulmonary capillary wedge pressure
(E) Heart rate

78. In evaluating this man's urine, which of the following findings is most consistent with the diagnosis of acute tubular necrosis (ATN)?

(A) Red blood cell (RBC) casts
(B) White blood cell (WBC) casts
(C) Double-refractile fat bodies
(D) Muddy-brown granular casts
(E) Hyaline casts

79. Which of the following values is an indication for renal replacement therapy (i.e., hemodialysis)?

(A) Serum creatinine that rises 1.0 mg/dL per day
(B) Serum BUN that rises >20 mg/dL per day
(C) Urine output <400 mL/day on total parenteral nutrition (TPN)
(D) Serum potassium = 5.9 mEq/L
(E) Serum sodium = 129 mEq/L

Setting: Satellite Clinic

Questions 80–83

A 24-year-old woman complains of irregular menses. She has not menstruated in 6 months. Previously, she had normal cycles. She is G_1P_0 after an abortive procedure that occurred approximately 12 months ago. On examination, skin, hair, breast development, and genitalia are within normal limits.

80. What is the next appropriate test?

(A) Thyroid-stimulating hormone (TSH)
(B) Luteinizing hormone/follicle-stimulating hormone (LH/FSH)
(C) 17-Hydroxysteroids
(D) Prolactin
(E) β-Human chorionic gonadotropin (β-hCG)

81. The woman undergoes several blood tests, and all the results are within normal limits. Based on the physical examination, which of the following procedures is the next appropriate test?

(A) Dehydroepiandrosterone sulfate (DHEAS)
(B) Testosterone
(C) Estrogen challenge
(D) Progestin challenge
(E) Ultrasound

82. Based on her history and physical examination, what is the likely cause of her complaint?

(A) Polycystic ovary syndrome
(B) Hyperprolactinemia
(C) Premature ovarian failure
(D) Asherman syndrome
(E) Hypothyroidism

83. Which of the following conditions is NOT associated with hypogonadotropic hypogonadism?

(A) Premature ovarian failure
(B) Sarcoidosis
(C) Sheehan syndrome
(D) Thyroid failure
(E) Hyperprolactinemia

Setting: Hospital

Questions 84–85

A 55-year-old man presents with several hours of substernal chest pain that radiates to his left arm and neck. The pain is associated with diaphoresis and shortness of breath. His medical history is significant for hypertension, elevated cholesterol, and type 2 diabetes mellitus. On physical examination, vital signs are: blood pressure, 150/70 mm Hg; heart rate, 98 beats/minute; and respiratory rate, 20/minute. Chest examination reveals bibasilar rales, and cardiac examination shows a regular rate and 2/6 systolic murmur radiating to the axilla. The rest of his examination is within normal limits. The ECG shows 1.5-mm ST-segment elevation in leads V_5 to V_6 and leads aVL and I.

84. Which of the following medications is NOT indicated in the initial treatment?

(A) Aspirin
(B) Metoprolol
(C) Tissue plasminogen activator (tPA)
(D) Intravenous heparin
(E) Verapamil

85. The patient is treated successfully and is admitted to the coronary care unit. His course during the next 2 days is uneventful. A submaximal stress test and echocardiogram are scheduled before discharge. Which of the following features is most associated with a poor prognosis during the first year after a myocardial infarction (MI)?

(A) Elevated cholesterol
(B) Ejection fraction of 35%
(C) Five premature ventricular contractions per hour during the first 24 hours post-MI
(D) Use of tPA over emergent revascularization
(E) Blood pressure of 110/70 mm Hg

Setting: Office

Questions 86–88

A 36-year-old woman presents after 2 days of generalized malaise and low-grade fever, along with severe dysuria and a clear vaginal discharge. She states that she had unprotected intercourse with a new boyfriend 6 days ago; he denied any history of sexually transmitted disease. She has no significant medical history and takes only multivitamins. On physical examination, the patient appears quite anxious, with a temperature of 38.9°C. On external vaginal examination, several small, ulcerative, exquisitely tender, and erythematous lesions are present on the labia, and several similar lesions are apparent in the vagina. Cultures are taken, and a wet mount examination reveals numerous white blood cells (WBCs).

86. You suspect that the woman has genital herpes. Which of the following statements regarding treatment with acyclovir is true?

(A) Early, high-dose therapy eradicates the virus and prevents recurrences
(B) Intravenous therapy is necessary for eradication of the virus
(C) Symptom reduction occurs in 3 to 5 days
(D) Symptom reduction occurs within 24 hours
(E) Drug therapy is effective in eradicating latent infection

87. The woman, who has experienced several recurrences of genital herpes during the past few years, returns several years later. She is now married and interested in pregnancy. She is concerned about the risk of herpes to the fetus. Which of the following statements about herpes viral infections during pregnancy is true?

(A) Transplacental transmission is thought to occur only during primary infection
(B) The rate of spontaneous abortions is higher in women with a history of previous infections
(C) Congenital infections are generally mild and can be treated with acyclovir at birth
(D) Cesarean section is not required when active lesions are present in the vaginal region
(E) The Papanicolaou (Pap) smear has a high sensitivity for detection of active viral infection of the cervix

88. The woman is concerned about her risk for cervical cancer. Which of the following statements concerning cervical cancer is correct?

(A) If she has had three, consecutive, Pap smears within normal results, she can have one Pap test every 5 years

(B) An epidemiologic association with herpes viral infections and cervical cancer exists

(C) Pap smears should be performed every 6 months

(D) No association with herpes viral infections and cervical cancer exists

(E) Human papilloma virus is the only known causative factor of cervical cancer

Setting: Hospital

Questions 89–92

A 26-year-old woman with a history of intravenous drug abuse presents on transfer from another hospital with fever, cough, and sore throat and complains of eye burning for 3 days. Diffuse erythema of her entire body develops, with conjunctival injection peeling of the mouth and lips. The skin rash has now progressed to include portions of the arms and legs and is indistinguishable from a severe burn.

89. Which of the following disorders is the most common cause of this disease?

(A) HIV

(B) Herpes simplex virus

(C) *Mycoplasma*

(D) Drug reaction

(E) Vasculitis

90. Which of the following measures is the most appropriate next step?

(A) Enzyme-linked immunosorbent assay (ELISA) for HIV

(B) Skin biopsy

(C) Steroids

(D) Blood cultures

(E) Silver sulfadiazine (Silvadene) cream

91. Within 2 days, the woman's oxygen requirements increase to 100% with a nonrebreather face mask, and her PaO$_2$ decreases to 50 mm Hg. Her chest radiograph reveals patchy alveolar infiltrates bilaterally. Which of the following conditions is the likely cause of this change?

(A) Congestive heart failure

(B) Interstitial pneumonitis

(C) Aspiration pneumonia

(D) Acute respiratory distress syndrome (ARDS)

(E) Pulmonary embolism

92. The woman's temperature decreases to 36.3°C, her blood pressure decreases to 80/50 mm Hg, and her heart rate increases to 124 beats/minute. Her extremities are cool. Which of the following conditions is the most likely cause of this change?

(A) Hypovolemia

(B) Sepsis

(C) Adrenal insufficiency

(D) Cardiogenic shock

(E) Neurovascular collapse

Setting: Office

93. A 59-year-old woman inquires about screening for cervical cancer. Her medical history is significant for menorrhagia secondary to fibroids, and she underwent a total abdominal hysterectomy 3 years ago. She is married and has two children. Her only medication is atenolol for hypertension. She does not smoke or drink alcohol. In response to her concern about cervical cancer screening, which of the following is most correct?

(A) She should have Papanicolaou (Pap) smears annually

(B) She should have Pap smears every 3 years

(C) She should have Pap smears every 5 years

(D) She only needs annual pelvic examinations

(E) She should have annual vaginal ultrasounds

Setting: Hospital

Questions 94–97

A 78-year-old man is referred to you secondary to severe pain and fatigue in his lower extremities. The pain, which began approximately 8 months ago, initially occurred only with activity. However, during the past 3 weeks, the man has experienced pain at rest and has noticed some skin ulceration and discoloration in his feet. Because the pain worsens with ambulation, he has significantly decreased his activity level. The man has a history of type 2 diabetes mellitus; coronary artery disease, with a myocardial infarction (MI) 3 years ago; and hypertension. He smoked cigarettes but quit 25 years ago. His current medications include insulin NPH 15 U 2 times a day, lisinopril 10 mg/day, aspirin 325 mg/day, and atorvastatin calcium 10 mg/day.

94. Which of the following physical examination findings would most support your diagnosis of the man's complaints?

(A) A diffuse, shallow ulcer on the left foot, just above the medial malleolus

(B) Pitting edema of the lower extremities

(C) Hyperesthesia of the feet

(D) A "punched out" ulcer on the dorsum of the foot that is painful, especially at night

(E) A harsh systolic ejection murmur in the aortic position

95. You measure the blood pressure at both the ankle and brachial regions to calculate the ankle-brachial index (ABI). Which of the following ABI values is indicative of severe arterial disease?

(A) 0.4

(B) 0.6

(C) 0.8

(D) 1.0

(E) 1.5

96. The man's ABI is 0.5. Which of the following measures is the next management step?

(A) Surgery to revascularize his lower extremities

(B) Angiography with possible angioplasty

(C) Increasing the dose of aspirin and beginning pentoxifylline

(D) Venography

(E) Digoxin for treatment of heart failure

97. Preoperative workup reveals obstruction of the superficial femoral artery on the right side and the popliteal artery on the left side. Which of the following procedures is most indicated?

(A) Aortobifemoral bypass
(B) Axillofemoral bypass
(C) Femoral-femoral bypass
(D) Femoral-tibial bypass
(E) Endarterectomy

Setting: Office

Questions 98–102

A 51-year-old woman presents for her annual physical examination. Her last menstrual period was 2 years ago. She has a history of hypertension and mild depression but no diabetes mellitus or coronary artery disease. A former cigarette smoker, she stopped more than 10 years ago. Her family history is significant for a father who had a myocardial infarction (MI) at 53 years of age. Her fasting lipid panel reveals:

Cholesterol	249 mg/dL
Low-density lipoprotein (LDL)	145 mg/dL
Triglycerides	190 mg/dL
High-density lipoprotein (HDL)	66 mg/dL

98. Which of the following measures is appropriate in patient management?

(A) Start simvastatin
(B) No therapy
(C) Diet therapy
(D) Start gemfibrozil
(E) Start niacin

99. The woman's current regimen for hypertension includes captopril and prazosin. She is normotensive today. What do you recommend?

(A) No change because she is normotensive
(B) Avoidance of β-blockers
(C) Change to an angiotensin receptor blocker
(D) Addition of a diuretic with plans to withhold prazosin
(E) Addition of a β-blocker

100. The woman asks you about screening tests. Which of the following is NOT a criteria for a good screening test?

(A) High sensitivity
(B) Acceptable test to patients
(C) Early detection of disease
(D) Availability of effective therapy if disease is discovered
(E) High specificity

101. The woman asks you about breast cancer screening. You show her study results finding a relative risk reduction of 0.75 when mammograms are performed annually for 10 years. The number-needed-to-screen based on this study is

(A) 25
(B) 33
(C) 75
(D) 333
(E) cannot be determined

102. The woman has not had colorectal cancer screening. You tell her that

(A) screening should commence at 65 years of age

(B) fecal occult blood testing (FOBT) has never shown a mortality benefit

(C) flexible sigmoidoscopy adds no benefit to FOBT alone

(D) screening begins at 50 years of age with FOBT annually and flexible sigmoidoscopy every 3 to 5 years

(E) digital rectal examination every 3 to 5 years and FOBT annually is adequate

Setting: Emergency Department

Questions 103–104

A 23-year-old African American man with no significant medical history presents with complaints of severe fatigue, "darkening color of my eyes," darkening of his urine, and shortness of breath with activity. For the past 5 days, he has been ill with an upper respiratory illness; for this condition, he has been taking trimethoprim-sulfamethoxazole that his mother had in the medicine chest. Physical examination is significant for blood pressure of 100/80 mm Hg and heart rate of 130 beats/minute. He has marked scleral icterus and a 2/6 systolic ejection murmur. The rest of the examination is within normal limits. Laboratory studies reveal:

Hematocrit	16%
Reticulocyte count	21%
Haptoglobin	Undetectable
Electrocardiogram (ECG)	Sinus tachycardia
Urinalysis	No red blood cells (RBCs), white blood cells (WBCs) on microscopic examination
	Positive hemoglobin on dipstick analysis

103. Which of the following abnormalities would you most expect to find on examination of the patient's peripheral blood smear?

(A) Hypersegmented neutrophils

(B) Heinz bodies

(C) Howell-Jolly bodies

(D) Schistocytes

(E) Target cells

104. Which of the following laboratory tests supports your leading diagnosis?

(A) Elevated serum creatinine

(B) Elevated unconjugated bilirubin

(C) Elevated conjugated bilirubin

(D) Normal serum lactate dehydrogenase (LDH)

(E) Elevated serum creatine kinase level

Setting: Office

105. A 36-year-old man is referred to you for evaluation of possible infertility. His wife, a 32-year-old woman, has two children from a previous marriage; he has no children of his own. Despite unprotected intercourse for 8 months, the woman has not become pregnant. An evaluation performed by her physician documented no abnormalities. The man has no medical history and takes only ibuprofen occasionally for back pain. He had a normal onset of puberty and had no significant childhood illnesses or surgeries. Review of symptoms is only notable for occasional headaches that have worsened recently.

Physical examination reveals a well-developed man, with well-developed musculature and a normal body hair pattern. Some suggestion of mild gynecomastia is evident. Testicular examination is notable for testes that are borderline small. Which of the following physical examination findings not mentioned in the case description is most consistent with the likely diagnosis?

(A) Temporal hair recession

(B) Presence of a varicocele

(C) One testis smaller than another

(D) Bilateral temporal visual field deficits

(E) Color blindness

Setting: Emergency Department

Questions 106–111

A 26-year-old man with hemophilia A presents with complaints of abdominal pain, nausea, and vomiting. The vomitus is dark in color and contains coffee-ground–like material. He states that his bleeding has been under control; he has not required a blood transfusion in years.

106. The most important next step is

(A) measurement of vital signs

(B) determination of the factor VIII level

(C) determination of prothrombin time/partial thromboplastin time (PT/PTT)

(D) performance of a complete blood count (CBC)

(E) performance of a rectal examination with guaiac testing

107. The man's blood pressure is 110/70 mm Hg both supine and standing. On rectal examination, he is guaiac-positive (occult only). Laboratory studies reveal:

Hemoglobin	10 g/dL
Hematocrit	30%
White blood cell	3,400/mm^3
(WBC) count	75% segs
	18% lymphocytes
Platelet count	168,000/mm^3
Prothrombin time (PT)	14.5 sec
Partial thromboplastin time (PTT)	43.2 sec

Transfusion of which of the following substances is the next appropriate step?

(A) Platelets

(B) Two units of red blood cells (RBCs)

(C) Cryoprecipitate

(D) Fresh frozen plasma

(E) Factor VIII-recombinant protein

108. While the man is in the hospital, he undergoes further testing, which reveals:

Alanine aminotransferase (ALT)	169 U/L
Aspartate aminotransferase (AST)	155 U/L
Alkaline phosphatase	115 U/L
Albumin	3.0 mg/dL
Total bilirubin	1.4 mg/dL

Which of the following conditions is the most likely cause of the laboratory abnormalities?

(A) Hepatitis B
(B) Hepatitis C
(C) Hemochromatosis
(D) HIV
(E) Budd-Chiari syndrome

109. One year later, the patient is brought to the ED after an episode of shaking with loss of consciousness. The family claims that it started suddenly without preceding trauma. Which of the following tests is most likely to yield a diagnosis?

(A) CT of the head
(B) Lumbar puncture
(C) MRI of the brain
(D) Serum cryptococcal antigen
(E) Toxoplasma titers

110. Which of the following measures is likely indicated?

(A) Pyrimethamine and sulfadiazine
(B) Trimethoprim and sulfamethoxazole
(C) Brain biopsy
(D) Amphotericin B
(E) Isoniazid, rifampin, pyrazinamide, and ethambutol

111. On recovery, the man complains of feelings of hopelessness, difficulty sleeping, and a complete loss of enjoyment from activities he formerly enjoyed. Which of the following measures is the next appropriate step?

(A) Prescription of an antidepressant
(B) Assessment of suicide risk
(C) Determination of thyroid-stimulating hormone (TSH) level
(D) Performance of a mini-mental state examination
(E) Determination of parathyroid hormone level

Setting: Office

Questions 112–113

A 60-year-old woman is referred to you for evaluation of a tremor, which began several months ago but has worsened during the past few weeks. She reports that the tremor is not present at rest but worsens with intended movement. A glass of brandy seems to reduce the tremor. She denies any other complaints. Her medical history is significant for hypertension and osteoporosis. Her medications include hydrochlorothiazide, verapamil hydrochloride, calcium carbonate, and calcitonin nasal spray. Her physical examination is within normal limits except for the tremor, which is most pronounced in the upper extremities. It is bilateral and symmetric, not present at rest, and aggravated by intentional movements.

112. Which of the following measures would you perform next?

(A) Thyroid function testing
(B) CT of the head with contrast
(C) Electroencephalogram (EEG)
(D) Nerve conduction velocity testing
(E) None (no further testing is necessary)

113. To improve the tremor, which of the following medications is indicated?

(A) L-Dopa
(B) Propranolol
(C) Haloperidol
(D) Bromocriptine mesylate
(E) Benztropine mesylate

Setting: Emergency Department

An 18-year-old teenager with a history of type 1 diabetes mellitus presents with a 1-day history of fevers, chills, and flank pain. In addition, she complains of dysuria and increased urinary frequency. She has been previously healthy. She is pregnant and reportedly at approximately 22 weeks' gestation. On review of symptoms, she has mild nausea and decreased appetite. Her medications include NPH insulin and sliding-scale regular insulin. Physical examination reveals:

General	Nontoxic appearing
Temperature	38.2°C
Blood pressure	110/70 mm Hg
Chest	Clear to auscultation
Heart	Regular rate and rhythm; no murmurs
Abdomen	Mild bilateral costovertebral angle tenderness; normal bowel sounds; suprapubic tenderness
Extremities	No edema

Laboratory studies reveal:

White blood cell (WBC) count	12,000/mm^3
Blood glucose	235 mg/dL
Blood chemistries	Normal
Liver function tests	Normal
Urinalysis	Large leukocyte esterase, trace red blood cells (RBCs)

114. Which of the following steps is the most appropriate after taking blood cultures?

(A) Oral nitrofurantoin 100 mg 4 times a day
(B) Oral trimethoprim-sulfamethoxazole 2 times a day
(C) Intravenous gentamicin 4.5 mg/kg per 24 hours
(D) Renal ultrasound and then intravenous ceftriaxone 1 to 2 g/24 hours
(E) Intravenous ceftriaxone 1 to 2 g/24 hours

Setting: Office

Questions 115–116

A 56-year-old woman presents with decreasing peripheral vision of several months' duration. Occasionally, she cannot make out objects on the periphery of her vision. Otherwise healthy, she has no other complaints. Physical examination is within normal limits except for the funduscopic examination, which demonstrates an enlarged cup-to-disc ratio.

115. Which of the following disorders is the most likely diagnosis?

(A) Cataracts
(B) Macular degeneration
(C) Papilledema
(D) Glaucoma
(E) Temporal arteritis

116. Which of the following medications is indicated for treatment of this condition?

(A) Timolol maleate 0.25% solution
(B) Pilocarpine 0.5% solution
(C) Prednisone
(D) Timolol maleate and pilocarpine
(E) Timolol maleate and prednisone

Setting: Office

Questions 117–121

A 42-year-old woman of Irish descent presents to her primary care physician with complaints of diarrhea. She has had loose stools up to 4 times per day for approximately 4 months; the condition is less severe when she fasts. She has had no significant abdominal pain and has no visible blood in her stool. One month ago, during a blood drive, she had a hematocrit of 30%.

117. Which of the following procedures is most likely to yield a diagnosis?

(A) Colonoscopy
(B) Barium enema
(C) Peripheral smear
(D) Intestinal biopsy
(E) Iron studies

118. On examination you note a bullous, violaceous skin eruption on both arms. The most likely cause is

(A) pemphigus vulgaris
(B) bullous pemphigoid
(C) epidermolysis bullosa
(D) dermatitis herpetiformis
(E) Stevens-Johnson syndrome

119. The most appropriate treatment for the skin eruption is

(A) prednisone
(B) psoralen ultraviolet-A range (PUVA)
(C) dapsone
(D) topical triamcinolone
(E) cefazolin sodium

120. If a blood chemistry panel is ordered, which of the following series of findings might you expect?

	Na$^+$ (mEq/L)	K$^+$ (mEq/L)	Cl$^-$ (mEq/L)	CO$_2$ (mEq/L)	Blood urea nitrogen (BUN) [mg/dL]	Creatinine (mg/dL)
(A)	125	4.5	90	30	40	2.0
(B)	136	3.3	105	21	14	0.8
(C)	138	4.0	100	13	20	1.0
(D)	145	2.5	85	45	5	0.9
(E)	150	3.7	115	25	20	1.8

121. You learn of two blood tests used to help diagnose this patient's diarrhea. Test 1 has a sensitivity of 89%, a specificity of 94%, and a cost of $100. Test 2 has a sensitivity of 92%, a specificity of 95%, and a cost of $500. You predict the woman's pretest probability to be 50%. You are concerned about her well-being and are eager to obtain an answer. Which of the following test(s) should you order?

(A) Test 1
(B) Test 2
(C) Test 1 followed by test 2
(D) Test 2 followed by test 1
(E) Test 2 must be given twice

Setting: Office

Questions 122–123

A 16-year-old girl who has never had a menstrual period but is otherwise healthy is referred to you. She has no siblings. She takes no medications and denies any drug use. Physical examination reveals a thin-appearing girl with normal vital signs but no breast development. Pelvic examination reveals a patent vagina.

122. Which of the following laboratory tests would be most helpful in the diagnosis of her condition?

(A) Follicle-stimulating hormone (FSH) level
(B) Karyotype analysis
(C) Serum testosterone
(D) Pelvic ultrasound
(E) Serum thyroid-stimulating hormone (TSH) level

123. Another 16-year-old girl with the same history and physical examination is referred to you. Her workup includes:

Pelvic ultrasound	Normal
Karyotype analysis	Normal
Serum follicle-stimulating hormone (FSH)	Slightly decreased
Serum testosterone	Normal
Serum thyroid-stimulating hormone (TSH)	Normal

Which of the following diagnoses is NOT likely to be a cause of primary amenorrhea in this patient?

(A) Anorexia nervosa
(B) Delayed puberty
(C) Müllerian agenesis
(D) Pituitary tumor
(E) Craniopharyngioma

Setting: Office

Questions 124–126

You are starting a cardiovascular prevention clinic as part of your group practice. The first patient you see is a 56-year-old man with a history of hypertension and a family history of premature cardiovascular disease. He has the following lipid profile:

Total cholesterol	310 mg/dL
Low-density lipoprotein (LDL)	180 mg/dL
High-density lipoprotein (HDL)	56 mg/dL
Triglycerides	459 mg/dL

124. Based on this man's risk profile, you decide to treat his hyperlipidemia. Which of the following therapeutic agents would you use first?

(A) Simvastatin 10 mg every night
(B) Gemfibrozil 600 mg 2 times a day
(C) Cholestyramine 4 mg 2 times a day
(D) Dietary therapy
(E) Colestipol 5 mg 2 times a day

125. You prescribe a medication for the man, who returns several weeks later with severe muscle aches. His serum creatine kinase is elevated. Which of the following therapeutic regimens is causally implicated in this situation?

(A) Simvastatin 10 mg every night
(B) Gemfibrozil 600 mg 2 times a day
(C) Cholestyramine 4 mg 2 times a day
(D) Dietary therapy
(E) Colestipol 5 mg 2 times a day

126. You modify the man's treatment, but he presents to the ED 2 weeks later with severe mid-epigastric abdominal pain that radiates to the back. His serum amylase is significantly elevated, and his serum triglyceride level is 1,400 mg/dL. Which of the following therapies is now causally implicated?

(A) Simvastatin 10 mg every night
(B) Niacin 500 mg 2 times a day
(C) Cholestyramine 6 mg 2 times a day
(D) Gemfibrozil 600 mg 2 times a day
(E) Dietary therapy

Setting: Hospital

Questions 127–132

A 36-year-old woman who is G_1P_0 is being followed-up by your practice. At 26 weeks' gestation she has a blood pressure of 150/90 mm Hg with peripheral edema and a 24-hour urine protein of 1 g. Except for the edema, she has no complaints. You decide to observe her closely with the recommendation of strict bed rest, a low-sodium diet, and frequent blood pressure monitoring. After 1 week, her blood pressure is 165/92 mm Hg, and her 24-hour urine protein is 2.5 g. Her 24-hour urine output is 1,500 mL.

127. Which of the following measures would you now recommend?

(A) Continued bed rest at home
(B) Emergent delivery
(C) Admission to the hospital for monitoring
(D) Admission to the hospital with magnesium sulfate infusion
(E) Initiation of outpatient antihypertensive therapy with a calcium channel blocker

128. You continue to follow the woman's case closely. At 28 weeks' gestation, her blood pressure is 162/110 mm Hg and her 24-hour urine protein excretion is 5.3 g. In the past 24 hours, her urine output was 375 mL. She is complaining of some blurring of her vision. An ultrasound examination of the fetus shows a normal biophysical profile. Which of the following measures would you now recommend?

(A) Control of blood pressure with hydralazine
(B) Emergent delivery
(C) Magnesium sulfate infusion
(D) Control of blood pressure with hydralazine, emergent delivery, and magnesium sulfate infusion
(E) Emergent delivery and magnesium sulfate infusion

129. On your order, the woman receives an infusion of magnesium sulfate (initial bolus of 7 g; then 2.5 g/hour). Your medical student awakens you and tells you that the woman's respiratory rate is 8/minute, and that she is now confused and lethargic. Which of the following measures would you next recommend?

(A) Emergent intubation
(B) Calcium gluconate 10 mL of a 10% solution
(C) Epinephrine 0.3 mL subcutaneously
(D) Naloxone
(E) Emergent delivery

130. In preparation for delivery, an amniocentesis is performed. Which of the following parameters is most useful in predicting lung maturity of the infant?

(A) Lecithin/sphingomyelin (L/S) ratio <2:1
(B) L/S ratio = 1:4
(C) L/S ratio = 4:1
(D) Type I alveolar cells in the amniotic fluid
(E) Type II alveolar cells in the amniotic fluid

131. A decision is made to deliver the infant. A neonatologist is called to attend the delivery secondary to the prematurity of the infant. A cesarean section is performed, and the infant is successfully delivered. However, the infant is in severe respiratory distress and is immediately placed in 100% oxygen. An arterial blood gas is obtained with a pH of 7.2, a PO_2 of 50 mm Hg, and a PCO_2 of 65 mm Hg. The next appropriate step in the management of this infant is

(A) intubation with mechanical ventilation
(B) exogenous surfactant instillation
(C) intravenous hydration
(D) intubation with mechanical ventilation and exogenous surfactant instillation
(E) intubation with mechanical ventilation and intravenous hydration

132. The infant is admitted to the neonatal ICU. The mother, who does well after delivery, is ready for discharge after 3 days. She is concerned about leaving her infant alone in the ICU, but realizes that she cannot stay in the hospital 24 hours a day. Which of the following measures is most helpful in maintaining a close bond between the parents and the infant?

(A) Strict enforcement of visiting hours to give structure to the parent's day

(B) Request that the parents leave the infant whenever any procedure is performed

(C) Strict enforcement of isolation of the infant to avoid microbiologic contamination

(D) Encouragement by the staff to allow the parents to partake in as much of the infant's care as medically feasible

(E) Weekly scheduled meetings with the health care team to provide updates on the infant's progress

Setting: Office

Questions 133–139

A 56-year-old man, a native of India, who has not seen a physician for over 10 years, comes in for a preemployment "physical." He has no complaints. His medical history is significant for hypertension, for which he takes metoprolol 25 mg 2 times a day. On review of symptoms, he notes cough productive of clear sputum for years. In addition, he has chronic dyspnea on exertion. He has smoked tobacco for 38 years; he does not use alcohol. He and his wife live together in a suburban community. They have two healthy children who were born in India. He formerly worked in a quarry for 30 years. His family history is unremarkable. Physical examination is notable for a blood pressure of 150/90 mm Hg and apical inspiratory rales. A chest radiograph finds a bilateral, apical reticular pattern with hilar calcifications. A purified protein derivative (PPD) measures 11 mm at 48 hours.

133. Which of the following measures is the most appropriate next step?

(A) Repeat the PPD

(B) High-resolution CT

(C) Tuberculosis prophylaxis

(D) Induced sputum samples

(E) Bronchoscopy

134. Which of the following conditions is NOT typically associated with an apical lung process?

(A) Silicosis
(B) Coal worker's pneumoconiosis
(C) Ankylosing spondylitis
(D) Asbestosis
(E) Eosinophilic granuloma

135. Pulmonary function tests reveal:

Forced expiratory volume in 1 second (FEV_1)	1.8 L (68% of predicted)
Forced vital capacity (FVC)	3.1 L (74% of predicted)
FEV_1/FVC	69%
Forced expiratory flow at 25% to 75% of FVC (FEF_{25-75})	40%
Carbon monoxide diffusion in the lung (DL_{CO})	72%

These values are most consistent with

(A) obstructive disease
(B) restrictive disease
(C) mixed obstructive and restrictive disease
(D) normal respiratory physiology
(E) diffusion abnormality

136. Metoprolol acts on which of the following chemicals?

(A) cGMP
(B) Inositol 1,4,5-triphosphate
(C) Diacylglycerol
(D) cAMP
(E) Nitric oxide

137. A routine lipid profile indicates:

Total cholesterol	246 mg/dL
Low-density lipoprotein (LDL)	181 mg/dL
High-density lipoprotein (HDL)	36 mg/dL
Triglycerides	245 mg/dL

Which of the following measures is the appropriate next step?

(A) No treatment
(B) 3-Hydroxy-3-methylglutaryl coenzyme A (HMG-CoA) reductase inhibitor
(C) Fibric acid
(D) Diet therapy
(E) Niacin

138. Which of the following measures is least necessary at this time?

(A) Fecal occult blood testing (FOBT)
(B) Prostate-specific antigen (PSA)
(C) Pneumovax
(D) Seasonal influenza vaccine
(E) Tetanus booster

139. You learn that the number-needed-to-screen for FOBT is nearly 1,000 to prevent colon cancer. Based on these data, what is the absolute risk reduction associated with FOBT?

(A) 0.1%
(B) 1%
(C) 10%
(D) 50%
(E) 100%

Setting: Hospital

Questions 140–142

A high-risk maternal–fetal service has started in your hospital. The following cases are seen in the first month of the new service.

140. An infant is born to an alcoholic mother. Which of the following abnormalities is NOT expected to result from the fetus's exposure to alcohol?

(A) Mental retardation
(B) Growth deficiencies
(C) Cleft palate
(D) Facial dysmorphism
(E) Increased risk of miscarriage

141. A mother delivers a healthy baby. She is worried because two of her sisters, a grandparent, and an uncle all have been diagnosed with cancer. She inquires about the risk of malignancy in her newborn. Which of the following inherited conditions is NOT associated with an increased risk of malignancy to the infant?

(A) Li-Fraumeni syndrome
(B) Von Hippel-Lindau syndrome
(C) Ataxia-telangiectasia
(D) Beckwith-Wiedemann syndrome
(E) McArdle syndrome

142. An infant is born with Down syndrome. Which of the following statements concerning this inherited condition is NOT true?

(A) The risk of having an infant with Down syndrome increases with increasing maternal age
(B) Cardiac defects occur in all cases
(C) Facial dysmorphism occurs in all cases
(D) Duodenal atresia can occur
(E) Developmental delay is characteristic

Setting: Emergency Department

Questions 143–146

A 20-year-old man is brought in by his friends following a snakebite, which he received while hiking in the Shenandoah Mountains. His friends are sure that the snake was a rattlesnake. On examination, right lower extremity swelling is evident. Within 1 hour, nausea, vomiting, and hypotension develop, and the man shows a decrease in level of consciousness.

143. Immediate therapy should include all of the following EXCEPT

(A) limb immobilization
(B) ice applied to the site of the bite
(C) measurement of vital signs
(D) determination of coagulation parameters
(E) admission to the ICU

144. The man continues to be hypotensive despite intravenous administration of 3 L normal saline. Which of the following relative measurements might be expected on examination with right heart catheter?

	Central Venous Pressure	Systemic Vascular Resistance	Cardiac Output	Pulmonary Capillary Wedge Pressure
(A)	Increased	Decreased	Decreased	Increased
(B)	Normal	Increased	Decreased	Increased
(C)	Decreased	Decreased	Increased	Decreased
(D)	Normal	Decreased	Decreased	Increased
(E)	Decreased	Increased	Decreased	Decreased

145. The man becomes unresponsive. At this time, the most important component of initial management is

(A) fluid repletion
(B) antibiotic administration
(C) inotrope administration
(D) antivenin administration
(E) airway management

146. The man's blood pressure improves after your intervention. Within 1 hour he is communicating and complaining of worsening pain in his right lower leg. The next management step is

(A) limb elevation
(B) antivenin administration
(C) measurement of intracompartmental pressure
(D) mannitol administration
(E) hyperbaric oxygen therapy

Setting: Emergency Department

Questions 147–150

A 51-year-old man complains of chest pain, which he describes as "gripping." The pain is substernal, and he has discomfort in his neck as well. He has never had this pain before; it came on suddenly while he was watching television. His medications include metformin hydrochloride, glyburide, and amlodipine. His ECG shows 1-mm ST-segment depression in the lateral leads (V_4 to V_6) with normal intervals and QRS complexes.

147. Which of the following agents is least likely to provide pain relief?

(A) Aspirin
(B) Metoprolol
(C) Captopril
(D) Heparin
(E) Tissue plasminogen activator (tPA)

148. The man receives several interventions and is pain free. The most appropriate next step is

(A) an immediate stress test
(B) an echocardiogram
(C) immediate catheterization
(D) a stress test in 48 to 72 hours
(E) thrombolysis

149. The man undergoes cardiac catheterization at a later date. Which of the following results would warrant consideration for coronary artery bypass surgery?

(A) 90% stenosis of the proximal left anterior descending coronary artery
(B) 60% stenosis of the left main artery
(C) 90% stenosis of the left anterior descending coronary artery, with an ejection fraction of 35%
(D) 90% stenosis of the left anterior descending coronary artery and 100% stenosis of the right coronary artery, with an ejection fraction of 35%
(E) 80% stenosis of the left circumflex artery and complete occlusion of the right coronary artery

150. After an ST-elevation myocardial infarction (MI), which of the following agents is least likely to decrease long-term mortality?

(A) Aspirin
(B) Nitroglycerin
(C) Simvastatin
(D) Propranolol
(E) Enalapril

ANSWER KEY

1-C	31-D	61-C	91-D	121-A
2-B	32-A	62-C	92-B	122-A
3-B	33-C	63-B	93-D	123-C
4-B	34-D	64-D	94-D	124-A
5-D	35-D	65-E	95-A	125-A
6-E	36-D	66-B	96-B	126-C
7-B	37-B	67-D	97-D	127-C
8-D	38-D	68-D	98-C	128-D
9-A	39-B	69-E	99-D	129-B
10-D	40-B	70-C	100-E	130-C
11-C	41-C	71-D	101-E	131-D
12-E	42-A	72-E	102-D	132-D
13-A	43-C	73-C	103-B	133-C
14-C	44-D	74-D	104-B	134-D
15-A	45-E	75-A	105-D	135-C
16-D	46-C	76-A	106-A	136-D
17-C	47-A	77-D	107-E	137-B
18-D	48-E	78-D	108-B	138-B
19-C	49-A	79-C	109-C	139-A
20-C	50-E	80-E	110-A	140-C
21-B	51-B	81-D	111-B	141-E
22-B	52-A	82-D	112-A	142-B
23-D	53-C	83-A	113-B	143-B
24-C	54-E	84-E	114-E	144-E
25-C	55-E	85-B	115-D	145-E
26-C	56-D	86-C	116-D	146-C
27-C	57-B	87-A	117-D	147-E
28-D	58-D	88-B	118-D	148-D
29-C	59-E	89-D	119-C	149-B
30-C	60-D	90-B	120-B	150-B

ANSWERS AND EXPLANATIONS

1–4. The answers are: 1-C, 2-B, 3-B, 4-B. (*Internal medicine*)
This patient has pheochromocytoma. The findings of severe, new-onset hypertension, flushing, diaphoresis, weight loss, headache, and palpitations should clearly suggest this diagnosis as the primary concern. The evaluation of pheochromocytoma involves confirmation of catecholamine excess and tumor localization. Laboratory studies include measurement of urinary vanillylmandelic acid and metanephrine levels, as well as urinary epinephrine and norepinephrine levels. Given such a clear-cut history, the other choices given in question 1 should not be diagnostic concerns. Radiologic assessment may involve CT or MRI of the abdomen (85% of pheochromocytomas are located in the adrenal medulla). Metaiodobenzylguanidine (MIBG) scanning is useful in locating extra-adrenal tumors. It is important to note that imaging of the adrenals should not be performed without functional evidence of increased catecholamine levels. The prevalence of incidental adrenal masses is high, and the diagnosis of pheochromocytoma relies on the presence of increased levels of catecholamines.

Medical treatment of the hypertension must precede surgical resection. Therapy must involve α-blockade with an agent such as phenoxybenzamine or prazosin. α-Blockade leads to reversal of vasoconstriction. Most patients also require a β-blocker, such as propranolol, to protect against arrhythmias. It is critical that β-blockers be added only after full α-blockade is established. In the absence of α-blockade, β-blockade results in unopposed α-stimulation and severe hypertension. Cardiac stress testing is not required without a history of angina. Diuresis should never be performed because these patients are usually volume-depleted at time of surgery.

Approximately, 10% of pheochromocytomas are malignant. These tumors tend to be more often seen in younger patients and tend to be extra-adrenal.

This patient's history of pheochromocytoma, as well as the family history of a thyroid tumor and death from stroke, should suggest a familial multiple endocrine neoplasia syndrome (MEN). Pheochromocytoma is associated with MEN types 2A and 2B. MEN 2A (Sipple syndrome) includes medullary thyroid carcinoma (100%), pheochromocytoma (50%), and parathyroid hyperplasia (40%). MEN 2B includes medullary thyroid carcinoma (100%), pheochromocytoma (50% to 90%), and mucosal neuromas (100%). Thus, screening for this patient should include serum calcium level and serum calcitonin levels.

5–9. The answers are: 5-D, 6-E, 7-B, 8-D, 9-A. (*Internal medicine, statistics*)
This patient's abrupt increase in abdominal girth and family history of liver disease should arouse a suspicion for cirrhosis with the subsequent development of ascites. At this time, liver function tests are the most appropriate test. His employment with a brake system manufacturer might have exposed him to asbestos, increasing his risk for mesothelioma or non–small cell lung cancer. When combined with asbestos exposure, his history of tobacco use further increases his risk of non–small cell lung cancer by nearly 100-fold. Although congestive heart failure can cause ascites, there is no evidence of this and an echocardiogram is unnecessary.

The ascites fluid albumin = 2.3 mg/dL, and the serum albumin = 3.8 mg/dL, which defines a serum albumin–ascites gradient (SAAG) of 1.5. A SAAG greater than 1.1 correlates well with portal hypertension as the cause for the ascites. Peritoneal carcinomatosis causes ascites exclusive of portal hypertension and is associated with a SAAG of less than 1.1. Hepatitis C causes ascites secondary to cirrhosis, which increases portal pressures. Budd-Chiari syndrome (hepatic vein thrombosis), veno-occlusive disease (commonly secondary to chemotherapy), and portal vein thrombosis all cause portal hypertension.

Hemochromatosis is a fairly common cause of liver disease in Caucasians, caused by aberrant absorption of iron through the gut. The definitive test for evaluation of hemochromatosis is the liver biopsy with calculation of the hepatic iron index (iron concentration ÷ patient's age in years). In individuals who are homozygous for hemochromatosis, the index is greater than 1.9. The presence of antimitochondrial antibodies identifies those with primary biliary cirrhosis, and ceruloplasmin is low in patients with Wilson disease. The HFE protein is most commonly aberrant as a C282Y translocation; evaluation of the HFE gene finds that 80% to 85% of cases are C282Y. The H63D translocation is less common; 5% are H63D. However, analysis of the

HFE gene misses many cases; therefore, the hepatic iron index is the gold standard. Anti–smooth cell antibody is seen in some patients with autoimmune hepatitis.

Hemochromatosis, which is rare in African American patients, increases the risk of hepatocellular carcinoma. An ophthalmology examination may help make the diagnosis in Wilson disease when Kayser-Fleischer rings are present.

To evaluate a new test, it is necessary to draw a 2 × 2 table:

		DISEASE	
		Present	Absent
TEST	**Positive**	a	b
	Negative	c	d

If the prevalence of disease is 50%, it helps to choose 100 patients arbitrarily, placing 50 in the "Present" column and 50 in the "Absent" column. The tests for sensitivity and specificity fill in the rest of the boxes; sensitivity = a/(a + c) and specificity = d/(b + d).

In this case, a = 40, b = 5, c = 10, and d = 45. If the man is free of disease, the test is negative in 90% of cases (specificity), and it is *not* more useful as a screening test where higher sensitivity is desired. If he has the disease, the test is positive in 80% of cases (sensitivity). If his test is negative, he has an 82% chance of *not* having the disease (negative predictive value) ([a + b]/[c + d] = 45/55).

10. The answer is D. (*Internal medicine, neurology*)
This patient has giant cell (or temporal) arteritis, a subacute granulomatous inflammation of large blood vessels, including the carotid artery, superficial temporal artery, and vertebral artery. This disorder, which is uncommon before 50 years of age, affects women twice as frequently as men. Nonspecific symptoms, such as fever, malaise, myalgia, weight loss, and arthralgia, are common. Headaches associated with the disease may be unilateral or bilateral and are characteristically localized to the scalp, over the temporal arteries. Pain or stiffness of the jaw, especially with chewing, is also characteristic.

A feared complication of giant cell arteritis is involvement of the ophthalmic artery, which can lead to permanent blindness. Diagnosis involves biopsy of the temporal artery. The erythrocyte sedimentation rate (ESR) is usually quite elevated, with levels greater than 100 mm/hour. Therapy with high-dose prednisone should be instituted at the moment the diagnosis is considered. The other complications listed do not occur in patients with giant cell arteritis.

11–12. The answers are: 11-C, 12-E. (*Obstetrics/gynecology*)
This patient has secondary amenorrhea, which is defined as cessation of menses for 3 or more consecutive months in a woman with previously normal cycles. Cessation of normal menses may occur as a result of a disturbance at any level of the regulatory pathway that controls normal menstrual cycles. It is possible to formulate a differential diagnosis by conceptualizing the pathways involved in normal menstrual cycles. For example, hypothalamic dysfunction leads to interruption of gonadotropin-releasing hormone secretion and loss of the midcycle luteinizing hormone (LH) surge. Causes of hypothalamic dysfunction include situational stress, anorexia nervosa, serious concurrent illness, excessive exercise and excess cortisol, androgens, and prolactin. Pituitary disorder can also lead to amenorrhea as a result of impairment in LH and follicle-stimulating hormone (FSH) release. These causes include pituitary neoplasms, pituitary infarction (Sheehan syndrome), and granulomatous diseases (e.g., sarcoidosis). Ovarian disorders leading to amenorrhea are marked by a hypergonadotropic response (i.e., marked increase in the concentrations of LH and FSH) secondary to removal of the

feedback inhibition by estrogens and progesterone secreted by the ovary. Ovarian causes of amenorrhea include menopause, polycystic ovary syndrome, and premature ovarian failure (e.g., from autoimmune diseases, radiation or chemotherapy, endometriosis). Endometrial scarring and adhesion formation may also lead to amenorrhea.

Evaluation of amenorrhea relies on a careful history and physical examination to provide clues to one of these causes. For instance, peripheral vision field defects should suggest a prolactinoma. In all instances, a pregnancy test should be performed. However, when the history, physical examination, and pregnancy test are unrevealing, further testing is required. One technique is to administer high-dose progestin therapy to test for the presence of withdrawal bleeding. In essence, this is a bioassay for FSH secretion, estrogen synthesis, and uterine responsiveness. Patients with the onset of withdrawal bleeding in response to progestin have inadequate progesterone synthesis and, probably, a problem with proper LH release from the pituitary. The two most common causes of this condition are polycystic ovary syndrome, which is distinguished by high levels of LH, and mild hypothalamic dysfunction, which is distinguished by low levels of LH. Primary ovarian failure is associated with high levels of FSH and LH and low levels of estrogen; prolactin levels are unaffected.

13–15. The answers are: 13-A, 14-C, 15-A. (*Internal medicine*)

The patient with HIV infection and fever is always a challenge. The cause of fever, diarrhea, or both correlates best with the CD4 count, which defines the degree of immunodeficiency. At a CD4 count of 350 to 400 cells/mm^3, herpes zoster, recurrent oral or vaginal candidiasis, or seborrhea may occur. At a CD4 count of 200 cells/mm^3, tuberculosis is a potential cause of fever. At a CD4 count of approximately 100 cells/mm^3, *Pneumocystis carinii*, histoplasmosis, coccidioidomycosis, *Cryptococcus,* toxoplasmosis, and *Cryptosporidium* may account for the fever. At a CD4 count of less than 50 cells/mm^3, HIV-associated dementia, cytomegalovirus, and *Mycobacterium avium-intracellulare* complex (MAC) develop.

MAC, the most common cause of fever in a patient with acquired immunodeficiency syndrome (AIDS) without other overt symptoms, is most often associated with the symptoms of fever with or without diarrhea. Laboratory tests usually find evidence of involvement of the biliary tree and bone marrow as evidenced by an increased alkaline phosphatase and pancytopenia, respectively. Blood cultures typically are of high yield, with a sensitivity of 85% in the febrile patient. An abdominal CT scan often finds hepatosplenomegaly and lymphadenopathy. Many other conditions may mimic or coexist with MAC, including abdominal lymphoma, HIV-wasting syndrome, *Salmonella, Campylobacter, Cryptosporidium, Microsporidium,* and *Isospora belli.* A large study in Haiti found that the three most common causes of diarrhea in patients with AIDS were *Cryptosporidium, Isospora,* and *Cyclospora.* AIDS-affected patients with *Cryptosporidium* may have biliary tract involvement, but they usually have right upper quadrant pain. *Isospora* and *Cyclospora* rarely present with these findings.

Treatment for MAC includes a macrolide antibiotic with ethambutol. Rifabutin is occasionally added, but it may cause uveitis in up to 40% of patients when used with clarithromycin. MAC can be prevented with weekly macrolide prophylaxis in AIDS patients with CD4 counts of less than 50 to 100 cells/mm^3.

16. The answer is D. (*Internal medicine*)

This patient presents with a constellation of anemia, renal failure, and proteinuria on a 24-hour collection, but not on dipstick analysis. She may also have rouleaux, the aggregation and clumping of red blood cells (RBCs) secondary to the presence of a paraprotein in the serum on a peripheral smear. It should be noted that the dipstick urinalysis displays only albuminuria, whereas the 24-hour collection and analysis determines total urine protein, including light chains.

The most likely diagnosis is multiple myeloma, the clonal proliferation of plasma cells. The median age at diagnosis is 68 years. Symptoms and findings include bone pain; pathologic fractures and lytic bone lesions; hypercalcemia; renal failure; anemia and fatigue; increased incidence of infections; and, occasionally, mass lesions with resulting organ damage. Renal failure may be secondary to hypercalcemia, amyloidosis, light chain deposition, or urate nephropathy. Diagnosis is established by finding high concentrations of light chains in the urine or serum, as well as plasmacytosis in the bone marrow. A thorough radiographic bone survey for lytic bone lesions is warranted.

17. The answer is C. (*Emergency medicine, neurology, internal medicine*)
The cause of this patient's hyponatremia is likely multifactorial and related to psychogenic polydipsia and volume depletion from vomiting. In the setting of seizures and severe hyponatremia (<110 mEq/L), acute and rapid treatment is indicated. Often, this requires the use of hypertonic (3%) saline to increase the sodium to a safer level at which seizures are no longer occurring (generally, about 120 mEq/L). However, rapid correction may also be harmful and can lead to the development of a central demyelinating lesion in the pons (central pontine myelinolysis). This condition is characterized by paraparesis or quadriparesis, dysarthria, dysphagia, and coma. In patients with severe hyponatremia, the serum sodium level should not rise more than 12 to 15 mEq/day. For this patient, rapid correction to a sodium of 120 mEq/L should be accomplished, followed by a slower normalization. The most important aspect of treatment is careful monitoring of the serum sodium through serial chemistries.

18–19. The answers are: 18-D, 19-C. (*Surgery*)
This patient clearly has an inguinal hernia. An indirect inguinal hernia originates at the deep inguinal ring and passes lateral to the inferior epigastric vessels. A direct inguinal hernia occurs directly through the abdominal wall without passing through the deep inguinal ring; it passes through the Hesselbach triangle, which is bounded by the lateral border of the rectus sheath, the inferior epigastric vessels, and the inguinal ligament. On physical examination, it is difficult to determine whether an inguinal hernia is direct or indirect. However, the finding of a mass in the scrotum clearly indicates that the hernia sac has traversed the superficial inguinal ring. A hernia through the femoral or obturator canal does not cause a groin mass on presentation.

The wound infection requires reexploration and removal of the synthetic mesh. Replacement of the mesh is not indicated in the setting of an infected surgical field; therefore, a repair that would not require mesh is appropriate. The other answer choices in question 19 do not provide adequate treatment.

20. The answer is C. (*Surgery*)
This patient has adhesive capsulitis, or frozen shoulder, a condition of unknown cause in which progressive restriction of the shoulder joint occurs in all directions. Often seen in individuals with diabetes, it also occurs in association with stroke, myocardial infarction (MI), cervical radiculopathy, and other conditions. It is more common in women and most often occurs in the fifth decade. Patients often complain first about overhead arm motions, such as hair combing. The common underlying factor is prolonged immobility of the arm. Thickening of the joint capsule with adhesion formation takes place.

Treatment of adhesive capsulitis involves pain relief, restoration of motion, and correction of any contributing cause. Patients recover in 2 to 3 years with analgesics alone. Recovery can be hastened to 6 to 8 weeks with steroid injections and physical therapy.

A classic impingement syndrome or subacromial bursitis would be most painful with abduction. Glenohumeral joint arthritis is relatively rare.

21–23. The answers are: 21-B, 22-B, 23-D. (*Internal medicine, obstetrics/gynecology*)
Hirsutism is defined as the excessive growth of androgen-responsive terminal hair in women. Dark, thick, terminal hair is found on the pubis, axilla, back, face, chest, and abdomen. Androgens, including dehydroepiandrosterone of the adrenal glands, androstenedione of the ovary, and testosterone of the ovary (primarily), cause an increase in the number and thickness of terminal hairs in these regions. Causes of hirsutism are classified as ovarian, adrenal, drug-related, idiopathic, or genetic. Ovarian disorders include polycystic ovary syn-

drome and ovarian tumors. Adrenal disorders include congenital adrenal hyperplasia, Cushing syndrome, and adrenal tumors. Drugs associated with hirsutism include cyclosporine, phenytoin, corticosteroids, and danazol. The presumed cause of idiopathic hirsutism is increased androgen-receptor sensitivity to normal androgen levels.

Polycystic ovary syndrome, the most common identifiable cause of androgen hypersecretion in women, is thought to be a luteinizing hormone (LH) hypersecretion abnormality. Patients present with obesity, anovulation, hirsutism, infertility, and enlarged cystic ovaries by ultrasound. Some patients have few or no symptoms. Laboratory tests often find an increased LH/follicle-stimulating hormone (LH/FSH) ratio. In polycystic ovary syndrome, the LH/FSH ratio is usually greater than 2.5; however, it can be lower.

History and physical examination should guide the workup. This 31-year-old patient is unlikely to have new-onset polycystic ovary syndrome, which typically begins between 15 and 25 years of age. However, polycystic ovary syndrome is still part of the differential diagnosis. The absence of hypertension and the normal body habitus argue against Cushing syndrome. The development of symptoms later in life and the rapid progression should prompt suspicion of a more serious underlying cause, such as an ovarian or adrenal tumor. To rule out an ovarian mass, which is found in about 50% of women with ovarian tumors, a bimanual pelvic examination is warranted. Testosterone levels of greater than 2.0 ng/mL suggest an androgen-secreting ovarian or adrenal tumor. In polycystic ovary syndrome, the total testosterone level is mildly elevated in 40% to 60% of patients. Dehydroepiandrosterone sulfate (DHEAS) levels of greater than 700 μg/dL suggest an adrenal tumor. In polycystic ovary syndrome, DHEAS is usually normal. For a patient with elevated testosterone levels but normal DHEAS levels, the search for an ovarian tumor should commence with ultrasound, CT, or MRI of the pelvis. CT of the abdomen would be inadequate. A dexamethasone suppression test is appropriate if Cushing syndrome is suspected.

Finasteride is a 5α-reductase inhibitor that inhibits the conversion of testosterone to dihydrotestosterone, the more "active" androgen. Leuprolide is a gonadotropic-releasing hormone agonist that can decrease LH and FSH levels when given continuously. Flutamide is an androgen receptor blocker, as is spironolactone and cyproterone. In addition, cyproterone effectively suppresses androgen secretion.

24. The answer is C. (*Obstetrics/gynecology*)
Postmenopausal bleeding should always prompt the suspicion of endometrial cancer. Nearly all women with endometrial cancer present with some form of vaginal bleeding. Important risk factors for the development of endometrial cancer include advancing age, history of a first-degree relative with endometrial cancer, obesity, diabetes mellitus, polycystic ovary syndrome, and postmenopausal estrogen use. There is also an association with breast and colon cancer. Of note, use of combined estrogen–progestin oral contraception protects against the development of endometrial cancer. Management of this patient next entails referral for endometrial sampling. A trial of progestin is useful in secondary amenorrhea to exclude abnormalities of the hypothalamic–pituitary axis. Pelvic ultrasound may show uterine abnormalities, but it is not a substitute for a biopsy in this case. A CA-125 level is elevated in ovarian cancer, not in endometrial cancer.

25. The answer is C. (*Obstetrics/gynecology*)
Recurrent vaginal yeast infections may often be a clue to an underlying medical condition. Cell-mediated immunity is critical in defending against fungal infections; such defects may be secondary to medications such as corticosteroids. Any impairment in this arm of the immune system may lead to recurrent fungal infections. In addition, the normal vaginal flora is important in the prevention of yeast infections, and any perturbation can lead to recurrent infections. A woman who is taking chronic antibiotics may be more prone to recurrent candidal infections. Other medical conditions that should be considered in women with recurrent yeast infections include diabetes mellitus and HIV. Except for diabetes mellitus, the conditions presented in the answer choices are not associated with recurrent yeast infections.

26–29. The answers are: 26-C, 27-C, 28-D, 29-C. (*Internal medicine*)

This patient has osteoarthritis and a history consistent with gout. Both of these conditions increase his risk of joint infection at some point in his life; his joint is not entirely normal. The most common causes of acute monoarthritis are trauma, gout, pseudogout, and infection. A warm joint should be presumed to be infected until proven otherwise. An infection can destroy a joint within hours, and immediate joint aspiration is essential to rule out infection. In addition, a cell count and culture should be obtained and the fluid evaluated for crystals. Negatively birefringent crystals are consistent with gout; positively birefringent crystals with pseudogout. Crystal arthropathy may occur in an infected joint. The presence of crystals does not rule out infection. Joint aspiration is necessary regardless of results on MRI or radiography. The rate of onset may provide a clue; infection and gout occur within hours to days, whereas pseudogout evolves during several days. Onset over weeks to months suggests an inflammatory arthritis such as Reiter syndrome or spondyloarthropathy. These diseases are often preceded by an inflammatory diarrhea or other infection.

The cell count is important. Normal synovial fluid contains less than 200 white blood cells (WBCs)/mm^3. With reactive arthritis or rheumatoid arthritis, the number of WBCs may be 20,000 to 50,000/mm^3. With a septic joint or gout, the WBC count is typically higher than 50,000/mm^3. A WBC count of higher than 100,000/mm^3 suggests infection. In addition, the higher the percentage of neutrophils (generally $> 75\%$), the greater the likelihood of infection.

Staphylococcus aureus is the most common pathogen isolated in native joint infectious arthritis. *Staphylococcus epidermidis* should be considered in prosthetic joints. Gram-negative rods, which occur most commonly in patients with chronic debilitating disease or those taking immunosuppressive agents, represent only 5% of infections. *Salmonella* can be seen in patients with sickle cell disease, while *Neisseria* is seen in those with C5 to C8 complement deficiency. Tuberculosis is now a rare cause; it often requires synovial biopsy to accurately make the diagnosis.

Because the suspicion of infection is high, antibiotics are the treatment of choice. The presence of *S. aureus* is important to recognize when choosing an antibiotic empirically. Colchicine is the most importance intervention for acute gouty arthritis; allopurinol should not be used in this setting because it may acutely exacerbate gouty flares. Prednisone is occasionally used in recalcitrant cases of gout. Naproxen, a nonsteroidal anti-inflammatory drug (NSAID), is also helpful in the treatment of crystal arthropathies.

30. The answer is C. (*Emergency medicine*)

In an individual with severe asthma, rapid tapering of corticosteroids can lead to addisonian crisis, which is typified by hypotension. This patient, recently in the ICU for asthma exacerbation, is likely still taking corticosteroids. The history of the patient throwing away her medications points to addisonian crisis as the most likely answer. A normal pulmonary examination and midline trachea exclude the diagnosis of a pneumothorax as a cause of the hypotension. The normal respiratory rate makes narcotic overdose unlikely. A patient with an acute intracerebral hemorrhage is usually hypertensive and bradycardic; thus a CT of the head does not have to be emergent. Broad-spectrum antibiotic therapy is indicated for the treatment of sepsis and the resulting hypotension.

31. The answer is D. (*Emergency medicine, internal medicine*)

The history, physical examination, and diagnostic studies are indicative of an aortic dissection. The chest radiograph demonstrates a widened mediastinum. Acute medical therapy is indicated to provide rapid control of blood pressure while the definitive diagnosis is being pursued. Antihypertensive therapy should control blood pressure as well as decrease cardiac contractility and shear force on the aorta. β-Blockers are ideal agents for this purpose. Often a more potent agent is required; a combination of a β-blocker with sodium nitroprusside or labetalol as a single agent is used. Sodium nitroprusside cannot be utilized alone because it leads to a reflex tachycardia and increased shear force. Definitive therapy is determined by whether the dissection is proximal or distal. Proximal dissections require prompt surgical intervention, whereas distal dissections can be initially managed medically.

32–33. The answers are: 32-A, 33-C. (*Statistics*)
This project is a cohort study. The starting point is the identification of subjects with an exposure of interest (in this case, blood transfusion). The researcher then checks for the occurrence of an end point (in this case, presence of hepatitis C) in exposed and unexposed groups at a later time. A case-control study is different: individuals with and without a disease are studied, and information is gathered about previous exposures. A randomized trial involves the random assigning of individuals to exposures or treatments. A retrospective trial involves following individual cases over time and looking for an end point.

The relative risk of a given individual developing hepatitis C if exposed to a blood transfusion can be determined by dividing the incidence rate of hepatitis C in both groups (12.6% ÷ 2.2% = 5.7%):

Incidence rate in transfused subjects	75/595 = 0.126
Incidence rate in nontransfused subjects	16/712 = 0.022

The result indicates that the incidence rate of hepatitis C is 5.6 times higher in those who received transfusions.

34–35. The answers are: 34-D, 35-D. (*Internal medicine*)
Male infertility generally occurs secondary to a limited number of factors. The most common causes include anatomic problems, such as obstruction of the seminal vesicles; adrenal disorders, with low testosterone levels; prolactinomas; and genetic abnormalities.

It is easy to diagnose obstruction by measuring the fructose level in semen. Typically, the secretions of the seminal vesicle are high in fructose, and a low fructose level indicates an obstructive process. Furthermore, no sperm should be present.

The finding of oligospermia, along with low follicle-stimulating hormone (FSH), luteinizing hormone (LH), and testosterone levels, suggests prolactinoma. Alcohol abuse can cause direct testicular damage resulting in low testosterone but high FSH and LH values. Primary hypothyroidism leads to an increase in thyrotropin-releasing hormone, which may cause hyperprolactinemia with low FSH, low LH, and low testosterone values. However, prolactinoma is a more common cause. Measurement of a prolactin level and MRI of the pituitary is the next management step.

36–39. The answers are: 36-D, 37-B, 38-D, 39-B. (*Internal medicine*)
This murmur is consistent with aortic stenosis. A loud systolic ejection murmur heard over the aortic position (second right intercostal space) is characteristic of this condition. In addition, an associated thrill is often present in the suprasternal notch or in the second right intercostal space. Aortic regurgitation is characterized by a high-frequency, early diastolic decrescendo murmur, which is best heard at the aortic position and left sternal border. Mitral regurgitation is characterized by a high-pitched holosystolic murmur heard loudest at the apex and radiating to the axilla. Mitral stenosis is characterized by a mid-diastolic murmur with a rumbling quality that has presystolic accentuation and is best heard at the cardiac apex. Tricuspid regurgitation gives rise to a soft holosystolic murmur heard along the right sternal border.

Aortic stenosis is commonly secondary to a congenitally bicuspid aortic valve, which becomes calcified and more rigid during the years and leads to outflow obstruction. Other causes of aortic stenosis include rheumatic fever, valve degeneration, and unicuspid valves. Often the physical examination can provide valuable clues to the severity of the valve lesion. The findings most indicative of more severe stenosis include a late-peaking murmur, a diminished A_2 component of the second heart sound (S_2), a delayed and weak carotid upstroke (pulsus parvus et tardus), and paradoxical splitting of the second heart sound (S_2). The loudness of the murmur does not correlate with the severity of the lesion. An early systolic ejection click is commonly heard when the valve is still mobile (i.e., early in the course of disease).

The ECG is usually normal until the stenosis becomes severe, at which time left ventricular hypertrophy may be seen. One of the ECG hallmarks of left ventricular hypertrophy is increased voltage in the limb leads. Supraventricular tachycardias are not specifically associated with aortic stenosis. Q waves are seen after transmural myocardial infarctions (MIs). Left axis deviation is more characteristic of left ventricular hypertrophy than right axis deviation.

Close follow-up (minimum: every 12 months) is essential in asymptomatic patients with aortic stenosis to determine whether symptoms secondary to the valve lesion, including angina, heart failure, and syncope, are present. Symptomatic patients should be referred for valve replacement. In addition, patients with aortic stenosis are at increased risk of bacterial endocarditis; they should receive antibiotic prophylaxis at the time of invasive procedures.

40–42. The answers are: 40-B, 41-C, 42-A. (*Emergency medicine, pediatrics*)
The rash is consistent with that seen in Henoch-Schönlein purpura, one of the hypersensitivity vasculitides. It usually affects children from 4 to 7 years of age but can occur in adults, in whom it has a worse prognosis. The disease is slightly more common in women and has a seasonal variation with a peak incidence in spring. It is believed to represent a hypersensitivity reaction to an antigenic stimulation from a substance such as an infection or drug.

Most patients with Henoch-Schönlein purpura have venulitis with inflammation of the postcapillary venules. The histopathologic hallmark of the disorder is leukocytoclasis, which refers to the occurrence of neutrophilic nuclear debris in and around the involved vessels. Palpable purpura (usually over the buttocks and down the legs), arthralgia, abdominal pain, and glomerulitis are also characteristic. IgA immune complexes are often seen on biopsy.

As with most inflammatory vasculitides, Henoch-Schönlein purpura results in an elevated erythrocyte sedimentation rate (ESR). Microscopic hematuria is evidence of renal involvement, and increased creatinine is a sign of overt renal failure. Anemia and liver involvement is not characteristic.

In children, Henoch-Schönlein purpura usually remits after approximately 1 week without therapy; however, it may recur for weeks to months. Occasionally, treatment consists of prednisone 1 mg/kg per day. Patients with renal involvement might benefit from plasmapheresis.

43–45. The answers are: 43-C, 44-D, 45-E. (*Emergency medicine, pediatrics*)
Anaphylaxis, a life-threatening multisystem disorder, results from exposure of a sensitized immune system to an allergen. The binding of IgE to activated mast cells leads to widespread release of histamine, leukotrienes, and other inflammatory mediators. Typical antigens that result in anaphylaxis include antibiotics, insect stings, foods, inhaled allergens, and other medications. The reaction incited by the antigen may elicit symptoms ranging from hives and local reaction to circulatory collapse and shock.

This patient, who presents with respiratory distress and early signs of shock, requires emergent therapy. Initial treatment should include epinephrine at a dose of 0.01 mg/kg (1:1,000 dilution). It is important to note the correct dose of epinephrine; the dilution of 1:10,000 is appropriate only in the setting of cardiac arrest, when 1 mg is given. The other agents listed as answer choices in question 43 are ancillary medications that should also be used, but only after epinephrine is given.

Clearly, this patient should be transported to an ED. Slowly released substances of anaphylaxis may lead to recurrence of symptoms in the next few hours. Therefore, all patients require monitoring for at least 4 to 6 hours. It is important to realize that the risks associated with anaphylaxis do not disappear after an initial response to epinephrine. Furthermore, treatment with diphenhydramine, H_2-receptor antagonists, and corticosteroids may prevent these later symptoms and lead to more rapid recovery. Intravenous hydration should also be given to any patient with hypotension. Antivenin plays no role in the treatment of anaphylaxis.

46–48. The answers are: 46-C, 47-A, 48-E. (*Internal medicine*)
In any patient older than 50 years with a fever of unknown origin, giant cell arteritis (temporal arteritis) must be considered. An erythrocyte sedimentation rate (ESR) is a good screening test. Typically, the ESR is

greater than 100 mm/hour. A history of headache, fever, and jaw claudication should further prompt suspicion. Immediate temporal artery biopsy is the gold standard. Prednisone 1 mg/kg per day is necessary immediately if any suspicion of disease exists (as in this patient) because ischemic optic neuropathy can be sight-threatening.

Generally, biopsy is necessary within 24 to 72 hours of initiation of steroids. However, some studies have found that temporal artery biopsy is useful up to 2 weeks following the initiation of steroids. It is important to note that a negative biopsy does not completely rule out giant cell arteritis. Because the vasculitis occurs in skip lesions, it may be missed. A 5-cm biopsy is optimal, and 1-mm cuts should be made when looking at the pathology. Bilateral biopsies are still only 70% to 80% sensitive, so a repeat biopsy is necessary.

The use of ESR is controversial other than in evaluation of vasculitides, such as temporal arteritis and polymyalgia rheumatica. Fibrinogen, the most abundant acute phase reactant, has the greatest effect on the elevation of ESR. Hyperalbuminemia only increases the ESR in conjunction with fibrinogen and immunoglobulins. Positively charged proteins such as paraproteins (as seen in myeloma and Waldenström macroglobulinemia) prevent the normal repelling action of the negatively charged red blood cells (RBCs), causing rouleaux formation and an increased ESR. The ESR increases with age alone. Macrocytic RBCs have a decreased surface-to-volume ratio and, thus, have less charge relative to their mass, which increases "aggregation" and the ESR. Hypoalbuminemic states also tend to increase the ESR.

49–51. The answers are: 49-A, 50-E, 51-B. (*Emergency medicine, pediatrics*)
Child abuse is all too common in society. The key to recognition of this devastating problem is a high degree of suspicion on the part of health care workers. Abuse may assume several forms: physical, emotional, psychologic, medical, or educational. Only with a careful history and physical examination can a practitioner obtain clues to the diagnosis. Often, an abused child is less than 4 years of age, handicapped or temperamental, and premature. Abusive parents often suffer from depression, low self-esteem, and substance abuse and may have a history of mental illness or criminal behavior. Financial problems and marital difficulties increase stress in the home in many cases.

Interestingly, because a child is more likely to be brought to the attention of a health care provider for an unrelated problem than a condition secondary to a complication of abuse, a high index of suspicion is imperative. Characteristics of the history that should lead to suspicion include injuries inconsistent with the history, patients reluctant to give information, and delay in seeking health care for serious injuries. In this case, the upper arm bruises are a key clue that should alert the physician to the possibility of abuse.

Careful observation makes it possible to determine the age of the bruise with a relatively high degree of accuracy. Bruises typically undergo a stereotypical transformation over time. In the first 24 hours, the bruise is typically red with some blue or purple discoloration. In the next 1 to 3 days, the bruise become blue to blue-brown. After 5 to 7 days, the bruise develops a green discoloration. Finally, after 10 days, the bruise becomes yellow. This information is important in obtaining objective verification of a parent's description of the injury. If the father's account of the injury is correct, the bruises should be red.

It is important to make sure that the bruising may not reflect an underlying medical condition. Coagulation defects, thrombocytopenia, and platelet disorders also can lead to bruises. Furthermore, it is important to rule out underlying fractures. A urinalysis would not provide any useful information.

With suspected child abuse, the correct action is to immediately notify protective services and a social worker. Admission to the hospital is indicated only if the condition of the child requires it. The other answer choices presented in question 51 are not appropriate responses.

52–54. The answers are: 52-A, 53-C, 54-E. (*Internal medicine*)
Colonic polyps come in many varieties. Tubular adenomas, which are common and occur in more than 10% of adults, are malignant in less than 10% of cases. Villous adenomas are more of a concern; they are malignant in approximately 33% of cases. Tubulovillous adenomas share characteristics of both tubular and villous polyps and are of intermediate malignant potential. Hamartomatous polyps, which are seen in juvenile poly-

posis and Peutz-Jeghers syndrome, are benign. Inflammatory polyps are seen primarily in inflammatory bowel disease and have no malignant potential. However, patients with inflammatory bowel disease are at increased risk for colon cancer (especially with ulcerative colitis).

Most polyps are either sessile (flat and extensively attached to the mucosa), or pedunculated (attached by a stalk). Tubular and tubulovillous adenomas are generally pedunculated. Villous adenomas are typically sessile, which is more worrisome for malignancy. The larger the adenoma, the more concern for malignancy.

Villous adenomas are usually located in the rectosigmoid colon and require segmental resection. Tubular adenomas can be removed endoscopically and require screening with colonoscopy within 3 to 5 years.

Of the polyposis syndromes, Gardner syndrome (multiple soft tissue tumors), Cronkhite-Canada syndrome (alopecia, fingernail dystrophy, and cutaneous hyperpigmentation), Cowden syndrome (polyposis with breast and thyroid cancers), and familial polyposis syndrome (associated with the adenomatous polyposis coli gene) have malignant potential. It should be noted that there is some controversy concerning whether the polyps in Cowden syndrome are premalignant; some studies do not support an increased risk of malignancy. In Peutz-Jeghers syndrome, the hamartomatous adenomas are associated with buccal mucosal hyperpigmentation.

55–57. The answers are: 55-E, 56-D, 57-B. (*Internal medicine*)
This patient has acne rosacea with an associated rhinophyma. Acne rosacea, which is rare in individuals younger than 30 years, is an inflammatory disorder that predominantly affects the face. Erythema, telangiectasias, and superficial pustules occur. Patients often describe worsening flushing after the ingestion of alcohol, exposure to heat, emotional stimuli, spicy foods, or hot drinks. With progression, the flushing can become permanent with subsequent connective tissue deposition of the nose (rhinophyma). Complications include iritis, keratitis, blepharitis, and chalazion.

Studies have shown that topical metronidazole is effective. Although oral tetracyclines may be beneficial, systemic treatment should be avoided if possible. Skin biopsy is rarely warranted. Fluorinated topical steroids may cause flares of rosacea. Trimethoprim-sulfamethoxazole is not a typical therapy for rosacea.

58–63. The answers are: 58-D, 59-E, 60-D, 61-C, 62-C, 63-B. (*Psychiatry, emergency medicine, internal medicine*)
This patient's constellation of symptoms should prompt the suspicion of schizophrenia as the cause of behavioral change. This devastating illness affects young adults, leading to severe impairment in thought, speech, and behavior.

It is essential to consider and rule out other conditions that may mimic schizophrenia before making the diagnosis. Bipolar disorder, especially in the manic phase of illness, may cause disordered thinking similar to that seen in schizophrenia. A key to distinguishing these disorders is that bipolar illness is generally intermittent with symptom-free periods, unlike schizophrenia. In addition, phencyclidine or hallucinogen use may also lead to symptoms nearly identical to that of schizophrenia. However, anxiety disorders do not share common features with schizophrenia. Anxiety disorders are typically characterized by excessive worry and tension and not by disordered thought processes.

In schizophrenia, the general level of functioning deteriorates over time. The *Diagnostic and Statistical Manual of Mental Disorders,* fourth edition (DSM-IV), lists characteristic symptoms of schizophrenia as follows:

Delusions
Hallucinations
Disorganized speech
Grossly disorganized or catatonic behavior
Negative symptoms such as affective flattening

Because family histories of mood disorders are relatively frequent and nonspecific, they provide no support to the diagnosis of schizophrenia. Symptoms in schizophrenia are progressive and not intermittent. Memory impairment and disorientation would support a medical cause for the patient's symptoms and are more typical of dementing illnesses.

Regarding the natural history of schizophrenia, it is clear that with each recurrence of severe illness, the prognosis worsens and impairment becomes more severe. The onset of schizophrenia generally occurs in the second or third decade of life, not the fourth. Most patients do suffer from prodromal symptoms before the full-blown disease becomes manifest, including depression, social withdrawal, suspiciousness, restlessness, and difficulty concentrating. In contrast to society's perceptions, the majority of persons with schizophrenia are not dangerous to others. However, the suicide rate in affected individuals is significantly elevated. Finally, it is believed that the acute, sudden onset of schizophrenic symptoms, especially when associated with a specific, identifiable stressor, may predict a better prognosis.

Typical neuroleptic drugs act to antagonize the D_2-dopamine receptor and are characterized by the unpleasant side effects of movement disorders (dystonias). These agents block the dopamine receptor, remove the negative effects of dopamine on the secretion of prolactin, and characteristically elevate prolactin levels. Generally, neuroleptic agents require 2 weeks to reach equilibration in body concentration, and thus, changes in medications should generally occur from 2 to 4 weeks after starting the drug. Psychosis usually resolves 2 to 6 weeks after the institution of treatment. The dosage that effectively controlled symptoms in the hospital should be continued in the outpatient setting, and major reductions in dosage are generally not appropriate until 3 to 6 months after discharge. One of the serious side effects of neuroleptics is tardive dyskinesia. This disorder, which is often irreversible after cessation of the medication, is typified by repetitive, involuntary movements of the mouth, tongue, and other body structures. Anticholinergic drugs may actually make this condition worse and certainly do not improve symptoms.

Neuroleptic malignant syndrome occurs in less than 1% of patients taking neuroleptic agents, but it has a mortality rate slightly higher than 10% and is a feared complication of the use of antipsychotic medications. Typical symptoms include hyperthermia, muscular rigidity, and altered consciousness. Drugs that block the D_2-receptor have the greatest potential for causing this disease. Rhabdomyolysis is common secondary to hyperthermia and muscle rigidity. Other complications include renal failure, seizures, cardiovascular collapse, disseminated intravascular coagulation (DIC), hepatic failure, aspiration pneumonia, and death. Serum sodium and serum calcium levels are typically in the normal range. Respiratory acidosis can occur but generally is seen in late stages and portends a high mortality. Thyroid-stimulating hormone (TSH) levels are within the normal range.

The goals of neuroleptic malignant syndrome treatment are to reduce temperature and muscle rigidity and to provide supportive care to ensure that complications such as pneumonia do not occur. Dantrolene, a commonly used therapeutic agent, reduces thermogenesis by uncoupling muscle contracture and may act to alter dopamine metabolism. Other agents that have been used successfully include muscle paralytics, bromocriptine, amantadine, and levodopa. The other agents listed as answer choices in question 63 are not effective in the treatment of neuroleptic malignant syndrome.

64–66. The answers are: 64-D, 65-E, 66-B. (*Pediatrics*)
An undescended testis (cryptorchidism) is the most common disorder of sexual differentiation in boys. In term infants, the incidence is 3.4%, and in premature neonates, the condition is more common. Cryptorchidism is bilateral in 10% to 20% of cases. Most undescended testes descend spontaneously by 3 months, but those that remain undescended by 6 months are unlikely to descend spontaneously. In an operation (orchiopexy), most testes can be brought down to the scrotum. This surgery is warranted at 9 to 15 months of age. Clinical trials have shown that hormonal treatment is not as effective.

Consequences of cryptorchidism include infertility, malignancy, torsion, and associated hernias. Following treatment for unilateral cryptorchidism, 85% of patients are fertile; with bilateral cryptorchidism, the value is

50% to 65%. The risk of malignancy, which is more common with bilateral cryptorchidism, is 4 to 10 times higher than that in the general population. The peak age for tumors is 15 to 45 years. The most common tumor is seminoma (65%). Although orchiopexy does not decrease the risk of cancer, it does decrease the proportion of cancers that are seminomatous to 30%.

67–68. The answers are: 67-D, 68-D. (*Internal medicine*)

This patient underwent splenectomy, which appeared to be effective initially, as it is in approximately 60% of patients with idiopathic thrombocytopenic purpura. However, the smear shows no Howell-Jolly bodies, which suggests an incomplete splenectomy. A radionuclide spleen scan could find evidence of an accessory spleen.

Patients with a history of splenectomy are at particular risk of infection by encapsulated organisms such as *Pneumococcus, Haemophilus influenzae,* and *Neisseria* species. Infection with *Babesia* or *Capnocytophaga canimorsus* puts patients at particular risk of increased mortality.

69–72. The answers are: 69-E, 70-C, 71-D, 72-E. (*Internal medicine*)

Malignant melanoma represents 3% to 5% of all skin cancers but accounts for up to 65% of all deaths from this disease. Affected patients are generally fair-skinned, have a history of becoming sunburned easily, and are younger than patients with other forms of skin cancers. One of the greatest risk factors for the development of malignant melanoma is intermittent, unaccustomed, sun exposure. Malignant melanoma is also associated with genetic conditions such as familial dysplastic nevi syndrome and xeroderma pigmentosum. Important factors in the evaluation of the skin lesions that should prompt suspicion of malignant melanoma can be easily remembered as the "ABCDs":

Asymmetry	Irregular elevation, nodularity, or indentation
Borders	Irregular borders or borders that blend or are difficult to visualize
Color	Variation of color across a lesion (rather than the actual color)
Degeneration	Ulceration, itching, bleeding, or rapid changes

In malignant melanoma, lesion location on the arms is a predictor of a somewhat better prognosis; perhaps this relates to earlier diagnosis and treatment. Poor prognostic factors include male sex, lesion location on the posterior neck and scalp, lesion ulceration, depth greater than 0.75 mm, and any invasion through the basement membrane into the papillary dermis or reticular dermis.

Cutaneous squamous cell carcinoma and basal cell carcinoma make up the bulk of nonmelanoma skin cancers. However, basal cell cancer occurs 3 to 4 times more frequently than squamous cell cancer. Because both types are related to chronic sun exposure, lesions often occur on parts of the body that commonly receive the most sun exposure. For squamous cell carcinoma, specific risk factors include immunosuppression, old scars and burns (Marjolin ulcers), venous stasis ulcers, and the presence of precursor lesions, such as those in actinic keratosis and Bowen disease. The lesions are typically red or brown, with crusted, hyperkeratotic surfaces and poorly defined borders. Squamous cell carcinomas do metastasize and do so *more* frequently than basal cell cancers. Poor prognostic factors include depth of penetration, overall size, older age, immunosuppression, and recurrent lesions.

According to the patient's description, his second lesion is basal cell carcinoma. This slow-growing malignancy rarely metastasizes but may lead to problems from local invasion and is often nodular, pearly, and translucent. Excision with wide local margins, which is associated with a 95% to 99% cure rate, is necessary.

73–76. The answers are: 73-C, 74-D, 75-A, 76-A. (*Internal medicine*)

The skin finding is consistent with erythema nodosum, an acutely tender and nodular skin eruption with marked erythema and bruising secondary to inflammation of subcutaneous fat (panniculitis). Erythema nodosum, which is more common in women, occurs commonly between 25 and 40 years of age. Triggers include infection, drugs, neoplasia, and autoimmune disorders. The most common cause is streptococcal infection, usually a pharyngitis, as in this patient. Other causes include tuberculosis, coccidioidomycosis, histoplasmosis, cytomegalovirus, Epstein-Barr virus, *Mycoplasma, Salmonella, Yersinia,* sarcoidosis, systemic lupus erythematosus, sulfonamides, penicillins, oral contraceptives, gold salts, and aspirin.

In erythema nodosum triggered by streptococcal infection, there is usually a preceding sore throat and a rise in the antistreptolysin O (ASO) titer. Given other possible causes of the disease, it would be reasonable to order a chest radiograph (sarcoidosis, infection), a skin biopsy (confirmatory of erythema nodosum), and an antinuclear antibody (ANA) (systemic lupus erythematosus). An erythrocyte sedimentation rate (ESR) is extremely nonspecific and not useful in this setting.

The nodules are exquisitely tender and are normally situated on the anterior tibial region. Initially, they are light red; later, they become dark red. The acute illness resolves in 6 to 8 weeks. Recurrence is unusual and should suggest lymphoma. Arthropathy, most commonly of the ankles, occurs in 50% of cases. Erythema nodosum is generally self-limited, and observation is appropriate initially. If the acute pain persists, a short course of steroids is indicated. A course of oral potassium iodide or hydroxychloroquine is an alternative to steroids.

The ANA is approximately 95% sensitive in making the diagnosis of systemic lupus erythematosus; 95 of 100 patients with systemic lupus erythematosus have a positive ANA. The anti-ssDNA antibody is positive in patients with cutaneous lupus. The anti-dsDNA antibody is not as sensitive (70%) as the ANA for systemic lupus erythematosus, but it is more specific and often correlates with disease activity. The anti-Smith antibody is approximately 30% sensitive for systemic lupus erythematosus but is also more specific than ANA for systemic lupus erythematosus. Finally, the anti-Ro antibody is seen in Sjögren syndrome and in cutaneous lupus.

77–79. The answers are: 77-D, 78-D, 79-C. (*Internal medicine, critical care medicine*)
Acute renal failure, which may lead to a mortality rate as high as 50% to 90%, is a common occurrence in severely ill patients. The renal failure generally results from acute tubular necrosis (ATN). The numerous causes of ATN include drugs (aminoglycosides), radiographic contrast agents, sepsis, and hypotension. Acute renal failure in patients in ICUs may also result from prerenal azotemia from hypovolemia, glomerular diseases, tubulointerstitial diseases, and postrenal (obstructive) failure. It is imperative to determine the patient's volume status in the process of determining the cause of the renal failure. Is oliguria (urine output <400 to 500 mL/24 hours) present as a result of dehydration or is it a result of ATN?

The determination of volume status in patients in the ICU may be extremely difficult. In this setting, placement of a pulmonary artery catheter may be helpful. The occurrence of a low pulmonary capillary wedge pressure supports volume depletion and may lead to a trial of intravenous fluids. Although the urine sodium is generally low in the presence of volume depletion, ATN from contrast agents may also cause a low urine sodium. Furthermore, diuretic therapy may lead to a falsely elevated urine sodium, as in this patient. The value of urine urea may sometimes be helpful; however, in ICU patients who are catabolic, this result is often difficult to interpret. Blood pressure and heart rate in the setting of sepsis and pressor support do not provide any indication of volume status.

Microscopic urinalysis can be invaluable when diagnosing the cause of renal failure. The finding of muddy-brown granular casts, which represent trapped tubular cells that have been sloughed from the injured renal tubules, support the diagnosis of ATN. Red blood cell (RBC) casts are typical of glomerulonephritis, white blood cell (WBC) casts are seen in pyelonephritis, and double-refractile fat bodies occur in the nephrotic syndrome.

Indications for hemodialysis in patients in the ICU include severe acidosis; severe hyperkalemia (not responsive to other therapies); volume overload; uremic pericarditis; and, according to some experts, serum creatinine greater than 10 mg/dL and serum blood urea nitrogen (BUN) greater than 100 mg/dL. In this patient, with oliguria, the institution of approximately 1 to 2 L of total parenteral nutrition (TPN) would rapidly lead to severe volume overload; therefore, hemodialysis would be necessary.

80–83. The answers are: 80-E, 81-D, 82-D, 83-A. (*Obstetrics/gynecology*)

Menstrual disorders are among the most common reasons that women seek medical attention. Secondary amenorrhea, the most common type, is defined clinically as the absence of menstruation for at least 6 months in women with previously normal cycles. Unexpected pregnancy is the leading cause of secondary amenorrhea in young women. Despite the lack of menses for 6 months, a β-human chorionic gonadotropin (β-hCG) level is the most important test to order initially. After pregnancy has been ruled out, levels of thyroid-stimulating hormone (TSH), glucose, and prolactin warrant checking; hypothyroidism, diabetes mellitus, and hyperprolactinemia are all treatable causes of secondary amenorrhea. A search for signs of virilization is warranted. Examination of the external genitalia and a pelvic examination might suggest hyperandrogenism (e.g., clitoromegaly). If found, a search for polycystic ovary syndrome (luteinizing hormone/follicle-stimulating hormone (LH/FSH), Cushing syndrome (cortisol), or congenital adrenal hyperplasia should begin.

No signs of virilization are evident in this patient. Thus, the next test is a progestin challenge, which tests for estrogen adequacy. Oral administration of medroxyprogesterone is given for 5 to 7 days. Abrupt withdrawal of this progestin should induce bleeding in women with adequate levels of estrogen. If there is no withdrawal bleeding, the FSH value should be checked. If the FSH level is low, it suggests a central deficiency of gonadotropic-releasing hormone (hypogonadotropic hypogonadism). If the FSH level is high, it suggests a hypergonadotropic hypogonadism (e.g., ovarian failure). Measurement of dehydroepiandrosterone sulfate (DHEAS) or testosterone would be appropriate if signs of virilization were apparent on physical examination. An ultrasound would be helpful if the pelvic examination suggested a mass.

This patient has a history of abortion, which means that she had a fully functional reproductive system 12 months ago. The manual abortion procedure can often cause adhesions within the uterus; this condition is referred to as Asherman syndrome. Because she had normal blood tests, it is unlikely that she has polycystic ovary syndrome, hyperprolactinemia, premature ovarian failure, or hypothyroidism.

Premature ovarian failure causes hypergonadotropic hypogonadism, which is associated with sarcoidosis and histiocytosis (granulomatous infiltration of the pituitary), Sheehan syndrome (ischemic pituitary disease secondary to labor), Kallmann syndrome (with anosmia), craniopharyngioma, hyperprolactinemia (causes low gonadotropic-releasing hormone), and hemochromatosis (pituitary infiltration with iron). In contrast, thyroid failure occurs with hypogonadotropic hypogonadism caused by panhypopituitarism.

84–85. The answers are: 84-E, 85-B. (*Internal medicine, emergency medicine*)

This patient presents with an acute anterior myocardial infarction (MI), and his ECG shows widespread ST-segment elevation indicative of transmural ischemia. The emergent treatment of MI is a true medical success story; dramatic improvements in survival have occurred in the past 20 years. Part of the improved survival is due to rapid recognition and treatment of the underlying pathophysiologic problem (i.e., plaque rupture and intracoronary artery thrombosis). The emergent treatment of MI in the ED must include aspirin, a β-blocker, antithrombin agent (heparin), and a means of obtaining coronary reperfusion (e.g., with a thrombolytic agent or percutaneous coronary angioplasty). The most important aspect of MI treatment is the rapid restoration of coronary perfusion—what particular method is used is of secondary significance. Generally, the use of calcium channel blockade in the setting of an acute MI is not indicated. Some data indicate that use of diltiazem may be beneficial in the setting of a non–Q wave MI. However, in the setting of ST-segment elevation and a transmural infarction, calcium channel blockade plays no role.

The most important prognostic feature post-MI is the ejection fraction. The long-term outcome of patients with significant decreases in ejection fraction (<40%) is significantly poorer. As noted previously, the particular method of opening an infarct-related artery does not matter. (Although percutaneous methods are more likely to be successful, outcomes are not significantly different as long as coronary reperfusion is obtained.) Elevated cholesterol does lead to increased risk for another MI or stroke, and treatment is appropriate. Ventricular ectopy is common in the first 24 to 48 hours after an MI and has no long-term prognostic significance. The patient's blood pressure would have no impact on survival.

86–88. The answers are: 86-C, 87-A, 88-B. (*Obstetrics/gynecology*)

Acyclovir, given by various routes, is effective in the treatment of initial and recurrent genital herpes infections. In initial episodes of genital herpes in outpatients, oral acyclovir 200 mg 5 times per day for 10 days leads to a reduction in viral shedding, symptoms, and time to healing. The decline in symptoms generally takes several days. Studies have shown that no initial acyclovir regimen results in consistent reductions in the development rate of recurrent disease.

Intravenous therapy is generally reserved for patients with severe or disseminated disease or in patients with underlying immunosuppression. In recurrent disease, acyclovir therapy initiated during the prodrome or at the first sign of lesions is associated with reduction in viral shedding and time to healing of 1.5 to 2 days, but no difference in the duration of pain.

Neonatal herpes infection may range from a mild localized infection to a severe, life-threatening systemic infection. Primary infection of the mother during pregnancy can lead to transplacental passage of virus, resulting in abortion, premature labor, skin lesions, chorioretinitis, microcephaly, or uterine growth retardation. Note that a history of maternal infection without active disease is not associated with an increased risk of abortion or prematurity. Congenital infection may manifest at the time of delivery with the previously mentioned signs along with hepatitis, jaundice, seizures, bleeding diathesis, and skin vesicles. Alternatively, neonatally acquired infections, which may be heralded by conjunctivitis with or without vesicles, may appear several days to weeks after birth. Neurologic signs generally predominate, and coma and death may occur if treatment with intravenous acyclovir is delayed.

The majority of neonatal infections occur from retrograde spread of the virus from the mother to the infant at the time of delivery as the infant passes through the infected genital tract. For this reason, it is strongly recommended that a cesarean section be performed in the setting of either active disease or complaints of symptoms consistent with a herpes viral syndrome prodrome. A Papanicolaou (Pap) smear is an insensitive screening test for active genital herpes infections and is not reliable.

Invasive cervical cancer is the second most common malignancy of the female reproductive tract. The Pap smear, which has led to dramatic decreases in mortality and morbidity from cervical cancer, is one of the greatest successes in screening for premalignant lesions. However, despite the use of this screening test, the incidence of cervical cancer has increased in younger women. The greatest contributing factor is the earlier age of participating in sexual activity. Infection with the human papilloma virus, a sexually transmitted disease, is related to cervical cancer. Various strains of the virus have displayed significant correlations with cervical cancer; women who become infected with human papilloma virus before 25 years of age are 40 times more likely to develop cervical cancer than women who are not infected. In addition, other viruses such as herpes simplex virus and Epstein-Barr virus have been implicated in cervical cancer. These viruses may act as tumor promoters or may simply be markers of high risk behavior.

As previously mentioned, the mainstay of cervical cancer control is the Pap smear. The typical false-negative rate for the Pap smear in the detection of cervical cancer is 20%. The suggested frequency of obtaining a Pap smear is controversial. Pap smears are not necessary in adolescents until they are sexually active (except for women who have been exposed to diethylstilbestrol in utero). However, all women 18 years of age and older should have a regular Pap smear even if they are not sexually active. This recommendation is based on the infrequent detection of adenocarcinoma of the cervix of such women. In women of reproductive age, the recommendation is generally for annual Pap smears, although some experts recommend screening intervals up to 2 to 3 years, especially if previous smears have been normal. There is no basis for screening every 6 months.

89–92. The answers are: 89-D, 90-B, 91-D, 92-B. (*Internal medicine, critical care medicine*)
This patient has toxic epidermal necrolysis, a clinicopathologic entity that is characterized by detachment of full-thickness epidermis. Toxic epidermal necrolysis, which has a female preponderance, occurs in older individuals and in those who use drugs. Other risk factors include HIV, bone marrow transplantation, and systemic lupus erythematosus. The primary cause of toxic epidermal necrolysis is an adverse drug reaction, although it is occasionally seen with hepatitis or *Mycoplasma* infection. (*Mycoplasma* is also a risk factor for erythema multiforme.) The most common drugs involved are sulfonamides, phenobarbital, phenytoin, carbamazepine, cephalosporins, quinolones, and allopurinol. The mean time between drug administration to the onset of symptoms is 14 days.

Toxic epidermal necrolysis usually begins with nonspecific symptoms, such as fever, cough, sore throat, and burning eyes, followed by skin and mucous membranes 1 to 3 days later. The rash, which begins on the face and upper trunk, extends rapidly. Sheet-like loss of the epidermis occurs in areas of confluent erythema. Mucosal involvement occurs in 85% to 95% of cases and usually precedes skin involvement. Extradermal involvement includes esophageal strictures, dysphagia from oropharyngeal involvement, hepatitis, pancreatitis, tracheobronchial erosions, acute respiratory distress syndrome (ARDS), anemia, lymphopenia, and sepsis. The other choices in question 91 are not immediate complications of toxic epidermal necrolysis.

Patients with toxic epidermal necrolysis should receive care in burn units. Fluid repletion is important. An early skin biopsy is important because patients with true toxic epidermal necrolysis should not receive steroids, which may benefit patients with erythema multiforme. An HIV enzyme-linked immunosorbent assay (ELISA) should be ordered but is not the most important test at this time. Silver sulfadiazine (Silvadene) should be avoided because it is a sulfonamide.

With the patient's increased oxygen requirement with a PaO_2/FIO_2 ratio of less than 250, ARDS should be suspected when the patient's temperature falls, and she becomes hypotensive, the criteria is satisfied for systemic inflammatory response syndrome, which is probably secondary to bacteremia. Sepsis, the most common cause of death in patients with toxic epidermal necrolysis, has developed. Hypovolemia, adrenal insufficiency, cardiogenic shock, and neurovascular collapse are all important causes of hypotension in critically ill patients. However, in this scenario, sepsis should be considered the most likely cause.

93. The answer is D. (*Obstetrics/gynecology, internal medicine*)
This patient, who has undergone a total hysterectomy, does not need a Papanicolaou (Pap) smear unless the surgery was for cervical cancer or dysplasia. In the majority of cases, the removal of the cervix is a common practice. Recently, some clinicians have questioned such removal. To check for the possible recurrence of cervical cancer in this case, a smear should be taken from the vaginal cuff. An annual pelvic examination is still important to screen for other reproductive tract disorders, such as ovarian cancer.

94–97. The answers are: 94-D, 95-A, 96-B, 97-D. (*Internal medicine, surgery*)
This patient, with intermittent claudication progressing to rest pain, gives a typical history of lower extremity arterial occlusive disease. He has significant risk factors for peripheral vascular disease, including coronary artery disease, elevated cholesterol, hypertension, and diabetes mellitus. The level of claudication, which is always below the level of arterial occlusion, may help localize the site of disease. Other important physical examination findings that may be present include reduced or absent pulses, dependent rubor, blanching of the skin on elevation, muscle atrophy, and hair loss. Skin ulcerations, a worrisome sign, signify impending gangrene. The location of ulcers secondary to arterial inflow disease is typically on the toes, heel, dorsum of the foot, or lower third of the leg. These ulcers are generally "punched out" in appearance and painful, especially at night. Venous ulcers are generally located on the ankle and are more diffuse and shallow, and those due to arterial disease often have a necrotic base. Ulcers due to diabetes are usually located on the plantar or lateral surface of the foot and are painless.

The ankle-brachial index (ABI), a comparison of blood pressures at the brachial artery with those at the ankle, is a rapid, easily performed screening test for arterial occlusive disease. Patients without significant arterial occlusive disease have ABI ratios of 0.9 to 1.0. In the setting of arterial ulcers and rest pain, the expected ratio is approximately 0.4, and this level of disease generally requires revascularization in order to salvage the limb.

The next management step is angiography, which determines the extent of arterial occlusive disease by careful examination of the degree and position of the occlusion. In addition, angioplasty provides good results for many lesions. The procedure involves examination of the entire infrarenal aorta, as well as arterial inflow to the vessels of the arch of the foot. A careful, thorough examination is required to provide a "road map" for possible revascularization by surgery.

This patient, who has occlusive disease in both the superficial femoral and popliteal arteries, would benefit most from a femoral-tibial bypass that would bring blood flow to the calf and foot. The other bypass procedures are not indicated. Femoral-femoral and axillofemoral bypasses are "extra-anatomic" bypass procedures designed to relieve inflow obstruction but do not require entering the abdomen. These procedures are indicated for high-risk surgical patients. Aortobifemoral bypass procedures are indicated for proximal arterial disease (i.e., iliac arteries). Endarterectomy, although usual for carotid artery disease, is typically not useful for lower extremity arterial occlusive disease because, while carotid disease tends to be localized, lower extremity arterial disease is more diffuse.

98–102. The answers are: 98-C, 99-D, 100-E, 101-E, 102-D. (*Internal medicine, statistics*)
The management of cholesterol is important in the primary care setting. The National Cholesterol Education Program (NCEP) guidelines recommend the screening of all individuals older than 20 years for total cholesterol and high-density lipoprotein (HDL). The desired cholesterol level is less than 200 mg/dL; for HDL, it is more than 35 mg/dL. Depending on an individual's low-density lipoprotein (LDL) value and risk factors for atherosclerotic disease, treatment may be appropriate. These risk factors include age (>45 years for men, >55 years for women [45 years if not taking estrogens]), family history of premature coronary artery disease (myocardial infarction [MI] or sudden death at <55 years for men, 65 years for women), current cigarette smoking, hypertension, diabetes mellitus, and low HDL. An HDL higher than 60 mg/dL is protective.

The presence of less than two risk factors, no heart disease, and an LDL greater than 160 mg/dL indicates that dietary therapy is necessary. Cholesterol-lowering medication is warranted if the LDL level exceeds 190 mg/dL. The presence of two or more risk factors means that dietary therapy should begin with an LDL of 130 mg/dL. Drug therapy is warranted with an LDL of 160 mg/dL. The occurrence of coronary artery disease or diabetes mellitus indicates that dietary therapy should begin with an LDL of 100 mg/dL and drug therapy with an LDL of 130 mg/dL.

In this case, the patient has three risk factors: age (she is postmenopausal), hypertension, and family history. However, her high HDL effectively makes this two risk factors. Her LDL of 145 mg/dL warrants dietary therapy only. If her LDL was greater than 160 mg/dL, drug therapy would be appropriate.

The Sixth Report of the Joint National Committee on Detection, Evaluation and Treatment of High Blood Pressure (JNC-VI) guidelines recommend β-blockers and diuretics as the first-line agents. Recently, the Antihypertensive and Lipid-Lowering Treatment to Prevent Heart Attack Trial (ALLHAT) suggested that α_1-blockers (e.g., prazosin) might be associated with increased mortality. The addition of a diuretic or β-blocker with plans to withhold this patient's prazosin might be appropriate. Prazosin is not a good choice for blood pressure control until other options have been exhausted. Angiotensin-converting enzyme (ACE) inhibitors are acceptable for individuals with diabetes and are clearly associated with decreased mortality in many settings. β-Blockers are acceptable in the setting of depression. Only propranolol with β_2-receptor blocking activity and more central nervous system (CNS) penetration are associated with depression, and no data suggest that metoprolol or atenolol are associated with depression.

In particular, a good screening test has high sensitivity. The test should be acceptable to patients. The disease should be fairly common or carry a significant burden of suffering to warrant screening. In addition, the screening test should detect disease early enough to benefit from treatment; early treatment should be more advantageous than late treatment. Specificity is more important as a confirmatory tool.

It is important to understand that the number-needed-to-screen (or treat) is the reciprocal of the *absolute risk reduction*. For example, studies often quote significant reductions in the risk of disease (e.g., 50%). If the risk decreases from 2% to 1%, the absolute risk reduction is only 1%, which might not be clinically important. The number-needed-to-screen takes this into consideration. This patient received data regarding relative risk reduction; from this, the number-needed-to-screen cannot be determined. To determine the number-needed-to-screen, the absolute risk reduction must be provided.

Because the lifetime risk of developing colorectal cancer is approximately 6%, screening is important. The American Cancer Society recommends annual fecal occult blood testing (FOBT) *and* a flexible sigmoidoscopy every 3 to 5 years after age 50 years of age. FOBT alone has been associated with a mortality benefit with a number-needed-to-screen of 339. If flexible sigmoidoscopy every 5 years is added, the number-needed-to-screen drops to 83 for men and 98 for women.

103–104. The answers are: 103-B, 104-B. (*Emergency medicine, internal medicine*)
This patient has glucose-6-phosphate dehydrogenase deficiency, an enzymatic defect that impairs the ability of red blood cells (RBCs) to defend themselves from oxidative stress. Normally, RBCs are able to detoxify oxidants produced in the setting of infection or by drugs. This detoxification relies on the production of glutathione, which in the setting of glucose-6-phosphate dehydrogenase deficiency cannot be produced in adequate amounts to prevent RBC destruction. As a consequence, oxidants damage the RBC and lead to hemolysis and precipitation of damage hemoglobin.

Numerous clinical and laboratory signs of active hemolysis are clearly apparent. The patient has jaundice secondary to the buildup of unconjugated bilirubin, a product of hemoglobin breakdown; hemoglobinuria secondary to massive release of hemoglobin in the blood and filtered in the urine; and dyspnea and tachycardia secondary to severe anemia. On a peripheral smear, Heinz bodies, or denatured and precipitated hemoglobin in RBCs, are often visible. Hypersegmented neutrophils are seen in vitamin B_{12} deficiency. Howell-Jolly bodies are RBC inclusions seen in asplenia. Schistocytes, which are seen in microangiopathic hemolytic anemias, indicate RBC shearing. Target cells, which occur with an increase in the surface-to-volume ratio of the RBCs, can be seen in a variety of conditions (e.g., thalassemia, liver disease, hemoglobin C).

Other laboratory results that occur in the setting of hemolysis include elevated lactate dehydrogenase (LDH), elevated unconjugated bilirubin, and low serum haptoglobin. There would be no reason to suspect an elevated serum creatinine or an elevate creatine kinase in this patient.

105. The answer is D. (*Internal medicine*)
The differential diagnosis of male infertility is extensive, as shown in the following list:

Varicocele
Obstruction
Infection (mumps)
Ejaculatory dysfunction
Hypogonadotropic hypogonadism
Autoimmune disorders
Psychologic conditions
Hyperprolactinemia
Cryptorchidism
Gonadotoxins (radiation, chemotherapy, drugs)
Developmental defects
Immotile cilia syndrome
Chromosomal abnormalities

The presence of gynecomastia and worsening headaches in this patient should lead to the suspicion of prolactinoma. The finding of bitemporal visual loss secondary to impingement of the tumor on the optic chiasm helps confirm this diagnosis. Further laboratory testing, including a serum prolactin level, and CT of the sella turcica would be indicated next. The other answer choices include common, benign findings that are not necessarily linked to infertility.

106–111. The answers are: 106-A, 107-E, 108-B, 109-C, 110-A, 111-B. (*Internal medicine, neurology*)
The hemophilias are X-linked coagulation disorders, which lead to the inadequate and inefficient generation of thrombin. Hemophilia A results from a deficiency in factor VIII, and hemophilia B results from a deficiency in factor IX. The clinical severity of these disorders correlates inversely with the circulating levels of plasma coagulant activity. Severe disease, with spontaneous bleeding in joints and soft tissues, results from less than 1% activity; moderate disease results from 1% to 5% activity; and mild disease, with excessive bleeding with trauma or surgery only, results from greater than 5% activity.

Severe hemophilia is manifested with bleeding typically between 18 and 21 months of age or, occasionally, at birth if labor is traumatic. The knees are the most prominent sites of spontaneous bleeding, followed by the elbows, ankles, shoulders, and hips. Bleeding from mucous membranes is due to the degradation of fibrin clots by proteolytic enzymes contained in the secretions. Bleeding of the tongue or retropharyngeal space can rapidly compromise the airway. Gastrointestinal (GI) hemorrhages typically originate from lesions proximal to the ligament of Treitz. Intracranial bleeds, the second most common cause of death after HIV/AIDS in individuals with hemophilia, occur secondary to trauma and are fatal in 30% of cases.

During episodes of minor bleeding, individuals should receive factor concentrate to reach 25% to 30% activity. When bleeding is life-threatening, the objective is a 100% level. Each unit of factor VIII concentrate/kg body weight increases activity level by 2% (1% per unit of factor IX).

This patient has coffee-ground vomitus, which prompts concern for upper GI bleeding. Assessment of vital signs is of utmost importance. This allows immediate assessment of the degree of bleeding; the hematocrit of 30% might not be reassuring in the setting of acute bleeding. Factor VIII concentrate should be given immediately. Cryoprecipitate and fresh frozen plasma are not the products of choice because of their potential to transmit bloodborne pathogens. Recombinant factor VIII avoids this problem.

The patient's liver function test abnormalities are most likely secondary to chronic hepatitis C. Virtually all individuals with hemophilia who received factor concentrate before 1985 were exposed to hepatitis C, which is more common than chronic hepatitis B in this setting. If the patient had received more blood transfusions, hemochromatosis might be a consideration.

When the patient returns with a seizure, intracranial hemorrhage, which may occur in 2% to 8% of patients, is a possibility. It is essential to consider HIV in the absence of trauma. In addition, the presence of HIV and a seizure should raise the suspicion for toxoplasmosis; 35% of affected patients present with seizure. MRI, the imaging modality of choice, usually shows bilateral lesions in the basal ganglia and corticomedullary junction. Treatment is pyrimethamine and sulfadiazine.

When the patient presents with symptoms suggestive of depression, the assessment of suicide risk is of paramount importance. Next, screening for hypothyroidism and treatment might be appropriate.

112–113. The answers are: 112-A, 113-B. (*Neurology*)
Information from the history and physical examination is used to classify a particular tremor. Several types of tremors may develop; generally, they are of three types: (1) essential, (2) Parkinson disease–associated, and (3) cerebellar disease–associated. An essential tremor is generally of 6 to 12 Hz in frequency, symmetrical, and worse with intention. Approximately 60% of patients with essential tremor have a family history of this type of tremor. A small amount of alcohol suppresses essential tremor. The tremor of Parkinson disease is a pill-rolling form with a frequency of 3 to 6 Hz that occurs at rest. Parkinson disease is also characterized by numerous other signs, such as masked facies and bradykinesia. A cerebellar tremor is present at rest and may worsen with intention; it has a slower frequency (3 to 5 Hz). Other cerebellar signs are often present.

It is important to remember that several medical conditions may lead to a tremor, most commonly hyperthyroidism and pheochromocytoma. The next step in this patient with characteristics of an essential tremor is thyroid function testing.

Treatment of essential tremor involves using nonselective β-adrenergic receptor blockers, such as propranolol. Other agents that may be effective include low-dose anxiolytics, such as diazepam and primidone. L-Dopa, bromocriptine, and benztropine are all acceptable treatments for Parkinson disease. Haloperidol, which may actually lead to dystonia, is not appropriate for the treatment of tremor.

114. The answer is E. (*Obstetrics/gynecology, emergency medicine*)
This patient has pyelonephritis, a condition that results from infection of the urinary bladder, with migration of bacteria up the ureters into the renal parenchyma. This disorder can be life-threatening in diabetes mellitus, pregnancy, or immunosuppression. Appropriate initial treatment generally involves intravenous antibiotics that cover the most likely pathogens, including *Escherichia coli, Staphylococcus saprophyticus,* and *Klebsiella pneumoniae.* Although oral antibiotics may be successful in some otherwise healthy patients with pyelonephritis, pregnant patients with diabetes mellitus, such as this one, require intravenous therapy and hospital admission. A renal ultrasound is not necessary unless there is clinical suspicion for nephrolithiasis or obstruction. Gentamicin alone would not be adequate antibacterial coverage.

115–116. The answers are: 115-D, 116-D. (*Neurology*)
The patient's funduscopic examination is typical for glaucoma, the leading cause of preventable blindness in the United States, where it affects two million people. The most common form is primary open-angle glaucoma, which leads to insidious asymptomatic vision loss that may not be detected until severe permanent vision loss occurs. The cause of glaucoma is increased intraocular pressure resulting from impaired outflow of aqueous humor. Both screening and diagnosis are simple and involve measurement of the intraocular pressure by tonometry. Assessment of the optic disc is also critical to the diagnosis, because elevated intraocular pressure leads to progressive loss of optic nerves and enlargement of the optic cup. An enlarged cup-to-disc ratio is characteristic.

Cataracts are opacities that develop in the lens of the eye that make funduscopic examination difficult but do not result in changes to the optic disc. Macular degeneration, another common cause of chronic vision loss, leads to deterioration of the retina. On funduscopic examination, changes in the macula, including the presence of hard exudates, may be apparent. There are no changes to the optic nerve. Papilledema is seen in the setting of raised intracranial pressure; this patient's history is not consistent with this condition. Temporal arteritis, an autoimmune condition, is characterized by numerous constitutional complaints and headaches that may, if untreated, lead to optic nerve ischemia and vision loss. The patient's history is inconsistent with this disorder.

Drugs that decrease aqueous humor production are the mainstay of therapy for glaucoma. These include β-adrenergic blocking agents (timolol) and carbonic anhydrase inhibitors. Other useful medications that facilitate the outflow of aqueous humor include parasympathomimetic agents, such as pilocarpine. Prednisone does not play a role in the treatment of this glaucoma; it may actually result in increased intraocular pressure.

117–121. The answers are: 117-D, 118-D, 119-C, 120-B, 121-A. (*Internal medicine, statistics*)
This patient has diarrhea that subsides while fasting, which suggests an osmotic diarrhea. One of the most common causes of osmotic diarrhea is celiac sprue, which should be considered in patients of English or Irish descent who present with diarrhea and iron deficiency anemia. A small bowel biopsy is the gold standard in making the diagnosis. The other diagnostic studies in question 117 do not aid in determining the cause of an osmotic diarrhea.

A bullous skin condition called dermatitis herpetiformis is associated with celiac sprue. Pemphigus vulgaris is a life-threatening disorder with suprabasilar epidermal separation. Bullous pemphigoid is an antibody-mediated separation of the epidermis just below the basal layer, which is most common in patients in their 60s to 70s and is usually not life-threatening. Epidermolysis bullosa is seen in children, where bullae form in areas of trauma. The best treatment for dermatitis herpetiformis is dapsone. Steroids, either oral or topical, are ineffective. Ultraviolet light–based therapies are effective in psoriasis but not in dermatitis herpetiformis. Antibiotics also play no role.

A non–anion gap acidosis may develop in a patient with diarrhea because diarrheal fluid is rich in both bicarbonate and potassium. The electrolytes should display a hypokalemic acidosis with no anion gap.

Question 121 illustrates an important concept. In choosing a test, it is essential to consider the sensitivity and specificity of the test. Recall that posttest odds of disease = pretest odds × likelihood ratio (likelihood ratio = sensitivity/[1 − specificity]). Test 1, which has a sensitivity of 89% and specificity of 94%, has a likelihood ratio of 14.8. The pretest odds = 0.5/(1.0 to 0.5) (pretest probability/[1 − pretest probability]). The posttest odds are 14.8. The posttest probability of disease = 14.8/(14.8 + 1); this is equivalent to a 93.6% chance of disease if the test is positive. Test 2, the more expensive test, which has a sensitivity of 92% and specificity of 95%, has a likelihood ratio of 18.4. For Test 2, the posttest probability of disease is 94.8%. However, this more expensive test offers a relatively small increase in probability of disease.

122–123. The answers are: 122-A, 123-C. (*Pediatrics, obstetrics/gynecology*)
This patient has primary amenorrhea, a relatively common problem with an extensive differential diagnosis, as shown in the following list:

Delayed puberty
Kallmann syndrome
Anorexia nervosa
Hypopituitarism
Hyperprolactinemia
Adrenal hyperplasia
Hypothyroidism
Pituitary tumor
Cushing disease
Craniopharyngioma

The first step in the diagnosis involves the determination of the presence of secondary sexual characteristics, such as breast development. If signs of breasts are absent, as in this adolescent girl, the first step is determination of a follicle-stimulating hormone (FSH) level. A high FSH level is indicative of gonadal dysgenesis, requiring a karyotype analysis to investigate for conditions such as Turner syndrome. A normal or low FSH is seen with hypogonadotropic hypogonadism. Hypothyroidism is rarely a cause of primary amenorrhea but can lead to secondary amenorrhea.

If signs of breast development are present, the next step is a pelvic sonogram to determine whether there is a uterus. An absent uterus is characteristic of both müllerian agenesis and androgen insensitivity. A serum testosterone value is used to distinguish between these conditions; it is elevated in androgen insensitivity. In question 123, müllerian agenesis would not be possible in the setting of a normal uterus on pelvic sonography. The presence of a uterus leads to a large differential diagnosis (see Table), and biochemical testing becomes important in determining the etiology of amenorrhea.

124–126. The answers are: 124-A, 125-A, 126-C. (*Internal medicine*)
Hypercholesterolemia is one of the most important risk factors for cardiovascular disease. Numerous clinical trials have demonstrated significant benefit (prevention of myocardial infarction [MI] and stroke) through re-

duction of low-density lipoprotein (LDL) cholesterol values and elevation of high-density lipoprotein (HDL) cholesterol values.

This patient is clearly at high risk for cardiovascular disease because of age, sex, family history, and hypertension. Ideally, his HDL should be greater than 35 mg/dL and LDL less than 130 mg/dL. However, his lipid profile indicates a mixed disorder, with a low HDL, elevated LDL, and elevated triglycerides. The 3-hydroxy-3-methyl-glutaryl coenzyme A (HMG-CoA) reductase inhibitors (e.g., simvastatin) offer the most benefit. These agents lower LDL and modestly lower triglyceride levels; they also increase HDL in some patients. Gemfibrozil is effective in lowering triglyceride levels and possibly raising HDL. However, this medication has only a negligible effect on LDL levels. Cholestyramine and colestipol, which are bile-acid binding resins, are effective in lowering LDL and raising HDL. However, these agents may significantly elevate triglyceride levels. Dietary therapy would be a useful adjunctive therapy but given such a high-risk profile, it would not be adequate alone.

Myopathy is a known complication of HMG-CoA reductase inhibitors. Its occurrence mandates discontinuation of simvastatin.

The subsequent development of severe hypertriglyceridemia results from the use of cholestyramine. Its occurrence mandates discontinuation of this agent.

127–132. The answers are: 127-C, 128-D, 129-B, 130-C, 131-D, 132-D. (*Obstetrics/gynecology, critical care medicine, pediatrics*)

Preeclampsia, or pregnancy-induced hypertension, is more common in primigravidas, especially in those younger than 20 years and older than 35 years. The pathogenesis is unknown but appears to be secondary to overvigorous vascular reactivity to endogenous pressor hormones. Risk factors for pregnancy-induced hypertension include elevated systolic blood pressure at the initial prenatal visit and obesity.

The presence of hypertension in conjunction with edema and proteinuria after the 20th week of gestation confirm the diagnosis. Hypertension is defined by two separate blood pressure readings in excess of 140/90 mm Hg at least 6 hours apart. Proteinuria is defined as a 24-hour urine protein excretion exceeding 500 mg/dL.

It is important to distinguish between mild and severe pregnancy-induced hypertension. Mild pregnancy-induced hypertension is blood pressure higher than 140/90 mm Hg but less than 160/100 mm Hg, with proteinuria of less than 5 g/24 hours. Severe pregnancy-induced hypertension is blood pressure higher than 160/110 mm Hg, with proteinuria of more than 5 g/24 hours. Other important characteristics include oliguria (<500 mL urine in 24 hours); vision changes (blurring, scotomas); and pulmonary edema.

Initially, this patient has mild pregnancy-induced hypertension and can be managed conservatively with bed rest and careful monitoring. If there is any question about ensuring close follow-up, hospitalization is necessary. If it is possible to deliver a mature infant safely, then delivery is appropriate.

In this patient, blood pressure and proteinuria worsen, despite conservative treatment. At this point, hospitalization is warranted. In the absence of oliguria and severe proteinuria, monitoring is appropriate. Emergent delivery of a premature infant at 26 weeks should be delayed as much as possible. Magnesium sulfate infusion has been shown in several studies to be useful in preventing seizures in severe pregnancy-induced hypertension. The patient clearly has severe pregnancy-induced hypertension at 28 weeks. Control of her blood pressure with an intravenous infusion of hydralazine is acceptable, a magnesium sulfate infusion is warranted, and emergent delivery of the infant is appropriate given the significant maternal risk of continuing the pregnancy.

Magnesium sulfate infusions are not without risk. High serum levels of magnesium lead to neuromuscular depression and ultimately respiratory depression and cardiac arrest. In the treatment of pregnancy-induced hypertension, the therapeutic maintenance range of magnesium levels is 4 to 7 mEq/L. The earliest sign of toxicity is the loss of patellar reflexes at 7 to 10 mEq/L; respiratory depression occurs at 10 to 15 mEq/L. The antidote for magnesium toxicity is calcium, which can be given as an intravenous infusion of 1 g of calcium gluconate. The other choices in question 129 are not appropriate; however, intubation may be necessary if the patient does not respond rapidly to the calcium infusion.

Amniocentesis may help predict lung maturity. Surfactant production generally begins during weeks 26 to 28, the terminal sac phase of lung development. At this time, the surface area of the lungs increases progressively. Surfactant is needed to decrease alveolar surface tension and increase lung compliance, preventing alveolar collapse at the end of expiration. The lecithin/sphingomyelin ratio (L/S) is predictive of lung maturity. An L/S ratio of more than 2:1 generally indicates lung maturity. It would be highly unlikely that an infant delivered at 28 weeks would have such a ratio.

The infant is in respiratory distress with a respiratory acidosis and hypoxemia. Emergent intubation, ventilation, and instillation of exogenous surfactant are required. In the absence of hypovolemia, intravenous hydration is not necessary acutely. In fact, there is a small risk of causing an intraventricular hemorrhage in such a premature infant by the overly aggressive introduction of intravenous fluids.

Difficulties in the formation of a bond between a critically ill infant and the parents often occur. The high degree of abuse that later occurs in children who were born prematurely is a reflection of this fact. Therefore, it is imperative that the medical care team be sensitive to this issue and encourage the formation of a strong family bond. It is important to ensure 24-hour visitation rights, allow the parents to be involved in the infant's care as much as is medically feasible, allow for direct skin-to-skin contact between the parents and infant, and provide counseling for the parents. Frequent discussions between the health care team and parents is essential in allowing the parents to be prepared for all possible outcomes.

133–139. The answers are: 133-C, 134-D, 135-C, 136-D, 137-B, 138-B, 139-A. (*Internal medicine, statistics*)

This patient, who was born in India and has worked in a quarry, has hypertension and a history of tobacco abuse. Findings on physical examination suggest interstitial lung disease, and the clinical picture is complicated.

A purified protein derivative (PPD) of 10 mm or more is considered positive in an individual who formerly lived in India, an endemic country for tuberculosis. Tuberculosis prophylaxis is warranted, and this patient should receive isoniazid to prevent the development of active tuberculosis. Isoniazid prophylaxis decreases that risk by 70% or more. The patient has no new symptoms or radiographic findings that suggest active tuberculosis, which would require isolation and induced sputum samples.

In addition, his employment in a quarry may suggest silicosis; the findings on the physical examination and the hilar calcifications seen on chest radiograph support this diagnosis. Silicosis is a high-risk comorbidity for tuberculosis; a PPD of 10 mm or more is positive.

Apical lung processes have a specific differential diagnosis, as shown in the following list:

Berylliosis
Eosinophilic granuloma
Sarcoidosis (variable)
Tuberculosis
Fungal infections
Chronic hypersensitivity pneumonitis
Silicosis
Coal worker's pneumoconiosis
Ankylosing spondylitis
Drugs (nitrogen mustard chemotherapy, gold, amiodarone)

Asbestosis more often involves the lung bases.

The patient's pulmonary function tests suggest an obstructive disease because the forced expiratory volume in 1 second/forced vital capacity (FEV_1/FVC) is less than 70%. In addition, the FVC is low, which also indicates a concomitant restrictive disease. Technically, it is necessary to obtain all lung volumes to be sure that the FVC is not low only secondary to an increased residual volume. The diffusion capacity (DLCO) is low, suggesting an interstitial disease other than emphysema, which can also have a low DLCO.

The man has been taking metoprolol for his hypertension. Recall that β-receptors stimulate the production of cAMP by activating adenylate cyclase. Metoprolol, a β-blocker, acts via the inhibition of cAMP. The other answer choices in question 136 are also second messenger systems involved in receptor-mediated processes; however, they are not involved in the action of β-blockers.

Primary care issues are also part of the overall examination. His high blood pressure, cigarette smoking, and age older than 45 years are three risk factors for atherosclerotic disease. His high-density lipoprotein (HDL), which is 36 mg/dL, is neither a negative nor a positive factor. With three risk factors but no known coronary artery disease, the threshold for diet therapy is a low-density lipoprotein (LDL) higher than 130 mg/dL, and for drug therapy, it is an LDL higher than 160 mg/dL. According to the National Cholesterol Education Program (NCEP) guidelines, a statin drug is most appropriate.

Disease prevention should also be a topic of discussion between the physician and the patient. His history of pulmonary disease should prompt recommendation for pneumococcal and influenza vaccine. He does not require Pneumovax again until he is 65 years of age, but he should have an annual influenza vaccine. In addition, because he has not seen a physician in longer than 10 years, he should have a tetanus-diphtheria booster, which is required every 10 years. There is no clear evidence that screening using prostate-specific antigen (PSA) is effective in improving the outcome in prostate cancer. However, discussion of the use of PSA with male patients is warranted. Some clinicians offer it to African American men with a family history of prostate cancer.

Screening for colon cancer with either endoscopy or fecal occult blood testing (FOBT) should also be a topic of discussion. Recall that, with FOBT, the number-needed-to-screen equals 1/(absolute risk reduction). A number-needed-to-screen of 1,000 represents an absolute risk reduction of 1/1,000, or 0.1%.

140–142. The answers are: 140-C, 141-E, 142-B. (*Pediatrics*)

Alcohol is probably the most common teratogen to which a fetus is exposed. The amount of alcohol ingested by the mother and the risk of fetal malformations are directly correlated. Because *no* amount of alcohol can safely be ingested during pregnancy, it should be avoided. Features of fetal alcohol syndrome can range over a wide spectrum but include facial dysmorphism, mental retardation, growth deficiency, and kidney malformation. Alcohol ingestion also results in an increased risk of miscarriages. Maternal alcohol use is associated with other milder neurodevelopmental abnormalities such as childhood hyperactivity. Cleft palate is not part of fetal alcohol syndrome.

The notion that individuals may have an inherited susceptibility to several forms of cancer is increasingly recognized. Some of these inherited syndromes include:

Syndrome	Features
Li-Fraumeni syndrome	Autosomally dominant inherited mutation in the tumor suppressor gene p53, leading to increased risk of osteosarcoma, breast cancer, and many other malignancies
Von Hippel-Lindau syndrome	Autosomally dominant inherited mutation, leading to increased risk of cerebellar hemangiomas and hemangioblastomas, as well as renal cell carcinoma and pheochromocytoma
Ataxia-telangiectasia syndrome	Autosomally recessive inherited mutation, leading to increased risk of breast cancer and leukemia
Beckwith-Wiedemann syndrome	Syndrome associated with increased risk of Wilms tumor, liver cancer, and renal cell carcinoma

McArdle disease, an inborn error in metabolism with deficient activity of skeletal phosphorylase, leads to impaired glycogen breakdown and symptoms of fatigue and muscle pain.

Down syndrome (trisomy 21) is the most common autosomal trisomy compatible with life. The risk of having a child with Down syndrome rises dramatically after a maternal age of 35 years. The reason for the increased risk with advancing maternal age is not known. Rarely does the extra chromosome come from the father. Down syndrome has many characteristics features, including short stature, microcephaly, dysmorphic facial features, duodenal atresia, Hirschsprung disease, short hands and fingers, mental retardation, and developmental delay. Cardiac defects are seen in approximately 35% of patients and include endocardial cushion defects and ventriculoseptal defects; up to 50% of these cardiac defects may be lethal.

143–146. The answers are: 143-B, 144-E, 145-E, 146-C. (*Emergency medicine, critical care medicine*)
About 375 of 3,500 species of snakes throughout the world are considered dangerous to humans. In the United States, 21 of approximately 120 species of snakes can be considered dangerous. Most commonly, snakebites are from rattlesnakes; copperheads; water moccasins; and, occasionally, cobras. Snake venom is a complex mixture of proteins designed to immobilize and kill prey. Most of its adverse effects are on the hematologic, cardiovascular, respiratory, and nervous systems. Rattlesnake envenomation results in alteration of vascular resistance and permeability, impairment of red blood cell (RBC) integrity and viscosity, induction of hypoperfusion, and decrease in neuromuscular transmission.

Several events occur after a rattlesnake bite. First, local swelling occurs secondary to transudation of fluid across damaged blood vessels. Edema of the face or muscle compartment can cause ischemic change by increasing compartment pressure and inhibiting arterial blood flow, which is referred to as compartment syndrome. This requires the measurement of intracompartment pressure. With pressures greater than 30 to 40 mm Hg, the compartment can be at risk of ischemia. Second, coagulopathy may develop, which resembles disseminated intravascular coagulation (DIC). Third, systemic changes occur, including nausea, vomiting, and mental status changes.

Standard management includes limb immobilization at heart level; measurement of vital signs; determination of prothrombin time (PT), partial thromboplastin time (PTT), and platelets; and admission to the ICU if hypotension is present or if a change in the level of consciousness occurs. Ice should not be used because the local vasoconstriction at the bite site decreases the rate of venom efflux.

In this case, hypotension occurs secondary to intravascular volume depletion caused by increased vascular permeability due to the venom. A right heart catheter (also known as a pulmonary artery catheter) detects decreased central venous pressure, increased systemic vascular resistance, decreased cardiac output, and a decreased pulmonary capillary wedge pressure. Although the vessels have increased vascular permeability, the systemic vascular resistance is usually maintained.

Management should include the "ABCs"—airway, breathing, and circulation; airway management should be first. Fluid repletion is the next intervention of most importance. If blood pressure cannot be maintained, the addition of a pressor (dopamine or phenylephrine) is appropriate. Antivenin is warranted if there is progression of pain, ecchymosis, swelling, hypotension, bleeding, mental status changes, or compartment syndrome. Because the effectiveness of antivenin decreases with time from envenomation, it should be used quickly.

The lower extremity pain at the site of envenomation is increasing, and the clinician should suspect compartment syndrome. Although the patient does have an indication for antivenin, the intracompartmental pressure should be measured first because fasciotomy may be required. Hyperbaric oxygen or mannitol play no role in this situation.

147–150. The answers are: 147-E, 148-D, 149-B, 150-B. (*Emergency medicine, internal medicine*)
When an individual presents with complaints of chest pain, certain features suggest a cardiac cause. The presence of "heaviness" or "gripping pain" is more typical for angina than sharp pain. This sensation often is associated with radiation to the neck, shoulders, or arms. A person may experience diaphoresis, shortness of

breath, or a sense of doom. In this case, the patient has pain suggestive of angina. His medications suggest a history of hypertension and diabetes mellitus, which are risk factors for coronary artery disease. Because the onset of pain occurred at rest, his condition is best classified as unstable angina. This scenario implies rupture of plaque with thrombus formation occluding a coronary artery.

The ECG shows ST-segment depression. At this time, there is no indication for reperfusion therapy with tissue plasminogen activator or cardiac catheterization. An International Study of Infarct Survival trial (ISIS-2) found that aspirin decreases mortality in this setting. β-Blockers have the same effect (Thrombolysis in Myocardial Infarction [TIMI] IIIB), as do angiotensin-converting enzyme (ACE) inhibitors. According to the Scandinavian Simvastatin Survival Study Group (4S) and the Carvedilol Arthrectomy Restenosis (CARE) trials, the statin medications decrease mortality in the setting of secondary prevention.

In the setting of unstable angina, many studies suggest that a conservative approach is associated with improved outcome if no high-risk features are associated with the unstable angina. These high-risk features include postinfarction angina, dynamic ECG changes, elevated troponin, arrhythmia, baseline ST-segment depression (without pain), and congestive heart failure. The Treat Angina With Aggrastat and Determine Cost of Therapy With an Invasive or Conservative Strategy–Thrombolysis in Myocardial Infarction (TACTICS–TIMI-18) trial found that these patients were better served by cardiac catheterization. In this case, the patient has no high-risk features and should be risk-stratified with a stress test after receiving 48 to 72 hours of heparin.

Whether coronary artery bypass surgery is warranted depends on the degree of stenosis in the coronary arteries. The Bypass Angioplasty Revascularization Investigation (BARI) found that patients with left main stenoses exceeding 50% *or* patients with three-vessel disease with an ejection fraction less than 40% derived a benefit from coronary artery bypass grafting.

Studies have shown that after a myocardial infarction (MI), several agents provide secondary prevention and decrease mortality. The most important of these are aspirin, cholesterol-lowering medications (e.g., simvastatin), β-blockers (e.g., propranolol), and angiotensin-converting enzyme (ACE) inhibitors (e.g., enalapril). Nitroglycerin is effective in reducing episodes of angina but has no mortality-associated benefit.

Test IV

QUESTIONS

DIRECTIONS: For each question, select the letter corresponding to the best answer. All questions have only one correct answer.

Setting: Emergency Department

Questions 1–3

A 76-year-old woman is rushed to the emergency department (ED) by her family when she is found unresponsive. The list of medications supplied by her daughter includes metformin hydrochloride, levothyroxine sodium, glipizide, and paroxetine hydrochloride. The patient has an electrocardiogram (ECG) (*below*) while other information is being gathered.

1. Which of the following is most likely to yield the diagnosis?

(A) Vital signs
(B) Thyroid-stimulating hormone (TSH)
(C) Blood glucose level
(D) Blood chemistries
(E) Creatine kinase

2. The woman's hemodynamic status declines. The most important initial intervention is

(A) hydrocortisone
(B) intravenous thyroxine
(C) rewarming
(D) saline infusion
(E) total parenteral infusion

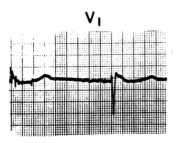
V₁

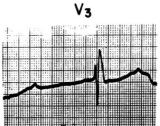
V₃

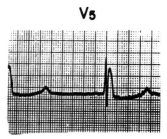
V₅

3. You learn that the woman has advanced directives stating that she does not want intubation or electrical shocks. You are concerned about her respiratory status. Her family insists on intubation. Which of the following actions do you take?

(A) Intubate the woman because she cannot confirm the "do not intubate" status
(B) Call the ethics department
(C) Abide by the advanced directives
(D) Ask the family to meet to make a decision regarding intubation
(E) Consult a psychiatrist to assess her competence

Setting: Satellite Clinic

Questions 4–8

A 26-year-old man presents with a 4-day history of frontal headache and purulent rhinorrhea. He had clear rhinorrhea and a sore throat 5 days earlier, with initial improvement followed by the presenting symptoms.

4. Which of the following tests/methods of evaluation is most sensitive for securing a diagnosis?

(A) Culture
(B) Radiograph
(C) CT scan
(D) Ultrasound
(E) History

5. Which of the following treatments do you recommend?

(A) Amoxicillin
(B) Azithromycin
(C) Observation
(D) Phenylephrine spray
(E) Surgery

6. On further history taking, you learn that he has suffered from multiple bouts of purulent rhinorrhea that have required treatment. He also reports that he is under considerable stress; he and his wife want children but are having difficulty conceiving. Which of the following conditions is the likely cause of his recurrent rhinorrhea?

(A) Wegener granulomatosis
(B) Vasomotor rhinitis
(C) Head and neck cancer
(D) Common variable immunodeficiency
(E) Ciliary dyskinesia (Kartagener syndrome)

7. A high-resolution CT scan of the chest might show which of the following findings?

(A) Mediastinal lymphadenopathy
(B) Bronchiectasis
(C) Pleural calcifications
(D) Ground glass infiltrates
(E) Pleural effusions

8. Which of the following organisms is least likely to be found on culturing of his sputum?

(A) *Staphylococcus aureus*
(B) *Haemophilus influenzae*
(C) Atypical mycobacteria
(D) *Aspergillus*
(E) *Pseudomonas*

Setting: Office

Questions 9–12

A 49-year-old woman with a history of hypothyroidism presents with complaints of frequent urination. Her medications include levothyroxine, aspirin, and many vitamins. Review of symptoms is otherwise unremarkable.

9. Which of the following causes is least likely?

(A) Hypercalcemia
(B) Hypokalemia
(C) Diabetes insipidus
(D) Diabetes mellitus
(E) Syndrome of inappropriate secretion of antidiuretic hormone (SIADH)

10. Which of the following drugs is the least likely to cause an inappropriate concentration of the urine?

(A) Ciprofloxacin
(B) Paroxetine
(C) Carbamazepine
(D) Chlorpropamide
(E) Clofibrate

11. Several laboratory tests are ordered. The results reveal:

Na^+	138 mEq/L
Cl^-	98 mEq/L
K^+	3.6 mEq/L
Ca^{2+}	10.5 mEq/L
Mg^{2+}	1.9 mEq/L
HCO_3^-	28 mEq/L
Phosphorus	3.0 mg/dL
Random glucose	168 mg/dL

Which of the following measures is the most appropriate next step?

(A) Oral glucose tolerance test
(B) Glycosylated hemoglobin
(C) Fasting glucose
(D) Urinalysis
(E) Check parathyroid hormone levels

12. Which of the following conditions is NOT associated with hypercalcemia?

(A) Sarcoidosis
(B) Lymphoma
(C) Hypothyroidism
(D) Vitamin A toxicity
(E) Hyperparathyroidism

Setting: Office

Questions: 13–17

A 46-year-old man with a history of hypertension and hyperlipidemia presents for an annual physical examination. Propranolol hydrochloride controls his blood pressure well, and pravastatin sodium controls his lipids levels effectively.

13. Which of the following measures is recommended at this time?

(A) Pneumovax
(B) Influenza vaccine
(C) Check of blood pressure
(D) Digital rectal examination
(E) Prostate-specific antigen (PSA) level

14. What laboratory test should be monitored?

(A) Alanine aminotransferase (ALT)
(B) Alkaline phosphatase
(C) Bilirubin
(D) Sodium
(E) Creatine kinase

15. Six months later, the man returns complaining of ankle swelling. On examination, ankle edema is evident bilaterally. He has no other complaints. Laboratory test results are remarkable for a sudden rise in low-density lipoprotein (LDL) cholesterol. Which of the following tests is least likely to yield a diagnosis?

(A) Urinalysis
(B) Thyroid-stimulating hormone (TSH)
(C) ALT
(D) CT of abdomen
(E) 24-hour urine free cortisol

16. Laboratory tests reveal:

Alanine aminotransferase (ALT)	50 mg/dL
Aspartate aminotransferase (ALT)	45 mg/dL
Thyroid-stimulating hormone (TSH)	2.4 μU/mL
Prostate-specific antigen (PSA)	2.5 ng/mL
Urinalysis	2 white blood cells (WBCs)/hpf
	2 red blood cells (RBCs)/hpf
	4+++ protein

Which of the following conditions is the most likely diagnosis?

(A) Hypothyroidism
(B) Liver failure
(C) Hodgkin lymphoma
(D) Membranous nephropathy
(E) Prostate cancer

17. Which of the following conditions is a complication of membranous nephropathy?

(A) Bleeding
(B) Exophthalmos
(C) Cardiomyopathy
(D) Pulmonary fibrosis
(E) Thrombosis

Setting: Office

Questions 18–22

A 51-year-old woman with a history of tobacco abuse has a recent history of hemoptysis. Although she "felt warm" several days go, she did not take her temperature. She describes her sputum as mucopurulent and streaked with blood.

18. Which of the following conditions is the most likely diagnosis?

(A) Bronchiectasis
(B) Malignancy
(C) Pulmonary embolus
(D) Bronchitis
(E) Tuberculosis

19. A chest radiograph reveals a 2.5-cm uncalcified density in the region of the right middle lobe. Which of the following procedures is the next step?

(A) Bronchoscopy
(B) CT scan of the chest
(C) Repeat plain film in 8 weeks
(D) Magnetic resonance imaging (MRI) of the chest
(E) High-resolution CT scan of the chest

20. After an extensive workup, it is determined that a lobectomy is the optimal treatment. Pulmonary function tests reveal:

Forced expiratory volume in 1 second (FEV_1)	50% predicted
Forced vital capacity (FVC)	75% predicted
FEV_1/FVC	60%

You interpret these results as

(A) obstructive disease
(B) restrictive disease
(C) mixed obstructive and restrictive disease
(D) restrictive disease; obstructive disease cannot be ruled out
(E) obstructive disease; restrictive disease cannot be ruled out

21. The woman has a forced expiratory volume in 1 second (FEV_1) of 1.2 L, and you are concerned about the proposed procedure. Which of the following measures do you recommend?

(A) Measurement of diffusion capacity (DLCO)
(B) Measurement of lung volumes
(C) Ventilation-perfusion ($\dot{V}/\dot{Q}$) scan
(D) CT angiogram
(E) Echocardiogram

22. Which of the following measures is least likely to improve patient outcome?

(A) Smoking cessation 2 weeks prior to the procedure
(B) Patient education regarding incentive spirometry
(C) Consistent use of chronic obstructive pulmonary disease inhalers prior to the procedure
(D) Use of epidural anesthesia
(E) Duration of surgery <3 hours

Setting: Emergency Department

Questions 23–24

A 74-year-old man complains of vision loss in his right eye. He has no pain. A funduscopic examination reveals a pale fundus with a red spot in the macular region.

23. Which of the following conditions is the most likely diagnosis?

(A) Central retinal artery occlusion
(B) Central retinal vein occlusion
(C) Acute angle-closure glaucoma
(D) Retinal detachment
(E) Iritis

24. Which of the following measures is the most important next step?

(A) Pilocarpine eyedrops
(B) Ocular massage
(C) Intravenous acetazolamide
(D) Fluorescein examination
(E) Emergency iridectomy

Setting: Satellite Clinic

Questions 25–26

A 14-year-old girl presents with a red eye. Pain in the right eye is exacerbated with light shone in either eye.

25. Which of the following measures is the most appropriate intervention?

(A) Topical steroids
(B) Sympathomimetic eyedrops
(C) Cholinesterase inhibitors
(D) Slit lamp examination
(E) Eye patch

26. Which of the following conditions is NOT associated with this disorder?

(A) Sarcoidosis
(B) Juvenile rheumatoid arthritis
(C) Colon cancer
(D) Crohn disease
(E) Tuberculosis

Setting: Emergency Department

Questions 27–31

A 12-year-old girl is brought in by her parents because she has acute onset of fever, nausea, vomiting, headache, and decreased concentration. Physical examination indicates that she is normotensive but has tachycardia. On her trunk and lower extremities are petechiae 1 to 2 mm in size.

27. Which of the following statements about this disease is NOT true?

(A) Fibrinogen levels are often low
(B) The degree of thrombocytopenia correlates with the severity of disease
(C) Focal neurologic findings are common
(D) It occurs most commonly in children and young adults
(E) Schistocytes may be seen on peripheral smear

28. You learn that the girl's family has a history of this clinical presentation. The most likely explanation is

(A) a dangerous family ritual
(B) common variable immunodeficiency disease
(C) sickle cell disease
(D) an autoimmune disease
(E) a terminal complement deficiency

29. Which of the following measures is the most appropriate intervention?

(A) Antibiotics
(B) Lumbar puncture
(C) Intravenous fluids
(D) Complete blood count (CBC)
(E) Fresh frozen plasma infusion

30. Severe hypotension develops within 24 hours. Which of the following measures do you recommend?

(A) Intravenous dexamethasone
(B) Bolus of normal saline; then check blood pressure
(C) Intravenous hydrocortisone
(D) A check of the cortisol level
(E) Infusion of packed red blood cells (RBCs)

31. Which of the following statements regarding prophylaxis for this disease is true?

(A) It protects patients from all serotypes of disease
(B) It is recommended for all adults older than 50 years with cardiopulmonary disease
(C) There is a live attenuated vaccine
(D) Patients with a family history of the disease derive little benefit from vaccination
(E) It is recommended for young adults living in close quarters, such as barracks and dormitories

Setting: Emergency Department

Questions 32–34

A 25-year-old man is brought in by his friends after passing out during a basketball game. He claims to have had recent chest pain and occasional palpitations. As a child he once had a high fever with a rash. His father has a history of a heart condition.

32. This man's disease is associated with

(A) no inheritance pattern
(B) autosomal dominant inheritance
(C) autosomal recessive inheritance
(D) X-linked recessive inheritance
(E) both autosomal dominant and spontaneous mutations

33. Which of the following findings might you expect on physical examination?

(A) A systolic murmur that increases with squatting
(B) A diastolic rumble
(C) An opening snap over the apex
(D) A systolic murmur that increases with Valsalva maneuver
(E) A systolic murmur that increases with firm handgrip maneuver

34. Treatment for this disorder includes all of the following agents EXCEPT

(A) metoprolol
(B) verapamil hydrochloride
(C) furosemide
(D) digoxin
(E) disopyramide

Setting: Satellite Clinic

Questions 35–36

A 17-year-old girl presents to the student health center in tears. She had sexual intercourse 12 hours prior without any contraception. Afraid of becoming pregnant, she is asking your advice.

35. Which of the following measures do you recommend?

(A) Waiting a few weeks and checking a pregnancy test
(B) Methylprednisolone acetate by injection today
(C) Two estrogen-containing oral contraceptive pills now and again in 12 hours
(D) Family planning counseling
(E) Prostaglandin analog

36. Which of the following statements regarding emergency contraception is true?

(A) Progestin-only pills are more effective
(B) Progestin-only pills are associated with more nausea and vomiting
(C) It is 100% effective
(D) It always works prior to fertilization
(E) It is less effective when given early after unprotected intercourse

Setting: Satellite Clinic

Questions 37–42

A sexually active 22-year-old woman presents for her routine Papanicolaou (Pap) smear for cervical cancer screening. The appearance of her cervix is within normal limits. Her pathology results return as "inflammatory with budding yeast."

37. Which of the following factors does NOT pose a risk for cervical cancer?

(A) Lower socioeconomic status
(B) Multiple sexual partners
(C) Smoking
(D) Immunocompromised state
(E) Positive family history

38. Which of the following measures is the most appropriate next step?

(A) Colposcopy
(B) Conization
(C) Pap smear, repeated in 6 weeks
(D) Treatment with antifungal agents, with Pap smear repeated in 4 months
(E) Interpretation of Pap smear as normal; repeated in 1 year

39. Which of the following findings on Pap smear is the least appropriate indication for colposcopy?

(A) Cervical intraepithelial neoplasia I
(B) Cervical intraepithelial neoplasia II
(C) Cervical intraepithelial neoplasia III
(D) Noninflammatory atypia
(E) Inflammatory atypia

40. Which of the following colposcopy results does NOT require biopsy?

(A) Acetowhitening epithelium
(B) Punctation
(C) Mosaicism
(D) Atypical vessels
(E) Nabothian cysts

41. Which of the following scenarios does NOT necessarily require conization?

(A) Transformation zone that cannot be seen
(B) Adenocarcinoma on Pap smear
(C) Negative endocervical curettage
(D) Microinvasion on biopsy
(E) Biopsy that is lower grade than Pap smear

42. Which of the following human papilloma virus serotypes is associated with the highest grade, fastest-progressing cervical cancer?

(A) 6
(B) 11
(C) 16
(D) 18
(E) 31

Setting: Satellite Clinic

Questions 43–45

A sexually active 23-year-old woman presents with an increased vaginal discharge. She complains of vaginal itching, burning with urination, and pain with intercourse. Pelvic examination reveals a frothy, yellow, odorous discharge, and petechial hemorrhages on the cervix.

43. Which of the following findings would you expect to see on wet mount/potassium hydroxide (KOH) preparation?

(A) Budding yeast
(B) "Fishy" odor
(C) Clue cells
(D) Motile trichomonads
(E) Low pH

44. Which of the following measures do you recommend?

(A) Clindamycin
(B) Metronidazole
(C) Miconazole
(D) Clotrimazole
(E) Cotton undergarments

45. The woman follows your advice but returns 6 weeks later with the same complaints. Only transient improvement has occurred. Which of the following measures do you now recommend?

(A) Repeat metronidazole with higher dose
(B) Treatment of the woman's sexual partner
(C) Oral ketoconazole
(D) Treatment of the woman and her sexual partner
(E) Ceftriaxone sodium and doxycycline

Setting: Hospital

Questions 46–48

A 50-year-old woman complains of a swollen leg. The swelling began approximately 48 hours ago. The woman has never had anything like this before. On examination, the right lower extremity is 4 cm larger than the left, with warmth and redness but no open cuts or lymphangitis. Lymphadenopathy of 1 cm is apparent in the inguinal regions bilaterally. Homans sign is negative.

46. Which of the following measures is the most appropriate next step?

(A) Penicillin G
(B) Radiography (plain films)
(C) MRI
(D) Ultrasound
(E) Amoxicillin-clavulanate

47. On further history taking, you learn that she has two cats at home that spend much of the time outdoors. While contemplating a potential infectious cause, you recall that a cat scratch can cause a limb infection. Which of the following pathogens is the infectious agent in this disease?

(A) *Pasteurella multocida*
(B) *Staphylococcus aureus*
(C) *Capnocytophaga felinis*
(D) *Bartonella henselae*
(E) *Toxoplasma gondii*

48. A diagnosis is made, and the woman is prepared for discharge. She asks about her prognosis. You tell her that

(A) she will recover and have an average risk of recurrence
(B) she is at increased risk for cancer and should have a CT scan of the chest, abdomen, and pelvis
(C) keeping the pets indoors will prevent future episodes
(D) her inguinal lymph nodes are a concern, and her case should be followed-up
(E) she should have routine cancer screening

Setting: Emergency Department

Questions 49–53

A 61-year-old Caucasian woman receives a diagnosis of deep venous thrombosis. Initially, she presented to the ED with 1 day of swelling of the left leg. She described no recent injuries or immobilization. She has begun no new medications.

49. Which of the following conditions is the most likely underlying risk factor?

(A) Protein C deficiency
(B) Antithrombin deficiency
(C) Factor V Leiden
(D) Homocystinemia
(E) Protein S deficiency

50. The woman has no complaints other than a slightly swollen left leg. An ultrasound finds a relatively small clot burden in her iliac venous system on the left side. Her vital signs, chest radiograph, and ECG are within normal limits. Which of the following measures do you recommend?

(A) Admission for unfractionated heparin
(B) Outpatient low-molecular-weight heparin
(C) Warfarin
(D) Outpatient low-molecular-weight heparin with warfarin
(E) Hirudin

51. The woman returns in 4 weeks with shortness of breath. Which of the following signs are you likely see on her chest radiograph?

(A) Normal findings
(B) Hampton hump
(C) Westermark sign
(D) Pleural effusion
(E) Cephalization

52. Which of the following findings are you likely to see on her ECG?

(A) $S_1Q_3T_3$ pattern
(B) Right bundle branch block
(C) Large r wave in V_1
(D) Right axis deviation
(E) Sinus tachycardia

53. On further discussion with the patient, you learn that her mother had a clot in her femoral artery when she was in her thirties. Which of the following conditions would be the most likely cause of her mother's clotting disorder?

(A) Protein C deficiency
(B) Protein S deficiency
(C) Antithrombin deficiency
(D) Antiphospholipid antibodies
(E) Factor V Leiden

Setting: Office

Questions 54–55

A 3-month-old boy is brought in by his mother with concerns regarding constipation. At birth he had delayed passage of meconium and now has poor feeding and bilious vomiting. On examination he has abdominal distension.

54. Which of the following conditions is least likely?

(A) Hypothyroidism
(B) Hypocalcemia
(C) Hypokalemia
(D) Botulism
(E) Hirschsprung disease

55. A barium enema, part of an extensive workup, demonstrates a distal segment of narrowed bowel with an abrupt transition to a dilated portion of proximal bowel. The next step is

(A) balloon dilatation
(B) botulinum toxin injection
(C) myomectomy
(D) high-fiber diet
(E) rectal biopsy

Setting: Hospital

Questions 56–57

56. A newborn is cyanotic. All of the following are potential causes EXCEPT

(A) truncus arteriosus
(B) tetralogy of Fallot
(C) ventricular septal defect (VSD)
(D) total anomalous pulmonary venous return
(E) transposition of the great vessels

57. Which of the following conditions is NOT associated with coarctation of the aorta?

(A) Turner syndrome
(B) Patent ductus arteriosus (PDA)
(C) VSD
(D) Klinefelter syndrome
(E) Bicuspid aortic valve

Setting: Satellite Clinic

Questions 58–61

A 3-year-old girl from inner-city Los Angeles presents to your clinic. Her mother reports that her daughter has had fever and cough for 3 days. On physical examination, she has a temperature of 39.7°C, injected conjunctiva, and red spots on her buccal mucosa. She is normotensive and communicative.

58. Which of the following agents is the cause of her disease?

(A) Varicella zoster virus
(B) Human herpes virus-6
(C) Paramyxovirus
(D) Parvovirus B19
(E) Rubella virus

59. This child's disease may be associated with a deficiency of

(A) vitamin A
(B) selenium
(C) vitamin B_6
(D) niacin
(E) vitamin E

60. Which of the following measures do you recommend?

(A) Acyclovir
(B) Immunoglobulin
(C) Penicillin
(D) Doxycycline
(E) Observation

61. You learn of a new test used to diagnose the girl's disease. The company that designed it shows you a study with 200 patients with a 50% prevalence of disease. There were 80 true-positive results, 20 false-negative results, 20 false-positive results, and 80 true-negative results. The sensitivity of the test is

(A) 20%
(B) 50%
(C) 80%
(D) 100%
(E) cannot be determined

Setting: Office

Questions 62–66

You are asked to see a 15-year-old boy for behavioral problems. After conducting intelligence tests, you determine that he has mild retardation. He is very tall for his age despite having parents of average height. On examination he has wide hips, little body hair, and small testes.

62. Which of the following physical findings might you also expect to see?

(A) Short arm span
(B) Splenomegaly
(C) Epicanthal folds
(D) Gynecomastia
(E) Flat nasal bridge

63. A buccal smear with karyotype is likely to reveal

(A) 45,XO
(B) 46,XX
(C) 47,XXX
(D) 47,XXY
(E) 47,XYY

64. The boy's parents are considering having another child. The risk of recurrence of this condition (in percent) is

(A) 0
(B) 25
(C) 50
(D) 100
(E) same as in the general population

65. While explaining genetic risk of inheritance, you give the parents a scenario to consider. If a man who is a carrier of an autosomal recessive disease marries a woman with the disease, the chance of their children having the disease, assuming 100% penetrance, is

(A) 0
(B) 25%
(C) 50%
(D) 100%
(E) cannot be determined

66. If a normal-appearing man marries a woman who is a carrier of an X-linked disorder, their children will be affected in what percentage of cases?

(A) 0
(B) 25
(C) 50
(D) 100
(E) More information is required

Setting: Office

Questions 67–70

A 2½-year-old boy whom you have never seen before is brought to your office because of reported belly pain. His mother claims that he has been complaining of left-sided abdominal pain for a few weeks. On examination, he is afebrile, but he has striking periorbital ecchymoses. A firm abdominal mass is evident on the left side.

67. Which of the following statements about this disease is true?

(A) Its incidence is higher in women
(B) Its incidence is higher in non-whites
(C) The median age at diagnosis is 5 years
(D) The disorder is found exclusively in the abdomen
(E) The disorder is associated with Beckwith-Wiedemann syndrome

68. You might seek all of the following physical findings EXCEPT

(A) subcutaneous nodules
(B) proptosis
(C) hepatomegaly
(D) varicocele
(E) coloboma

69. This disease is associated with

(A) p53 suppressor gene
(B) N-*myc* proto-oncogene
(C) RB gene
(D) BRCA1 gene
(E) WT-1 gene

70. Which of the following measures is the most appropriate next step?

(A) Urine free cortisol level
(B) Dexamethasone suppression test
(C) Urine vanillylmandelic acid
(D) Aldosterone level
(E) Plasma renin activity

Setting: Emergency Department

Questions 71–72

A 56-year-old woman with a long-standing history of atrial fibrillation is brought by the rescue squad to the ED after an episode of syncope at home. Her medications include quinidine, aspirin, metformin, and hydrochlorothiazide. Recently she had an upper respiratory infection for which she was seen at a local walk-in clinic.

71. Which of the following conditions is the likely cause of the syncope?

(A) Hypoglycemia
(B) Ventricular tachycardia
(C) Atrial fibrillation
(D) Situational syncope
(E) Aortic stenosis

72. Treatment for the woman's recent upper respiratory infection likely involved which of the following agents?

(A) Cefuroxime
(B) Amoxicillin
(C) Amoxicillin-clavulanate
(D) Fluoroquinolone
(E) Clarithromycin

Setting: Office

Questions 73–75

The family of a 74-year-old woman expresses concern. Twelve hours ago, the woman experienced the sudden loss of speech production, as well as right-sided weakness. Within 1 hour, she had returned to baseline.

73. Which of the following conditions was the likely cause of this event?

(A) Seizure
(B) Myocardial infarction (MI)
(C) Cardioembolic event
(D) Transient ischemic attack
(E) Subarachnoid hemorrhage

74. Physical findings are most remarkable for blood pressure of 169/85 mm Hg, S_4 heart sound without murmurs on cardiac examination, and carotid bruit on the left side. Which of the following measures is the most appropriate next step?

(A) Echocardiogram
(B) Angiogram
(C) Duplex ultrasound
(D) Electroencephalogram (EEG)
(E) CT scan of the head

75. The best indication for endarterectomy in this patient is stenosis of the carotid artery of what degree?

(A) 20%
(B) 40%
(C) 60%
(D) 80%
(E) 100%

Setting: Office

Questions 76–78

A 54-year-old woman who wishes to establish primary care with your practice comes to the office. She has no specific complaints at this time but is interested in preventive care. Her past medical history is significant for two uncomplicated full-term pregnancies, a benign breast nodule that was removed 3 years ago, and an appendectomy at 16 years of age. She is currently taking a multivitamin and calcium supplements. She recently quit smoking after using 1 pack per day for 15 years. Review of symptoms indicates several results of note: no menses for 1 year, occasional hot flashes, moderate fatigue, and rare bifrontal headaches.

76. All of the following conditions may be attributed to an absence of estrogen EXCEPT

(A) osteoporosis
(B) increased risk of cardiovascular disease
(C) hot flashes
(D) vaginal dryness
(E) increased risk of endometrial cancer

77. The woman is interested in pursuing estrogen replacement therapy (ERT), which may lead to an increased risk of all of the following disorders EXCEPT

(A) gallbladder disease
(B) deep venous thrombosis
(C) breast cancer
(D) endometrial cancer
(E) pancreatitis

78. Which of the following regimens of ERT is most appropriate?

(A) Conjugated estrogen 0.625 mg once a day
(B) Micronized estrogen 1 mg once a day
(C) Conjugated estrogen 0.625 mg once a day with medroxyprogesterone 5 mg once a day
(D) Transdermal estrogen patch
(E) Transdermal estrogen patch with medroxy-progesterone 10 mg given only on the last day of the month

Setting: Office

Questions 79–81

A 38-year-old man comes to see you regarding the recent onset of some unusual symptoms. During the past 6 to 8 months he has noted progressively worsening irritability, moodiness, and cognitive decline. An antidepressant initially helped, but lately he has noted worsening memory loss. Along with this, he has noted increased fidgetiness and restlessness. For the past month, he also reports that he has had unpredictable muscle jerks of his upper extremities, as well as facial grimacing. Secondary to these motor problems, he has stopped socializing in large groups. He is not taking any medications and denies any illicit drug use.

79. Which of the following measures would be most helpful in determining the cause of this man's symptoms?

(A) CT scan of the brain with contrast
(B) Formal cognitive testing
(C) Complete blood count (CBC)
(D) Family history
(E) Drug screen

80. Physical examination reveals a well-developed individual; pulmonary, cardiac, ophthalmic, and gastrointestinal (GI) systems and vital signs are within normal limits. On neurologic examination, mini-mental status testing reveals impaired short-term memory and difficulty naming objects. Motor examination shows normal strength, and sensory examination is normal. You note occasional facial grimacing, and the patient's voluntary movements are sometimes interrupted by involuntary muscle jerks. Routine laboratory tests, including liver function studies, are in normal limits. Which of the following conditions best explains the patient's condition?

(A) Wilson disease
(B) Huntington disease
(C) Parkinson disease
(D) Sydenham chorea
(E) Focal torsion dystonia

81. The man is concerned about his prognosis. Which of the following occurrences is most likely?

(A) A slow, irreversible progression to dementia and death within 10 to 20 years
(B) Good control with treatment using antidopaminergic drugs
(C) No prognostic information is available because the course of the disease is so variable
(D) Remitting and relapsing features and a normal life span
(E) Rapid progression to dementia and death within 1 to 3 years

Setting: Office

Questions 82–85

During a routine prenatal examination of a pregnant woman at 30 weeks' gestation, you note that the uterus is significantly larger than expected for the estimated gestational date and that it is difficult to palpate the fetus. You review the chart and recalculate the estimated gestational date; the date remains at 30 weeks.

82. Your next step should be

(A) auscultation of fetal heart tones with a fetoscope
(B) reassurance and reexamination in 1 to 2 weeks
(C) complete blood count (CBC) and metabolic profile
(D) examination for cervical effacement
(E) ultrasound of the fetus and uterus

83. You institute your plan. One of the conditions in your differential diagnosis is hydramnios. Which of the following conditions may lead to hydramnios?

(A) Potter syndrome (absence of fetal kidneys)
(B) Diabetes mellitus
(C) Intrauterine growth retardation
(D) Ruptured membranes
(E) Congenital toxoplasmosis

84. Workup reveals the presence of hydramnios. A detailed fetal examination shows no clear abnormalities, and maternal examination is within normal limits. Which of the following conditions is NOT a possible complication of hydramnios?

(A) Maternal discomfort
(B) Preterm labor
(C) Uteroplacental insufficiency
(D) Respiratory compromise
(E) Premature rupture of the membranes

85. It is decided that therapy to decrease the amount of amniotic fluid is warranted. Which of the following agents decreases the production of amniotic fluid?

(A) Propranolol
(B) Dexamethasone
(C) Indomethacin
(D) Magnesium sulfate
(E) Folic acid

Setting: Office and Emergency Department

Questions 86–89

A 54-year-old man, an automobile mechanic in a brake repair shop, presents for evaluation of worsening dyspnea. During the past 12 months, he has become short of breath with increasingly less activity; he now becomes dyspneic after walking up one flight of stairs. He denies cough, wheezing, chest pain, or lower extremity edema. He has smoked 1 pack of cigarettes a day for 35 years. His father died of a pulmonary disease.

Physical examination reveals a thin man in no distress. He is afebrile, with a blood pressure of 110/80 mm Hg and a respiratory rate of 18/minute with oxygen saturation of 89% on room air. No lymphadenopathy or jugular venous distension is evident. Pulmonary examination reveals distant breath sounds, few rales at the lung bases, and occasional expiratory wheezes.

86. Pulmonary function tests reveal:

Value	Predicted (%)
Spirometry	
Forced vital capacity (FVC)	45
Forced expiratory volume in 1 second (FEV_1)	31
FVC/FEV_1	53 (actual %)
Forced expiratory volume at 25%–75% of FVC ($FEF_{25\%-75\%}$)	15
Lung Volumes	
Total lung capacity (TLC)	142
TLC/residual volume (RV)	214
Diffusion capacity (DL_{CO})	40

Which of the following diagnoses is most consistent with these values?

(A) Asthma
(B) Silicosis
(C) Asbestosis
(D) Chronic obstructive pulmonary disease (COPD)
(E) Idiopathic pulmonary fibrosis

87. An arterial blood gas reveals:

pH	7.39
P_{CO_2}	62 mm Hg
P_{O_2}	59 mm Hg

Which of the following therapies would have the greatest impact on this man's survival?

(A) Digoxin
(B) Albuterol nebulizer treatments
(C) Corticosteroids
(D) Supplemental oxygen by nasal cannula
(E) Theophylline

88. Which of the following findings would be most expected on echocardiography?

(A) Normal right and left ventricular function
(B) Severely decreased left ventricular function
(C) Decreased right ventricular function and right ventricular strain
(D) Severe aortic stenosis
(E) Severe mitral regurgitation

89. You begin treatment with initially excellent results. However, 6 months later you are called to see the man in the ED secondary to increased shortness of breath, as well as purulent and increased sputum production. His chest radiograph is unchanged, and his oxygen saturation on 3 L oxygen by nasal cannula is 90%. Which of the following therapies is indicated?

(A) Albuterol nebulizer treatments
(B) Albuterol nebulizer treatments and prednisone
(C) Albuterol nebulizer treatments, prednisone, and azithromycin
(D) Albuterol nebulizer treatments, prednisone, and amoxicillin
(E) Albuterol nebulizer treatments, prednisone, and theophylline

Setting: Emergency Department

Questions 90–91

A 34-year-old man presents to the ED after injuring his right knee playing football with his friends. After catching a pass, he planted his right leg, and it twisted inward and forward. He heard a "pop," and within minutes swelling and a blue discoloration developed. He has no medical history. On examination, he is unable to bear weight, and there is a large knee effusion with a blue hue. Radiographs of the knee show some anterior displacement of the patella and no fractures.

90. Which of the following injuries is the most likely diagnosis?

(A) Lateral cruciate ligament tear
(B) Posterior cruciate ligament tear
(C) Medial cruciate ligament tear
(D) Anterior cruciate ligament tear
(E) Multiple cruciate ligament tears

91. An orthopedic surgeon is not immediately available. Which of the following measures, along with nonsteroidal anti-inflammatory agents (NSAIDs), would be the most appropriate initial care of this man?

(A) Full-leg casting and crutches
(B) Knee immobilizer and crutches
(C) Compression bandage (Ace wrap) and crutches
(D) Aspiration of the effusion, knee immobilizer, and crutches
(E) Aspiration of the effusion, full-leg casting, and crutches

Setting: Office

Questions 92–93

The mother of a 4-year-old boy brings him to see you because the boy's teacher reports that the child has attention deficit hyperactivity disorder. Apparently, during school, the boy is easily distracted, fidgets constantly, is unable to wait his turn, and frequently interrupts the other children in class. The mother says that she has noted similar problems at home. The boy, who is very forgetful, is unable to follow through on his chores. Several parents have also complained that her son is impulsive and very hyperactive.

92. Which of the following physical examination findings can be seen more frequently in patients with attention deficit hyperactivity disorder?

(A) Cleft palate
(B) Café-au-lait spots
(C) High arched palate
(D) Blue sclera
(E) Albinism

93. Which of the following treatments is NOT a possible treatment for attention deficit hyperactivity disorder?

(A) Methylphenidate hydrochloride

(B) Dextroamphetamine sulfate

(C) Behavioral therapy

(D) Lorazepam

(E) Imipramine

Setting: Emergency Department

Questions 94–95

A 13-year-old girl is hit by a car while riding her bicycle. Her helmet is thrown off during the collision. On arrival at the hospital, her blood pressure is 60/40 mm Hg; she is unconscious and becomes apneic. She is intubated, has her cervical spine stabilized, and receives intravenous fluid resuscitation. As a result, her vital signs stabilize. An emergent CT scan of the head demonstrates massive cerebral edema without acute hemorrhage and small-sized ventricles. An intracranial pressure monitor records elevated pressures.

94. Which of the following therapies would NOT be effective in lowering the intracranial pressure?

(A) Intravenous mannitol

(B) Hyperventilation to lower the P_{CO_2}

(C) Elevation of the head of the bed to 30 degrees

(D) Pentobarbital sodium

(E) Removal of cerebrospinal fluid (CSF) by ventriculostomy

95. The girl receives aggressive treatment with pentobarbital, mannitol, and hyperventilation. Despite these measures, there is no improvement for several days, and brain death evaluation is initiated. Which of the following statements regarding this evaluation is true?

(A) The Glasgow Coma Score should not be used to document brain death

(B) Use of barbiturate medications does not affect the ability to diagnose brain death

(C) MRI of the brain can often be helpful in difficult situations

(D) Brain death cannot be diagnosed with a cerebral angiogram

(E) Brain death cannot be diagnosed while a patient remains on artificial ventilation

Setting: Hospital

Questions 96–98

A 45-year-old woman undergoes an abdominal hysterectomy for fibroids and excessive menstrual bleeding. The procedure is uneventful but is complicated by some postoperative nausea and vomiting. She is treated with intravenous fluids (5% dextrose and 0.5 normal saline at 200 mL/hour) and admitted to your service. Overnight, she continues to complain of nausea and incisional pain. Promethazine hydrochloride (Phenergan) and morphine sulfate have good results. On morning rounds, she is confused and somnolent with stable vital signs. Physical examination is remarkable only for incisional tenderness. Laboratory work reveals a serum sodium of 110 mEq/L.

96. The cause of her hyponatremia is

(A) syndrome of inappropriate secretion of antidiuretic hormone (SIADH)
(B) primary polydipsia
(C) hypothyroidism
(D) Addison disease
(E) heart failure

97. Which of the following laboratory results confirms the diagnosis?

(A) Urine osmolality <100 mOsm/L
(B) Urine osmolality >150 mOsm/L
(C) Elevated thyroid-stimulating hormone (TSH)
(D) Urine sodium <10 mEq/L
(E) Fractional excretion of sodium <1%

98. Which of the following measures would be the most appropriate treatment for this patient?

(A) Change intravenous fluids to normal saline
(B) Furosemide
(C) Fluid restriction
(D) Hypertonic saline infusion
(E) Demeclocycline hydrochloride

Setting: Hospital

Questions 99–100

A 65-year-old man is admitted to the hospital after developing fevers, chills, and hypotension during dialysis, which he began 2 weeks ago. The dialysis occurs through a temporary catheter placed in the right internal jugular vein. He states that he noted some redness and pain around the catheter yesterday, and he had a shaking chill before dialysis this morning. During dialysis, his temperature rose to 39°C, and rigor developed; in addition, his blood pressure fell from 140/90 to 90/60 mm Hg. On examination, there is some purulence and erythema around the catheter site. Blood cultures are obtained and arrangements are made to admit the man to the hospital.

99. Which of the following organisms would be most likely to grow from this patient's blood cultures?

(A) *Streptococcus pneumoniae*
(B) *Streptococcus pyogenes*
(C) *Klebsiella pneumoniae*
(D) *Candida albicans*
(E) *Staphylococcus aureus*

100. Which of the following agents is appropriate initial treatment of this man?

(A) Gentamicin
(B) Cefazolin sodium
(C) Ceftriaxone
(D) Vancomycin
(E) Imipenem

Setting: Hospital

Questions 101–105

A 45-year-old man with acute leukemia is admitted with a hematocrit of 12%. A type and screen is performed, and a transfusion of packed red blood cells (RBCs) is started. The first unit of blood is administered without complications. However, during the infusion of the second unit of blood, the patient's temperature rises to 38.9°C. The infusion is stopped, and the blood is sent back to the blood bank, where it is confirmed that the blood typing is correct.

101. What is the likely cause of this febrile reaction to the blood transfusion?

(A) Incompatible blood transfusion
(B) Bacterial contamination of the unit of blood
(C) Viral contamination of the unit of blood
(D) Response secondary to donor white blood cells (WBCs)
(E) Response to plasma proteins

102. The man requires another transfusion several days later. During the infusion of the first unit of blood, itching and urticaria develop, followed by wheezing. The transfusion is halted. What is the likely cause of *this* transfusion reaction?

(A) Incompatible blood transfusion
(B) Bacterial contamination of the unit of blood
(C) Viral contamination of the unit of blood
(D) Response secondary to donor WBCs
(E) Response to plasma proteins

103. Which of the following measures would be appropriate therapy for *this* transfusion reaction?

(A) Acetaminophen
(B) Intravenous hydration and furosemide
(C) Diphenhydramine
(D) Methylprednisolone acetate, diphenhydramine, and epinephrine
(E) Albuterol nebulizer and diphenhydramine

104. The man returns after his first cycle of chemotherapy complaining of severe fatigue. His hematocrit is 14%. A blood transfusion is begun. Severe back pain, temperature to 39°C, blood pressure of 70/40 mm Hg, and nausea develop within 30 minutes of initiation of the transfusion. The transfusion is stopped immediately. What is the likely cause of *this* transfusion reaction?

(A) Incompatible blood transfusion
(B) Bacterial contamination of the unit of blood
(C) Viral contamination of the unit of blood
(D) Response secondary to donor WBCs
(E) Response to plasma proteins

105. Which of the following rapid diagnostic tests would yield the correct diagnosis for *this* transfusion reaction?

(A) Complete blood count (CBC)
(B) Centrifugation of whole blood and inspection of the supernatant
(C) Urinalysis
(D) Chest radiograph
(E) Blood cultures

Setting: Emergency Department and Hospital

Questions 106–110

A 65-year-old man presents with several weeks of generalized fatigue and malaise. He had not seen a physician in the past 30 years and is unaware of any prior medical problems. Occasionally, he takes acetaminophen or ibuprofen; they are his only medications. He usually drinks 2 or 3 beers every day, and he has smoked 1 pack of cigarettes per day for the past 42 years. Review of symptoms is notable for polyuria and polydipsia, intermittent nausea, and constipation.
   Physical examination reveals:

General appearance	Thin man with normal vital signs
Cardiac	Regular rate with no murmurs
Lungs	Rales at left base
	Decreased breath sounds at right base with associated dullness to percussion
Abdominal	Hypoactive bowel sounds, no masses, and no hepatosplenomegaly
Extremities	No edema or cyanosis
	Clubbing on both hands

106. Which of the following laboratory tests/procedures, in addition to a complete blood count (CBC) and a chemistry panel, is indicated in the initial workup of this man's symptoms?

(A) Hepatic panel and chest radiograph
(B) Hepatic panel and thyroid panel
(C) Hepatic panel
(D) Chest radiograph
(E) Chest radiograph and serum protein electrophoresis

107. Which of the following conditions should NOT be included in the initial differential diagnosis of this man's complaints?

(A) Liver disease
(B) Hypercalcemia
(C) Malignancy
(D) Major depression
(E) Tuberculosis

108. Laboratory work reveals:

Na^+	140 mEq/L
Cl^-	100 mEq/L
$H_2CO_3^-$	27 mEq/L
Ca^{2+}	12.1 mEq/L
Phosphorus	3.1 mg/dL
Blood urea nitrogen (BUN)	45 mg/dL
Creatinine	2.1 mg/dL

The man's hypercalcemia is most likely mediated by

(A) elevated vitamin D levels
(B) elevated parathyroid hormone levels
(C) elevated parathyroid-related hormone levels
(D) skeletal invasion by the tumor
(E) renal insufficiency

109. Which of the following findings would most likely be apparent on the man's chest radiograph?

(A) Normal
(B) Hyperinflation and bullous emphysema
(C) Hilar lymphadenopathy and bullous emphysema
(D) Pleural effusion and hilar adenopathy
(E) Granulomas

110. Which of the following measures would be the appropriate treatment at this point?

(A) Intravenous hydration
(B) Corticosteroids
(C) Pamidronate disodium
(D) Plicamycin
(E) Calcitonin

Setting: Emergency Department

Questions 111–113

A 22-year-old man with AIDS presents with severe headache, nausea, vomiting, blurry vision, and fever of 24 hours' duration. He has had headaches and low-grade fevers for the past week. The patient is taking only trimethoprim-sulfamethoxazole. Currently cared for at a local hospice, he has suffered from AIDS for the past 6 years; his course has been marked by *Pneumocystis carinii* pneumonia, Kaposi sarcoma, *Candida* esophagitis, and severe wasting.

Physical examination indicates:

Vital signs	
Temperature	39°C
Blood pressure	180/100 mm Hg
Respiratory rate	20/min
General	Marked distress with photophobia
Neck	Moderately rigid to movement
Oropharynx	Within normal limits
Chest	Clear bilaterally
Heart	Tachycardia, regular rate
Abdominal	Normal bowel sounds, no masses
Neurologic	
Cranial nerves	Intact
Motor and sensory examination	Within normal limits
Funduscopy	As shown

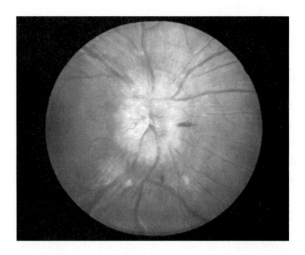

111. The funduscopic examination is most consistent with which of the following diagnoses?

(A) Advanced diabetes mellitus
(B) Optic neuritis
(C) Retinal detachment
(D) Episcleritis
(E) Papilledema

112. To make the appropriate diagnosis and institute appropriate therapy, which of the following should be performed immediately?

(A) CT of the brain
(B) Lumbar puncture
(C) Intravenous mannitol
(D) Intravenous dexamethasone
(E) Intravenous ceftriaxone alone

113. Which of the following is the most likely diagnosis?

(A) Bacterial meningitis
(B) Toxoplasmosis
(C) Lymphoma
(D) Cryptococcal meningitis
(E) Metastatic Kaposi sarcoma

Setting: Emergency Department

Questions 114–115

A 34-year-old woman, pregnant with her first child, presents to the ED with fever, nausea, back pain, and dysuria of several hours' duration. She is currently at 26 weeks' gestation, and so far, her pregnancy has been uncomplicated. For the past several hours, she has had several shaking chills and dull pain on the right side of her back. Last night, she had some burning with urination and awoke every 1 to 2 hours to urinate. On examination, she is febrile to 39°C and has marked right-sided costovertebral angle tenderness. Urinalysis reveals white blood cells (WBCs) and WBC casts.

114. Which of the following conditions is the most likely diagnosis?

(A) Nephrolithiasis
(B) Abruptio placentae
(C) Glomerulonephritis
(D) Preeclampsia
(E) Pyelonephritis

115. Which of the following measures is the most appropriate course of action?

(A) 5-day outpatient treatment with oral ciprofloxacin
(B) 7-day outpatient treatment with nitrofurantoin
(C) Overnight admission and treatment with a 7-day course of nitrofurantoin
(D) Hospital admission and initial treatment with intravenous ceftriaxone
(E) Renal biopsy

Setting: Emergency Department

Questions 116–117

A 2-year-old boy is brought to the ED by his parents. Reportedly, he has been ill with a "viral syndrome" for the past 2 days, with fever, anorexia, and rhinorrhea. However, during the past 6 to 8 hours, he has become extremely lethargic, and he has started to vomit and complain of diffuse abdominal pain. His father is sure his son has appendicitis and requests that a surgeon attend to him immediately. On physical examination, a firm mass in the right upper quadrant is palpable.

116. Your next step should be to

(A) call a surgeon immediately
(B) obtain a complete blood count (CBC), blood chemistries, and liver enzymes
(C) obtain a plain film of the abdomen
(D) obtain a CT scan of the abdomen
(E) obtain an ultrasound of the abdomen

117. Which of the following procedures is indicated in the care of this child?

(A) Appendectomy
(B) Barium enema
(C) Intravenous antibiotics
(D) Lumbar puncture
(E) Colonoscopy

Setting: Emergency Department and Hospital

Questions 118–120

A 34-year-old woman with a long history of depression presents after ingesting approximately 60 mL of drain cleaner during a suicide attempt. Physical examination reveals ulcerations of the lips and oropharynx, with surrounding erythema and blistering. The remainder of the examination is within normal limits. A chest radiograph is normal without evidence of free mediastinal air.

118. Which of the following procedures is indicated?

(A) Nasogastric tube placement
(B) Induction of vomiting
(C) Broad-spectrum antibiotics
(D) Early upper endoscopy
(E) CT of the chest and abdomen

119. The patient undergoes a procedure and is placed on parenteral nutrition for 2 weeks while her esophagus heals. She is then able to tolerate oral feeding and is discharged home. Which of the following complications can she expect in the future?

(A) Gastroesophageal reflux
(B) Sclerosing mediastinitis
(C) Esophageal strictures
(D) Gastric carcinoma
(E) Oral cancer

120. The woman does well for the next 6 months. Then acute hematemesis develops; it is intermittent initially but soon becomes profuse. The rescue squad is called, but by the time they arrive she is unconscious. She is resuscitated en route to the ED, where the profuse hematemesis continues. Ultimately, she becomes hypotensive followed by a pulseless electrical activity code. Efforts to resuscitate her are unsuccessful. An autopsy is requested by the woman's family. The most likely cause of death is

(A) cirrhosis with an esophageal variceal bleed
(B) a Mallory-Weiss tear of the esophagus
(C) a bleeding gastric ulcer
(D) an aortoesophageal fistula
(E) a bleeding esophageal carcinoma

Setting: Office

Questions 121–123

A 56-year-old man, who presents after a recent conviction for driving under the influence of alcohol, is interested in stopping his alcohol consumption. He states that he has abused alcohol for nearly 30 years, drinking from 12 beers to 1 quart of hard liquor per day. He began to drink socially in college, and his consumption has subsequently increased. He has tried to remain sober several times; his longest period of abstinence was 2 weeks. Reportedly, he has never suffered withdrawal symptoms or blackouts. He currently works as a sales executive for an electronics company. At present, he is married with two children, and his wife is supportive of his decision.

121. The man is interested in using disulfiram (Antabuse) to help him remain abstinent. Which of the following statements regarding this agent is NOT true?

(A) Its primary action is to block aldehyde dehydrogenase
(B) Myocardial infarctions (MIs) may occur with its use
(C) Patients must continue to use it for prolonged periods (i.e., years) to obtain full benefit
(D) Patients may suffer reactions after drinking alcohol as long as 1 to 2 weeks after they stop using it
(E) Patients who take it may develop reactions to medications containing alcohol

122. Which of the following conditions would NOT be expected to occur during the acute phase of alcohol cessation?

(A) Tachycardia
(B) Hallucinations
(C) Rhinorrhea
(D) Seizures
(E) Suicidal ideation

123. Which of the following statements about alcoholics and alcoholism is NOT true?

(A) There is a high percentage of underlying depression in these patients
(B) Many alcoholics drink to avoid anxiety
(C) Outpatient rehabilitation programs are more successful than inpatient units
(D) Controlled consumption is a validated alternative to complete abstinence
(E) Alcoholics Anonymous has success rates comparable to those of specialized treatment programs

Setting: Hospital

Questions 124–125

A 72-year-old woman is admitted to the psychiatry service with severe depression. During the past 6 weeks, she has stopped eating and does not talk to others. Her primary care physician has attempted trials of numerous antidepressants without success. The woman, who has been speaking to people who are not present, has recently become increasing paranoid. Physical examination and laboratory work have been unrevealing, and she is currently refusing all medications.

124. Which of the following therapies would be most likely to offer significant benefit?

(A) Intensive psychotherapy
(B) Behavioral therapy
(C) Electroconvulsive therapy
(D) Lorazepam
(E) High-dose trazodone hydrochloride

125. Which of the following is NOT a side effect of electroconvulsive therapy?

(A) Memory loss
(B) Seizures
(C) Myocardial infarction (MI)
(D) Mania
(E) Myalgias

Setting: Office

Questions 126–127

A 65-year-old man and his 62-year-old wife, who both have type 2 diabetes mellitus, are planning a trip to Latin America. Their glycemic control is excellent. The husband, who also suffers from atrial fibrillation, is taking atenolol and warfarin. Both the man and his wife are concerned about the possibility of traveler's diarrhea, and they have read that a prophylactic treatment is available.

126. Which of the following regimens would you recommend?

(A) Cholera vaccine
(B) Drinking only bottled water during the trip
(C) Ciprofloxacin for 3 to 5 days after the onset of diarrhea
(D) Cephalexin for 7 days after the onset of diarrhea
(E) No prophylaxis is indicated

127. The couple decides against your recommendation and takes bismuth subsalicylate (Pepto-Bismol; 2 tablets 4 times daily) during their trip. The husband notes that his gums bleed whenever he brushes his teeth and a minor scrape on his leg is still bleeding long after the injury. Which of the following is implicated in the man's prolonged bleeding?

(A) Overdosage of warfarin
(B) Potentiation of warfarin effect secondary to bismuth
(C) Inhibition of warfarin absorption by bismuth
(D) Effect of Pepto-Bismol on platelet function
(E) Interaction of warfarin and new diet in Latin America

Setting: Office

Questions 128–130

A 49-year-old woman presents for routine care. For the past several visits, her blood pressure has consistently been 160/90 mm Hg. Her medications include conjugated estrogens 0.625 mg/day. She denies alcohol use, over-the-counter cold preparation use, and illicit drug use, and she smokes 1 pack of cigarettes per day. Both her mother and father have hypertension. You have a discussion with her about the possibility of initiating antihypertensive therapy. Before initiating therapy, you ask the woman to have her blood pressure checked outside the office. She calls with the following blood pressures: 120/70 mm Hg, 123/80 mm Hg, and 126/76 mm Hg.

128. Which of the following measures would you recommend?

(A) Repeating the blood pressure measurements after discontinuing estrogen
(B) Daily exercise and repeating blood pressure measurements in 2 to 3 months
(C) Begin hydrochlorothiazide 25 mg
(D) 24-hour ambulatory blood pressure monitoring
(E) Begin atenolol 25 mg

129. After instituting your recommendation, the woman returns with a blood pressure of 162/90 mm Hg, and you advise treatment. Before doing so, you obtain some screening laboratory tests; her serum potassium is 3.1 mEq/L. All of the other laboratory tests are within normal limits. Which of the following conditions could account for these findings?

(A) Primary hyperaldosteronism
(B) Cocaine abuse
(C) Essential hypertension
(D) Addison disease
(E) Hyperthyroidism

130. To confirm the diagnosis you are considering, which of the following laboratory tests would be most helpful?

(A) CT of the abdomen
(B) MRI of the abdomen
(C) Thyroid-stimulating hormone (TSH)
(D) Renin/aldosterone ratio
(E) Urine drug screen

Setting: Outpatient Clinic

Questions 131–134

131. You are rotating through the urology clinic. The first patient you are asked to see is a 45-year-old woman with multiple sclerosis who has developed urinary incontinence of recent onset. She complains that she often loses large volumes of urine and has started to use adult diapers. Post-void residual volume of urine is 80 mL. Which of the following measures is a reasonable treatment strategy?

(A) Long-term, indwelling Foley catheter
(B) Intermittent Foley catheter
(C) Pelvic muscle exercises
(D) Scheduled voiding
(E) Prompted voiding

132. Your next patient is a 70-year-old woman who complains of urinary incontinence after physical activity (especially gardening) and after coughing or laughing. On examination you note a prolapsed cystocele and a postvoid residual urine volume of 350 mL. The woman is opposed to any surgical procedures. Which of the following measures is a reasonable treatment strategy?

(A) Long-term, indwelling Foley catheter
(B) Intermittent Foley catheter
(C) Pelvic muscle exercises
(D) Scheduled voiding
(E) Prompted voiding

133. The next patient, who is referred from the local nursing home, is an 80-year-old woman with a history of a stroke and dementia. Every morning, the nursing home staff finds that she has urinated in bed. Furthermore, during the day she has required adult diapers secondary to incontinence. Because of this problem, she has developed recurrent candidal skin infections. A postvoid residual urine volume is 60 mL. Which of the following measures is a reasonable treatment strategy?

(A) Long-term, indwelling Foley catheter
(B) Intermittent Foley catheter
(C) Pelvic muscle exercises
(D) Scheduled voiding
(E) Prompted voiding

134. The last patient of the day is a 78-year-old man who complains of urinary urgency and the inability to make it to the bathroom before wetting himself. He is not taking any medications. On physical examination, he has a symmetrically enlarged prostate without nodules. A postvoid residual urine volume is 150 mL. Which of the following measures is a reasonable treatment strategy?

(A) Long-term indwelling Foley catheter
(B) Intermittent Foley catheter
(C) Pelvic muscle exercises
(D) Scheduled voiding
(E) Prompted voiding

Setting: Hospital

Questions 135–136

A recent journal article reports the sensitivity of chest radiograph findings in the diagnosis of pneumonia in patients with acute respiratory distress syndrome (ARDS). The paper reports that the finding of asymmetrical infiltrates on chest radiography has a sensitivity of 57% and a specificity of 70% for the diagnosis of nosocomial pneumonia.

135. Which of the following is the best definition of positive predictive value?

(A) Probability that a test or procedure will be positive when disease is present
(B) Probability that disease is present when the test or procedure is positive
(C) The value that separates a positive from a negative for a given test
(D) The number of true-positive tests in all patients tested
(E) The number of true-positive tests divided by the number of false-positive tests

136. In the ICU, pneumonia develops in 10% of patients with ARDS. In this situation, what is the positive predictive value of finding asymmetrical infiltrates on chest radiograph?

(A) 17%
(B) 25%
(C) 75%
(D) 82%
(E) 94%

Setting: Office

Questions 137–138

A 59-year-old man with a long history of poorly controlled type 2 diabetes mellitus presents with the acute onset of double vision. He noted onset of pain behind his left eye on awakening followed shortly thereafter by diplopia. His medical history is significant for hypertension, tobacco abuse, obesity, and coronary artery disease.

On physical examination, the man's blood pressure is 180/98 mm Hg. The left eye is unable to adduct on gaze to the right, but gaze to the left is intact. Both pupils react normally to light, and mild left eyelid ptosis is present. The rest of the neurologic examination is notable only for a dense peripheral neuropathy that affects both legs up to midcalf. Cardiac examination is notable only for an S_4 heart sound. The remainder of the physical examination is within normal limits.

137. Which of the following lesions accounts for his symptoms?

(A) Lesion in cranial nerve (CN) II
(B) Lesion in CN III
(C) Lesion in CN VI
(D) Occipital lobe stroke
(E) Retinal detachment

138. Which of the following conditions is the most likely cause of this man's complaint?

(A) Myasthenia gravis
(B) Horner syndrome
(C) Multiple sclerosis
(D) Diabetes mellitus
(E) Cerebrovascular accident

Setting: Satellite Clinic

Questions 139–142

You are rotating through a sexually transmitted disease clinic at the local health department. The first patient is an 18-year-old woman with complaints of a 2-month history of a white, creamy, vaginal discharge with foul odor. She has mild dysuria and pruritus. Over-the-counter treatments for *Candida* vaginitis have not yielded success. She is sexually active but has not had intercourse for the past 6 weeks. On examination, you note a vaginal pH of 6.5 and a strong odor when potassium hydroxide (KOH) is applied to a slide of the discharge.

139. Which of the following would you expect to see on the wet mount slide of the vaginal discharge?

(A) Budding yeast
(B) Numerous white blood cells (WBCs)
(C) Benign appearance with a few squamous cells
(D) Clue cells
(E) *Trichomonas* organisms

140. Which of the following treatment measures is appropriate?

(A) Oral fluconazole
(B) Intravaginal miconazole for 7 days
(C) Metronidazole orally for 7 days
(D) Topical estrogen cream
(E) Intramuscular ceftriaxone, single dose

141. Your next patient is a 30-year-old woman with a recent diagnosis of HIV infection. She is complaining of severe vulvar pruritus and erythema, as well as a white vaginal discharge. She has used over-the-counter creams to self-treat similar conditions during the past year. Currently, she is not sexually active. She recently took cephalexin for a urinary tract infection. On examination, severe vulvar irritation with erythema and edema is event. The pH of the thick, white discharge is 3.5. Which of the following would you expect to see on the wet mount slide of the vaginal discharge?

(A) Budding yeast
(B) Numerous white blood cells (WBCs)
(C) Benign appearance with a few squamous cells
(D) Clue cells
(E) *Trichomonas* organisms

142. Which of the following measures would be an appropriate treatment for this condition?

(A) Oral fluconazole
(B) Intravaginal miconazole for 7 days
(C) Metronidazole orally for 7 days
(D) Topical estrogen cream
(E) Intramuscular ceftriaxone, single dose

Setting: Hospital

Questions 143–145

Three patients share the following characteristics:

1. Admission to the ICU with temperatures to 39.5°C
2. Hypotension that requires intravenous dopamine for maintenance of mean arterial pressure above 60 mm Hg
3. Obtundation, or obtunded sensorium, that requires intubation, with arterial blood gases that show mild, metabolic acidosis and respiratory alkalosis

143. A 24-year-old woman is receiving treatment for acute myelocytic leukemia with intensive chemotherapy. On the day of transfer to the ICU, her absolute neutrophil count is less than 50 cells/mm³. She does not have a central venous catheter. Which of the following antibiotic regimens is most appropriate?

(A) Vancomycin
(B) Cefoxitin and doxycycline
(C) Cefepime
(D) Piperacillin/tazobactam and gentamicin
(E) Ceftriaxone and azithromycin

144. A 48-year-old man is admitted from the ED with a dense, right middle lobar pneumonia. Which of the following antibiotic regimens is most appropriate?

(A) Vancomycin
(B) Cefoxitin and doxycycline
(C) Cefepime
(D) Piperacillin/tazobactam and gentamicin
(E) Ceftriaxone and azithromycin

145. A 38-year-old female prostitute presents with vaginal discharge, cervical motion tenderness, and a tender right adnexa. Which of the following antibiotic regimens is most appropriate?

(A) Vancomycin
(B) Cefoxitin and doxycycline
(C) Cefepime
(D) Piperacillin/tazobactam and gentamicin
(E) Ceftriaxone and azithromycin

Setting: Hospital and Emergency Department

Questions 146–147

A 48-year-old woman is admitted with a complete small bowel obstruction and emergently taken to surgery, where a large leiomyoma is found to be obstructing the terminal ileum. The tumor is removed along with the terminal ileum. The woman recovers uneventfully. Several months later, she presents with fatigue, and her hematocrit is 27%.

146. Which of the following findings might you expect to see on her peripheral smear?

(A) Microcytosis
(B) Spherocytosis
(C) Schistocytes
(D) Hypersegmented neutrophils
(E) Thrombocytosis

147. During the next few months, the woman begins to have severe, foul-smelling diarrhea that is positive for fecal fat. She presents to the ED with severe right-sided flank pain and hematuria. Ultrasound demonstrates a large kidney stone in the right renal pelvis. The composition of the kidney stone would likely be

(A) cystine
(B) calcium oxalate
(C) struvite
(D) uric acid
(E) none of the above

Setting: Satellite Clinic

148. A 25-year-old woman, who has recently given birth to a healthy male infant and begun to breast-feed, presents with a 2-day history of left breast tenderness and erythema, along with a low-grade fever. On examination, she is currently afebrile and has a 2×3-cm^2 area of erythema just under her left nipple. No purulent drainage or abscess is felt. An ultrasound confirms that there is no fluid collection. Which of the following treatment measures is appropriate?

(A) Warm compresses and nonsteroidal anti-inflammatory agents (NSAIDs)
(B) Antistaphylococcal antibiotics and continuation of breast-feeding until her condition improves
(C) Antistaphylococcal antibiotics and cessation of breast-feeding until improved
(D) Topical steroids and NSAIDs
(E) Suppression of lactation with bromocriptine

Setting: Hospital

149. A 46-year-old man suffers a spinal cord injury in a motor vehicle accident. His course in the ICU is prolonged; eventually, he is extubated. However, several hours after extubation he suffers from respiratory distress and becomes hypotensive. A chest radiograph shows bilateral pulmonary edema. Despite diuretics, the man continues to deteriorate and requires emergent intubation. The attending physician decides that the intubation is extremely difficult because the patient is in a neck collar and the clinician is unable to visualize the uvula. Furthermore, the respiratory therapist comments that it is difficult to ventilate the patient by mask. Which of the following airway management strategies is most appropriate?

(A) Emergent cricothyrotomy
(B) Rapid-sequence intubation with propofol and succinylcholine chloride
(C) Rapid-sequence intubation with propofol and pancuronium
(D) Nasal intubation with propofol and succinylcholine chloride
(E) Topical anesthesia with lidocaine to the airway followed by nasal intubation

Setting: Hospital

150. You are asked to chair a committee to investigate the use of antibiotics in your hospital. One of the primary concerns has been the recent increase in the use of vancomycin by all physicians. You wish to publish guidelines that restrict the use of vancomycin to those situations in which it is absolutely indicated. Which of the following clinical scenarios constitutes an appropriate use of vancomycin?

(A) Primary therapy for *Clostridium difficile* colitis
(B) Primary therapy as part of a regimen for infective endocarditis
(C) Convenient home therapy for a strain of *Staphylococcus aureus* that is sensitive to oxacillin
(D) Therapy for a β-lactam–resistant *Staphylococcus epidermidis* infection
(E) Primary therapy for peritonitis in a patient with end-stage renal disease who is receiving peritoneal dialysis

ANSWER KEY

1-A	31-E	61-C	91-B	121-C
2-C	32-E	62-D	92-C	122-C
3-C	33-D	63-D	93-D	123-D
4-C	34-D	64-E	94-E	124-C
5-A	35-C	65-C	95-A	125-D
6-E	36-A	66-E	96-A	126-C
7-B	37-E	67-E	97-B	127-D
8-D	38-D	68-E	98-C	128-D
9-E	39-E	69-B	99-E	129-A
10-A	40-E	70-C	100-D	130-D
11-D	41-C	71-B	101-D	131-D
12-C	42-D	72-E	102-E	132-B
13-C	43-D	73-D	103-D	133-E
14-A	44-B	74-C	104-A	134-B
15-D	45-D	75-D	105-B	135-B
16-D	46-D	76-E	106-A	136-A
17-E	47-D	77-E	107-D	137-B
18-D	48-E	78-C	108-C	138-D
19-A	49-C	79-D	109-D	139-D
20-E	50-D	80-B	110-A	140-C
21-C	51-A	81-A	111-E	141-A
22-A	52-E	82-E	112-A	142-A
23-A	53-D	83-B	113-D	143-D
24-B	54-B	84-C	114-E	144-E
25-D	55-E	85-C	115-D	145-B
26-C	56-C	86-D	116-C	146-D
27-C	57-D	87-D	117-B	147-B
28-E	58-C	88-C	118-D	148-B
29-A	59-A	89-C	119-C	149-E
30-A	60-E	90-D	120-D	150-D

ANSWERS AND EXPLANATIONS

1–3. The answers are: 1-A, 2-C, 3-C. (*Emergency medicine, internal medicine*)
The electrocardiographic (ECG) findings are consistent with Osborne waves, or J waves, which are seen in hypothermia. Classically, there is a deflection inscribed between the QRS complex and the beginning of the ST segment. In the left ventricular leads, the polarity of the wave is positive, and its amplitude is inversely related to body temperature. The physiologic mechanism of the Osborne wave is still unknown.

Because this patient has evidence of hypothermia on ECG, her vital signs, including temperature, are the most direct way to elucidate her problem. In the emergency department (ED), the next question is the source of the hypothermia. The differential diagnoses include environmental exposure; malnutrition; hypothyroidism; adrenal insufficiency; hepatic failure; hypoglycemia; sepsis; uremia; hypothalamic dysfunction; and ethanol, lithium, opiate, benzodiazepine, phenothiazine, and barbiturate toxicity. To narrow the list of possible diagnoses, further history taking is necessary. A thyroid-stimulating hormone (TSH) level is warranted; however, the result would not be available in a timely fashion. A glucose level, which should be rapidly obtained in any unresponsive patient, would not account for the ECG findings. Although blood chemistries are necessary, it is unlikely that the results would explain the patient's unresponsiveness. Creatine kinase would be useful as a check for rhabdomyolysis in a patient found unconscious for an unknown period of time.

The primary management is rewarming via active, passive, internal, or external measures. Passive rewarming involves the use of blankets and a warm environment allowing endogenous heat production to rewarm the patient. It is important to keep the head covered. Body temperature increases 0.5° to 2.0°C/hour. Active external warming uses heating blankets, heat lamps, and warm water immersion to rewarm at a faster rate. However, blood pressure may drop if the direct warming causes peripheral vasodilation in a dehydrated patient. In addition, the peripheral vasodilation allows cooler peripheral blood to enter the core circulation, causing core temperature "after drop." Active internal warming involves the use of warm intravenous saline infusion, warm humidified air, warm pleural or peritoneal lavage, or warm colonic or bladder lavage. The most efficient method of rewarming is extracorporeal warming by hemodialysis or cardiopulmonary bypass. This method can increase core temperature 1° to 2°C every 3 to 5 minutes.

If rewarming is already underway, intravenous saline is the most important measure for correcting hemodynamic compromise. Isotonic fluids should be used; however, lactated Ringer solution should be avoided because hypothermia inhibits lactate metabolism in the liver.

With regard to intubation or "code" status, a patient's advanced directives should be followed unless the patient directly states that there be a change. However, it is always prudent to involve the hospital's ethics group in difficult situations. Families often have other desires, but the patient's wishes must be followed.

4–8. The answers are: 4-C, 5-A, 6-E, 7-B, 8-D. (*Internal medicine*)
This 26-year-old man has sinusitis, which is an inflammation of the paranasal sinuses surrounding the eye. In this common condition, it is often difficult to distinguish between bacterial sinusitis, which requires treatment, and viral or allergic sinusitis, which is usually self-limited. The use of antibiotics in the treatment of bacterial sinusitis is controversial. Acute sinusitis is usually self-limited, but it can occasionally lead to life-threatening central nervous system (CNS) complications such as infection or thrombosis.

CT studies of patients with "viral" upper respiratory infections reveal that more than 85% have a self-limited paranasal sinusitis that resolves without treatment. The typical symptoms are rhinorrhea and nasal stuffiness. In 0.5% to 2.0% of cases, bacterial sinusitis may follow, resulting in purulent nasal discharge, facial pain, fever (50%), teeth pain, frontal headache, or fatigue. In this situation, patients have experienced a previous upper respiratory infection followed by worsening of symptoms, including purulent rhinorrhea. This suggests bacterial sinusitis. The three most common causal organisms are *Streptococcus pneumoniae, Haemophilus influenzae,* and *Moraxella catarrhalis.* Occasionally, anaerobes are involved in the setting of dental infections or recurrent infections. Rhinoviruses can be isolated concomitantly with bacteria.

The diagnosis of sinusitis is primarily clinical, but imaging can be useful. Plain radiographs of the sinuses are sufficiently sensitive to rule out frontal and maxillary sinusitis, but their ability to detect sinusitis in ethmoidal or sphenoidal sinuses is poor. CT is extremely sensitive, but it may often "overcall" sinus disease (i.e., lead to a false-positive result). To decrease the false-positive rate, as with any test, CT is necessary only in patients with a high pretest probability. Ultrasound has a lower sensitivity than radiography or CT but has good specificity. Sinus and nasal culture has a high rate of false-negative and false-positive results.

The optimal treatment remains controversial. In the few existing randomized controlled trials, antibiotics show some benefit over decongestants alone; however, cure rates without antibiotics are also high (nearly 70%). The best first agents are amoxicillin and trimethoprim-sulfamethoxazole. Amoxicillin-clavulanate and cefuroxime should be reserved for sinusitis that does not resolve. However, random controlled trials have not found clear benefit of amoxicillin-clavulanate over amoxicillin alone. Because azithromycin and clarithromycin are less useful against penicillin-resistant *S. pneumoniae,* they are not optimal choices. Phenylephrine is a useful adjunctive therapy, but its use should not exceed 3 days.

Secondary causes of recurrent sinusitis include Kartagener syndrome (immotile cilia syndrome), head and neck cancer (causing obstruction), Wegener granulomatosis, and common variable immunodeficiency. This patient, who is having difficulty fathering a child, may have sperm motility abnormalities suggestive of Kartagener syndrome; which includes recurrent upper and lower respiratory infections such as sinusitis, otitis media, and bronchiectasis in combination with situs inversus. Wegener granulomatosis, a small-vessel vasculitis, manifests with head and neck, lung, and kidney disease. Common variable immunodeficiency is a disorder in which patients have deficient production of all major immunoglobulin classes. Affected individuals present with frequent pulmonary infections, bronchiectasis, chronic giardiasis, splenomegaly, and generalized lymphadenopathy.

A high-resolution CT scan might find bronchiectasis secondary to frequent infections related to poor ciliary function. Pleural calcifications are seen in patients with asbestos exposure. Ground glass infiltrates are common with any inflammatory interstitial disease of the lungs. Pleural effusions can be seen with numerous inflammatory lung conditions or with heart failure.

Examination of the sputum in patients with bronchiectasis (dilated, patulous bronchi) often shows *Streptococcus pneumoniae, Haemophilus influenzae, Pseudomonas* species, *Staphylococcus aureus,* and atypical mycobacteria. *Aspergillus* occurs primarily in association with allergic bronchopulmonary aspergillosis, in which bronchiectasis is found centrally and apically.

9–12. The answers are: 9-E, 10-A, 11-D, 12-C. (*Internal medicine*)

This woman appears to be describing polyuria. However, this is a difficult diagnosis to make by history alone because the patient might be describing many episodes of urination with scant production of urine. Thus, a 24-hour urine collection is essential; 3 L/day is considered the threshold for polyuria.

The approach to polyuria also involves checking urine osmolality. A high osmolality suggests a solute diuresis secondary to glucose, mannitol, radiocontrast, urea (if high protein feeding), medullary cystic disease, or resolving acute tubular necrosis or obstruction. A low osmolality suggests primary polydipsia, phenothiazines, hypothalamic disease, central diabetes insipidus, or nephrogenic diabetes insipidus. Both hypercalcemia and hypokalemia result in concentrating defects at the level of the kidney tubules. Diabetes mellitus causes polyuria secondary to glucose solute diuresis. Syndrome of inappropriate secretion of antidiuretic hormone (SIADH) would not cause polyuria; patients inappropriately reabsorb water.

Drugs are a frequent cause of SIADH. The most common agents are chlorpropamide; vincristine; cyclophosphamide; carbamazepine; selective serotonin reuptake inhibitors, including paroxetine; clofibrate; narcotics; and tricyclic antidepressants. Ciprofloxacin is not a common cause of SIADH.

The result of this patient's random glucose test prompts the concern for diabetes mellitus; however, this result is not diagnostic of diabetes. To diagnose diabetes mellitus, any *one* of the following three criteria is necessary: (1) a random glucose level of more than 200 mg/dL in the setting of symptoms consistent with diabetes mellitus, including polyuria, polydipsia, and polyphagia; (2) a fasting glucose level of more than 126 mg/dL; and (3) a positive oral glucose tolerance test. A fasting glucose test is indicated. However, urinalysis provides the urine osmolality via the specific gravity and also looks for glucose in the urine. It is the most logical next step. Glycosylated hemoglobin is a reasonable clinical choice because it helps guide treatment decisions, but it is not the standard of care for diagnostic purposes. A parathyroid hormone level would be useful if the patient was clearly hypercalcemic, and an albumin level would be useful to ascertain if the corrected calcium is actually higher.

Hypercalcemia can cause polyuria by downregulating the aquaphorin 2 channels in the collecting duct system of the kidneys, causing nephrogenic diabetes insipidus. Causes of hypercalcemia include hyperparathyroidism, hyperthyroidism, immobility, milk-alkali syndrome, Paget disease, Addison disease, acromegaly, lymphoma, renal carcinoma, squamous cell carcinoma, sarcoidosis and other granulomatous diseases and vitamins A and D excess. Hypothyroidism is not a typical cause of hypercalcemia.

13–17. The answers are: 13-C, 14-A, 15-D, 16-D, 17-E. (*Internal medicine*)
This patient appears fairly healthy and is taking two medications. In primary care medicine, health maintenance including vaccines can have the greatest impact on patients. Several organizations have their own primary care guidelines, including the American College of Physicians, United States Preventive Services Task Force, the National Cholesterol Education Program (NCEP), and the American Academy of Family Physicians. For any given preventive medicine topic, each organization recommends various measures, which are often similar. All organizations recommend blood pressure checks at all visits, particularly for patients with hypertension.

The Centers for Disease Control and Prevention (CDC) recommends Pneumovax, a 23-polyvalent pneumococcal vaccine, for any individual with cardiopulmonary disease, no spleen, or otherwise immunocompromised status. This vaccine is given a second time at 65 years of age for these patients and to all patients at 65 years of age. It should be given every 5 to 7 years for those at high risk. This patient does not require Pneumovax at this time. The influenza vaccine is warranted for the same high-risk population for whom Pneumovax is beneficial, and all individuals older than 50 years should receive it.

Most organizations do not recommend a digital rectal examination for the purpose of colorectal cancer screening until 50 years of age unless the individual is at high risk (e.g., inflammatory bowel disease, familial adenomatous polyposis). However, the American Cancer Society does recommend digital rectal examinations at 40 years of age. This patient is not known to be at high risk for colorectal cancer, so age 50 years is a reasonable cutoff. At the patient's current age, prostate-specific antigen (PSA) screening in the absence of symptoms would not be warranted.

Because this patient is taking pravastatin, a 3-hydroxy-3-methylglutaryl-CoA (HMG-CoA) reductase inhibitor, he should undergo screening for liver toxicity. This includes the measurement of alanine aminotransferase (ALT). Creatine kinase would be important should signs and symptoms of rhabdomyolysis, a rare complication of this class of medications, develop. When given with a fibric acid or cyclosporine, all HMG-CoA reductase inhibitors ("statins") cause rhabdomyolysis more commonly.

When the patient returned months later with ankle swelling, consideration of the differential diagnosis for edema is appropriate. Possibilities include liver failure, hypothyroidism, lymphatic obstruction, corticosteroid use, Cushing syndrome, congestive heart failure, and hypoalbuminemia secondary to liver failure or nephrotic syndrome. The sudden rise in low-density lipoprotein (LDL) evokes another differential diagnosis, which includes hypothyroidism, nephrotic syndrome, liver disease, addition of a β-blocker, addition of a thiazide diuretic, corticosteroid therapy, Cushing syndrome, as well as other more obscure causes. A urinalysis, thyroid-stimulating hormone (TSH), ALT, and 24-hour urine free cortisol would all be useful. CT of the abdomen is unlikely to yield the diagnosis for the increasing LDL cholesterol.

The patient's laboratory results are within normal limits except for a significant amount of protein in the urine. This may be due to nephrotic syndrome, which is defined as proteinuria of more than 3 g/24 hours. The six most common causes of this condition include membranous nephropathy, minimal-change disease, membranoproliferative glomerulonephritis, focal segmental glomerulosclerosis, amyloidosis, and diabetes mellitus. Membranous nephropathy is the most likely diagnosis because it is the most common cause of nephrotic syndrome in adults without diabetes mellitus. The normal TSH and liver function tests rule out hypothyroidism and liver disease as causes of the patient's edema. Neither Hodgkin disease nor prostate cancer leads to edema.

Thrombosis, particularly of the renal veins, is a complication of membranous nephropathy. This is thought to occur secondary to loss of antithrombin, protein C, and protein S in the urine. The prothrombic molecules are larger and generally not lost in the urine as significantly.

18–22. The answers are: 18-D, 19-A, 20-E, 21-C, 22-A. (*Internal medicine*)
The workup of hemoptysis can be difficult because the list of causes is so extensive. The causal conditions include upper airway bleeding, gastrointestinal (GI) bleeding, bronchogenic carcinoma, bronchitis, bronchiectasis, lung abscess, pneumonia, tuberculosis, mycetoma, Goodpasture syndrome, Wegener granulomatosis, lupus pneumonitis, pulmonary embolism, mitral stenosis, and systemic coagulopathy. History taking can often narrow the list. In this case, the patient reports mucopurulent sputum streaked with blood, a classic description of the hemoptysis associated with bronchitis, which is the most common cause of hemoptysis in the outpatient setting. Documented fevers, chills, or shortness of breath suggest pneumonia, whereas a putrid smell suggests an abscess. The chronic production of copious amounts of sputum suggests bronchiectasis. Of course, a history of exposure to tuberculosis with weight loss and fevers would indicate tuberculosis. Coexisting renal disease might suggest Wegener, Goodpasture, or Churg-Strauss syndromes. The acute onset of shortness of breath with pleuritic chest pain might indicate a pulmonary embolism.

When a chest radiograph reveals a solitary pulmonary nodule, the clinician must risk stratify the patient for significant disease. Granulomas and hamartomas account for the majority of these nodules, but certain features suggest a more worrisome diagnosis, such as primary or metastatic lung cancer. An old chest radiograph is one helpful clue because a lesion that does not change in size for 2 years is benign. Age is important; the probability of malignancy is 2% if a patient is younger than 30 years, and it increases by 10% to 15% with each successive decade. A history of smoking, plus weight loss, hemoptysis, headache, and bone pain increases the likelihood of malignancy. The calcification pattern can be helpful because an eccentric pattern of calcium within the nodule suggests malignancy. A lesion with a "popcorn" appearance suggests a hamartoma. The larger the nodule (>1 cm), the more worrisome for malignancy.

This 51-year-old woman has a smoking history, hemoptysis, and a large mass without calcifications, which means she is at high risk for having a bronchogenic malignancy. A bronchoscopy with the intent to biopsy the lesion is necessary. A tissue diagnosis is needed and, therefore, more imaging is unnecessary. Waiting 8 weeks for repeat films is unreasonable.

The patient's forced vital capacity (FVC) is low (<80%), suggesting restrictive disease, although the FVC could be low secondary to air trapping with a high residual volume. The FEV_1/FVC is less than 70%, suggesting a concomitant obstructive process. It is impossible to distinguish between these conditions without having lung volumes.

An estimated postoperative FEV_1 of 800 mL or more is required before considering lung resection surgery. Patients with a forced expiratory volume in 1 second (FEV_1) of less than 2 L require preoperative ventilation-perfusion studies to estimate the postoperative FEV_1. The patient's FEV_1 measurement of 1.2 L means that the ventilation-perfusion ($\dot{V}/\dot{Q}$) scan is necessary.

The indicators for increased surgical risk from pulmonary complications include smoking, obesity (controversial), surgical procedure close to the diaphragm, age (controversial), FEV_1 less than 2 L, and PCO_2 greater than 45 mm Hg. Measures that can be taken to diminish the chance of pulmonary complication include smoking cessation at least 8 weeks prior to the surgery (less than 8 weeks of increased complications), bronchodilator use in patients with chronic obstructive pulmonary disease, patient education regarding incentive spirometry, use of epidural anesthesia when possible, duration of surgery of less than 3 hours if possible, use of continuous positive airway pressure postoperatively, use of laparoscopic procedures if possible, and the use of antibiotics preoperatively if a respiratory infection is present (with a delay of surgery). Research has shown that paradoxically, the risk of a perioperative pulmonary complication is higher in patients who stop smoking less than 8 weeks prior to surgery than in those who continue to smoke.

23–24. The answers are: 23-A, 24-B. (*Neurology*)
Painless monocular loss of vision in older persons is most commonly secondary to an embolic event that causes central retinal artery occlusion. The classic funduscopic examination finds a pale fundus with a "cherry-red spot" representing the blood supply of the macula from the uncompromised choroid beneath it.

Although central retinal vein occlusion may present similarly to central retinal artery occlusion, the appearance of the fundus is much different. Venous engorgement with hemorrhages, often described as a "blood and thunder," are apparent. This may be associated with hypercoagulable states. Both iritis and glaucoma present with a painful eye. Retinal detachment presents with floaters or a particular pattern of partial vision loss.

The primary treatment is ocular massage to try to dislodge the clot. It is also possible to improve perfusion by lowering the intraocular pressure. The patient should be referred emergently to an ophthalmologist. Later he will need a cardiovascular workup to search for an embolic source.

Pilocarpine eyedrops are used in the setting of acute angle-closure glaucoma. Although intravenous mannitol or acetazolamide might decrease intraocular pressures, which could increase perfusion to the retina, ocular massage and emergent referral to an ophthalmologist is the treatment of choice. A fluorescein examination is used to look for corneal trauma. Iridectomy is used prophylactically for individuals at risk for narrow-angle glaucoma.

25–26. The answers are: 25-D, 26-C. (*Pediatrics*)
The most common causes of a red eye include conjunctivitis (bacterial, viral, or allergic), uveitis (iris, ciliary body, or choroid), corneal injury, or acute glaucoma. The patient's photophobia suggests an anterior uveitis (iritis); the pain in the right eye when light is shown in the left eye supports an iritis of the right eye that is exacerbated by the consensual light reflex with movement of the iris. On physical examination, the affected eye has a small pupil that is poorly responsive to light. A slit lamp examination discloses cells in the anterior chamber, which are referred to as "cell and flare."

Once the diagnosis is confirmed, the patient receives treatment with topical steroids and a pupil-dilating agent to prevent posterior synechiae formation between the iris and the lens of the eye. A sympathomimetic drop with a topical steroid is useful after confirmation by slit lamp examination. A cholinesterase inhibitor is parasympathetic and is not the treatment of choice.

Many systemic diseases are associated with uveitis, including ankylosing spondylitis, celiac sprue, tuberculosis, sarcoidosis, juvenile rheumatoid arthritis, Behçet disease, inflammatory bowel disease, and Reiter syndrome. Uveitis is not associated with colon cancer.

27–31. The answers are: 27-C, 28-E, 29-A, 30-A, 31-E. (*Pediatrics, emergency medicine*)
Neisseria meningitidis, the second most common cause of community-acquired adult bacterial meningitis in the United States, is now the leading cause of bacterial meningitis in children and young adults, with a mortality rate of 13%. The acute clinical presentation can vary from transient fever and bacteremia to overwhelming sepsis with death. Classically, there is an acute onset of fever, nausea, vomiting, headache, and myalgia and an inability to concentrate. Many cases are initially mistaken for severe "flu." Focal neurologic signs and seizure are rare.

On physical examination, hypotension with tachycardia is often evident. Petechiae and ecchymoses are found most commonly at sites of pressure, such as belt and strap areas. Kernig and Brudzinski signs are often absent. The rash appears as discrete lesions 1 to 2 mm in diameter on the trunk and lower portions of the body.

Hemorrhages may occur on the mucous membranes of the soft palate, ocular, and palpebral conjunctiva. The petechiae, which correlate with the degree of thrombocytopenia, are a clinical indicator of the potential for disseminated intravascular coagulopathy (DIC) and bleeding. DIC is not uncommon, and thus, often fibrinogen is low, D-dimer is high, prothrombin time (PT) is high, partial thromboplastin time (PTT) is high, and schistocytes can be seen on a peripheral smear.

Patients with a deficiency in complement levels are at increased risk for meningococcal disease. This can be seen in patients with C3 deficiency, properdin deficiency, or late complement component (C5 to C9) deficiency. Such patients tend to manifest meningococcal disease later in life and have milder cases, except for the properdin-deficient group, who have an increased incidence of fatal disease.

Immediate antibiotics can be lifesaving. Two sets of blood cultures are warranted, and an age-appropriate empirical antibiotic should follow. A lumbar puncture should follow immediately thereafter (within 15 to 30 minutes of antibiotics), and the fluid should be sent for Gram's stain and culture.

In this case, the patient became more hypotensive, which should raise the suspicion of adrenal hemorrhage (Waterhouse-Friderichsen syndrome). Intravenous dexamethasone can be given immediately; it does not interfere with a cortisol assay that should follow. (Hydrocortisone interferes with that assay.) It is reasonable to give fluids and check a complete blood count (CBC) for DIC or bleeding.

The use of the meningococcal vaccine is controversial. It is not cost-effective for all patients, but it is recommended for those at high risk, including students and military personnel living in close quarters. The vaccine, which consists of four bacterial polysaccharides, is 90% effective in studies of children. It is effective for complement-deficient patients because it covers Y and W-135 serotypes, the most common types infecting these patients. However, although the vaccine covers serotypes A, C, and Y, it does not cover serotype B, which accounts for nearly all isolates in the United States.

32–34. The answers are: 32-E, 33-D, 34-D. (*Emergency medicine, internal medicine*)
This patient had an episode of syncope. The differential diagnosis of syncope is extensive; causal conditions can essentially be classified as cardiac or noncardiac. In most young individuals, the cause is noncardiac, but this patient has a family history of heart condition, which should raise the suspicion for hypertrophic cardiomyopathy, a leading cause of sudden death in young adults. The patient's history of fever with a rash as a child might prompt consideration of rheumatic fever, but he is too young to have the clinical manifestations of rheumatic valvular disease.

Hypertrophic cardiomyopathy results from one of many mutations of the myosin, tropomyosin, or troponin genes. Although it generally has an autosomal dominant inheritance pattern, it may occur spontaneously.

Most commonly, patients present between 20 and 40 years of age. Cardinal features include marked, often asymmetric, left ventricular hypertrophy involving the septum, causing outflow tract obstruction. Pathologically, the myocytes show disarray and disorganization. There is marked noncompliance, which increases filling pressures, causing dyspnea during exercise or even angina despite the lack of coronary artery disease. Outflow obstruction is present in 25% of cases. Maneuvers that decrease the left ventricular volume, such as vasodilation or the Valsalva maneuver or increased contractility, accentuate the murmur, and maneuvers that increase the left ventricular volume (e.g., squatting or handgrip maneuver) and separate the septum from the anterior mitral valve leaflet, diminish it. In this case, the patient's syncope likely occurred secondary to an increased outflow tract gradient causing decreased cardiac output, from elevated filling pressures activating vagal reflexes, or a ventricular arrhythmia arising within the areas of abnormal myocyte organization.

Who should receive treatment is the subject of controversy. Therapy is not encouraged in asymptomatic patients unless severe hypertrophy (an equivalent adult wall thickness >35 mm) or an outflow tract gradient is present. The initial treatment is β-blockers, followed by verapamil if necessary. Other methods of treatment include dual-chamber pacemakers, septal reduction procedures, and mitral valve replacement. Loop diuretics, such as furosemide, are used because of the diastolic dysfunction seen in these patients; however, these agents should be used judiciously to prevent "overdiuresis." Disopyramide is useful because it decreases the inotropic state, but it can increase atrioventricular conduction in the event that atrial fibrillation occurs and should be used with caution. Digoxin exacerbates the outflow tract gradient by increasing contractility and decreasing left ventricular volume.

35–36. The answers are: 35-C, 36-A. (*Pediatrics, obstetrics/gynecology*)
In the United States, three million unintended pregnancies occur each year, accounting for 48% of all pregnancies. Nearly 50% of women between the ages of 15 and 44 years have had an unintended pregnancy. Emergency contraception, which has the potential to reduce this number significantly, works in many ways, including inhibition of ovulation, trapping of sperm in thickened cervical mucus, inhibition of egg tubal transport, interference of fertilization, or prevention of implantation by disrupting the uterine lining. Emergency contraception consists of either combined estrogen–progestin pills or progestin-only preparations, and they are most effective when taken up to 12 hours after intercourse.

The combined pill used most commonly is Ovral, which consists of ethinyl estradiol 100 μg and levonorgestrel 0.5 mg. A woman should take two Ovral pills within 72 hours of intercourse, followed by two more pills 12 hours later. She should use the same schedule with other regimens; with Levlen, Levora, Lo/Ovral, or Nordette, she should take four pills at a time, and with Alesse or Levlite, five pills at a time.

The progestin-only preparations are more effective; a recent study has found that they are 88% efficacious, whereas combined preparations are 75% efficacious. A recently released product named Plan B consists of 0.75 mg of levonorgestrel. A woman should take one pill within 72 hours of intercourse, followed by another pill 12 hours later. The progestin-only preparations are associated with less nausea and vomiting.

37–42. The answers are: 37-E, 38-D, 39-E, 40-E, 41-C, 42-D. (*Obstetrics/gynecology*)
In the United States, the annual incidence of invasive cervical cancer exceeds 15,000 cases annually, with an annual mortality of 5,000 cases. For an American woman, the lifetime incidence of cervical carcinoma in situ is greater than 2%. The asymptomatic period, during which cytologic detection is possible, is long, and thus, the Papanicolaou (Pap) smear can be lifesaving. The primary risk factors for invasive cervical carcinoma are sexual activity, particularly with multiple partners; smoking; immunocompromised status (e.g., HIV infection); and lower socioeconomic status. A positive family history is not a risk factor for cervical cancer.

How frequently Pap smears are necessary has been a subject of controversy. Most authorities recommend commencement of Pap smears when a woman reaches the age of 18 years or when she becomes sexually active. If she has two annual smears that are negative, screening every 3 years is acceptable. For patients at high risk (early age of first intercourse, multiple sexual partners, HIV, history of sexually transmitted disease), recommendations call for annual Pap smears.

The scoring of Pap smears is confusing. There are three commonly used systems: World Health Organization (WHO), Papanicolaou, and Bethesda systems.

WHO	Papanicolaou	Bethesda
Normal		
Atypical	Inflammatory (bacteria, yeast)	
	Noninflammatory (HPV)	LGSIL
Dysplasia	Mild (CIN I)	LGSIL
	Moderate (CIN II)	HGSIL
	Severe (CIN III)	HGSIL

CIN = cervical intraepithelial neoplasia; HGSIL = high-grade intraepithelial lesion; HPV = human papilloma virus; LGSIL = low-grade squamous intraepithelial lesion.

The Pap smear is considered unsatisfactory if no endocervical cells are seen. The designation "atypia of squamous cells of undetermined significance" is controversial; this condition "lies between" inflammatory atypia and low-grade squamous intraepithelial lesions (LGSILs). It is important because 3% to 10% of all smears have the "atypia of squamous cells" designation; of these, 60% to 88% are normal, 8% to 30% represent LGSILs, and 4% to 10% represent high-grade squamous intraepithelial lesions (HGSILs).

In this case, the patient is sexually active, and the result of her screening Pap smear is "inflammatory with budding yeast." The standard of care is treatment with an appropriate medication followed by a repeat Pap smear in 4 months; this woman should receive antifungals for *Candida.* Until she receives treatment for the inflammatory condition, further invasive procedures (colposcopy, conization) should not be performed.

The indications for colposcopy are any result with LGSIL or "worse," and the patient with inflammatory atypia that does not resolve after treatment with appropriate antibiotics.

Colposcopy is essentially a screening test for biopsy in which the cervix is visualized and washed with acetic acid. The classic criteria for biopsy are acetowhitening epithelium, punctation, mosaicism, and atypical vessels. A nabothian cyst is merely glandular tissue in the transformation zone that did not appropriately convert to squamous epithelium. It is not premalignant.

Next, an endocervical curettage is performed in the search for criteria for conization. These include:

- Transformation zone that cannot be seen (high-risk region)
- Pap smear "worse" than the biopsy (implying "missed" biopsy)
- Pap smear showing adenocarcinoma
- Positive endocervical curettage
- Biopsy showing microinvasion

It is well known that human papilloma virus is a risk factor for cervical cancer. Serotypes 6 and 11 are associated with condyloma acuminata, and serotypes 16, 18, 31, 33, and 35 are more carcinogenic. Human papilloma virus serotype 18 is associated with the most rapid progression to invasive cervical cancer, often within 1 year, and it is also associated with adenocarcinoma.

43–45. The answers are: 43-D, 44-B, 45-D. (*Obstetrics/gynecology*)
Vaginal discharge is a common presenting complaint in women in the United States. Some vaginal infections put women at risk for upper genital tract disease or a complication of a present or future pregnancy. Therefore, the approach to this complaint is important. The vaginal microflora of healthy, asymptomatic women contains many unclumped, rod-like organisms dominated by *Lactobacillus.* The normal pH of vaginal secretions is 3.5 to 4.1.

The most common cause of an abnormal discharge is infection with bacteria, yeast, or parasites. The most common cause of an increased number of leukocytes in the vaginal fluid, or "vaginitis," is *Trichomonas vaginalis* or *Candida albicans.* The most common cause of increased discharge is a bacterial overgrowth referred to as "vaginosis" (40% to 50%), in which inflammation is not a feature. *Candida,* which may be a commensal organism in the vagina, is the second most common agent (20% to 25%), followed by *Trichomonas* (15% to 20%). The character, amount, and odor of the discharge help distinguish between these causes.

T. vaginalis, a small motile protozoan, is sexually transmitted and is often present with other infections. Because it can survive in hot tubs, tap water, and chlorinated swimming pools, sexual contact may not be the only means of transmission. The most common symptoms of trichomoniasis include a yellow, frothy, malodorous discharge; pruritus; dyspareunia; dysuria; and, occasionally, vulvar erythema. (However, 10% to 50% of women are asymptomatic.) Pelvic examination occasionally finds petechial hemorrhages of the external genitalia and cervix (strawberry cervix). A wet mount finds motile trichomonads in approximately 25% of cases.

In symptomatic candidiasis, patients most often complain of vulvar irritation and burning. Potassium hydroxide (KOH) preparations show budding yeast. In bacterial vaginosis, patients complain of a thin, white-gray, malodorous discharge but rarely of burning or itching. The wet mount shows clue cells, which are vaginal epithelial cells with a stippled appearance due to the adherence of bacilli on their surfaces. The addition of KOH to a sample of discharge produces amines and a "fishy" odor (whiff test).

The treatment of choice is metronidazole 500 mg 2 times a day for 7 days. A one-time dose of 2 g is less efficacious but is associated with greater compliance. The other answer choices in question 44 are not effective therapies against trichomoniasis. If the patient relapses after successful treatment, both the woman and her sexual partner require treatment. Patients should be instructed to avoid alcohol intake because of the disulfiram (Antabuse)-like effect of metronidazole.

46–48. The answers are: 46-D, 47-D, 48-E. (*Internal medicine*)

A unilateral swollen leg with warmth and redness but no evidence of open wounds or lymphangitis prompts suspicion of deep venous thrombosis. Inguinal lymphadenopathy up to 1 cm is considered normal; however, if this lymphadenopathy is new, fixed, or tender, it is more likely to be pathologic. The use of Homans sign, which is 10% to 50% sensitive for deep venous thrombosis, is poor physical evidence for ruling out this condition. With a high suspicion of deep venous thrombosis, a Doppler ultrasound study of the lower extremity is more than 90% sensitive. Antibiotics may ultimately be required to treat this condition (penicillin or amoxicillin-clavulanate). However, a diagnosis should be made before treatment is prescribed. A plain film or MRI would not aid in diagnosis of possible deep venous thrombosis.

The optimal treatment for deep venous thrombosis is still controversial. The use of low-molecular-weight heparin is gaining acceptance based on a number of clinical trials finding equivalent efficacy when compared with unfractionated heparin. In addition, research has shown that the length of hospital stay is significantly decreased. Patients should receive warfarin (Coumadin) on day 1 and continue it for at least 6 months; a recent study suggested that longer periods of treatment may be optimal.

Catscratch disease (*Bartonella henselae*) most commonly occurs as a result of a kitten scratch. A papule forms 1 to 2 weeks after a scratch, with subsequent persistent lymphadenopathy in a draining lymph node region. In more than 50% of cases, only one lymph node is involved, most often the axillary nodes. Biopsy finds granulomas and stellate abscesses. Most cases are self-limited, but severe cases can be treated with azithromycin. *Capnocytophaga felinis* and *Pasteurella multocida* can be acquired by a cat bite and lead to a local cellulitis. *Toxoplasma gondii* can be obtained from exposure to infected cat feces. Such exposure may lead to congenital malformations and serious central nervous system (CNS) infections in immunocompromised hosts.

Deep venous thrombosis is a chronic disease; recurrence is more likely than in the general population. In addition, one study found that the incidence ratio (risk) of developing cancer within the first year after a thromboembolic event is as high as 6.7. The most common cancers are ovarian, pancreatic, liver, lung, kidney, brain, and lymphoma. Despite this, most organizations recommend diligent routine screening. Aggressive screening, including full-body CT, is not recommended.

49–53. The answers are: 49-C, 50-D, 51-A, 52-E, 53-D. (*Emergency medicine, internal medicine*)

Deep venous thrombosis (DVT) is a common disorder, but it is difficult to determine when a hypercoagulable workup is necessary. The most accepted indications are an age between 40 and 60 years, no clearly definable risk factor, family history of thrombosis, recurrent events, or thrombosis at an atypical site (e.g., cerebral vein, mesenteric vein). Of the hypercoagulable disorders, few present before the age of 50 years. Conditions such as antithrombin (III) deficiency, protein C deficiency, and protein S deficiency, which affect 0.003% to 0.4% of the population, are rare. Factor V Leiden, a common disorder, is carried by up to 14% of the Caucasian population; it occurs much less often in non-Caucasian individuals. Affected patients, like the woman in this case, present with their first thromboembolic event at an age older than 50 years. Factor II mutations, which also affect Caucasians older than age 50, are associated with a twofold to sevenfold increased risk of thromboembolic events.

After an ultrasound confirms a small, deep venous thrombosis, initiation of an anticoagulation regimen is necessary. There is mounting evidence to suggest that low-molecular-weight heparin is at least equivalent to unfractionated heparin for the purpose of deep venous thrombosis treatment. Therefore, the optimal treatment is an outpatient regimen of low-molecular-weight heparin with warfarin initiated simultaneously. With the concomitant administration of low-molecular-weight heparin, the theoretical risk of a hypercoagulable state associated with the initiation of warfarin is rarely significant. Hirudin is a direct thrombin inhibitor used primarily in patients with heparin-induced thrombocytopenia.

The return of the patient 4 weeks later with acute onset of shortness of breath prompts concern for pulmonary embolus. Chest radiography is normal. A Hampton hump is a region of infarcted lung most commonly in the periphery, and a Westermark sign is a hypolucent region of oligemia. These findings are rare. Pleural effusions can be seen in the setting of pulmonary embolus. They are exudative in two thirds of cases and are rarely greater than one third of the lung hemithorax. They are seen in fewer than 50% of cases of pulmonary embolism.

The ECG findings are most commonly that of a sinus tachycardia. The $S_1Q_3T_3$ is evidence of right heart strain, which is present in 5% to 15% of cases. Right bundle branch block, right axis deviation, and large r wave in V_1 are all signs of right heart strain that occur in a minority of cases. Atrial fibrillation may also be evident.

Arterial clots are associated with antiphospholipid antibody syndrome (e.g., lupus anticoagulant, anticardiolipin antibody), homocystinemia, heparin-induced thrombocytopenia, and factor II abnormality. The other answer choices in question 53 are associated with an increased risk of venous, not arterial, thromboses.

54–55. The answers are: 54-B, 55-E. (*Pediatrics*)
This patient's chief complaint is constipation. Most of these children have no underlying disorder and can be treated solely for the symptom; fewer than three bowel movements per week is considered abnormal. A formal evaluation should be undertaken for children with constipation at birth or with unrelenting symptoms.

The differential diagnosis includes:

---

* Structural lesions, including anal fissures, bowel stenosis, proctitis, extrinsic compression of bowel
* Neuromuscular disorders, including smooth cell disorders, spinal cord defects, Hirschsprung disease
* Medications, including anticholinergics and opiates
* Metabolic causes such as hypothyroidism, hypercalcemia, hypokalemia, uremia, dehydration
* Lead intoxication
* *Clostridium botulinum* infection
* Psychosocial factors, including sexual abuse

Hypocalcemia is not associated with constipation. (However, hypercalcemia may lead to this problem.)

In this clinical scenario, the history of delayed passage of meconium and poor feeding with bilious vomiting should raise the suspicion of Hirschsprung disease. There are several theories concerning its pathogenesis; however, it appears to be secondary to failed migration of ganglion cells into the myenteric plexuses of the distal colon. As a result, the abnormally innervated distal colon remains tonically contracted and obstructs the distal passage of feces. Disease is restricted to the rectosigmoid area in 80% of patients.

The diagnosis is usually made within the first 3 months of life; the neonate presents with delayed passage of meconium, poor feeding, bilious vomiting, and abdominal distension. A barium enema demonstrates a transition zone between the abnormally narrowed segment and the dilated normal proximal bowel. A rectal biopsy confirms no ganglionic cells or hypertrophied nerve trunks. Biopsy is the only method available for the diagnosis of Hirschsprung disease.

Initial treatment consists of a diverting colostomy with segmentectomy at age 6 months to 1 year. A reanastomosis procedure is undertaken at a later time. A patient with a small segment of involvement may respond to an anorectal myomectomy.

56–57. The answers are: 56-C, 57-D. (*Pediatrics*)

Some congenital heart defects cause cyanosis at birth and some do not become evident until later in life. The defects that manifest as cyanosis at birth have right-to-left shunts. These include tetralogy of Fallot (most common cause of cyanotic congenital heart disease), tricuspid atresia, transposition of the great vessels, total anomalous pulmonary venous return, and truncus arteriosus (the five *T*s). The more common defects, including ventricular septal defect (VSD) (most common congenital heart disease overall), atrial septal defect (ASD), and patent ductus arteriosus (PDA), have left-to-right shunts initially that can eventually cause pulmonary vascular damage and hypertension, reversing the shunt (Eisenmenger syndrome).

Coarctation of the aorta results from constriction of the aorta most commonly at the junction of the ductus arteriosus with the aortic arch, just distal to the subclavian artery. This condition, which accounts for 6% of congenital heart disease cases, is 2 to 3 times more common in the male sex. The clinical presentation varies according to the degree of constriction. Most affected patients present with symptoms related to low cardiac output, including irritability, lethargy, poor feeding, and growth failure. Findings on physical examination include decreased or absent lower extremity pulses; skin mottling; a single, loud, S_2 heart sound; and hepatomegaly. Patients with milder cases, who live into early adulthood, display rib notching on chest radiograph secondary to thoracic collateral blood flow. An earlier radiographic finding is the "3" sign, consisting of prestenotic and poststenotic dilatation of the aorta with a dilated left subclavian artery. Congestive heart failure may develop in infancy or later in childhood.

Coarctation of the aorta is associated with PDA (66%), VSD (30%), and bicuspid aortic valves. In addition, the incidence is increased in patients with Turner syndrome (XO) but not in those with Klinefelter syndrome (XXY).

58–61. The answers are: 58-C, 59-A, 60-E, 61-C. (*Pediatrics, statistics*)

Measles (rubeola) is a highly contagious viral disease that occurs primarily in children living in densely populated areas. Still a major problem worldwide, measles is less common in the United States because of vaccination efforts. The cause of the disease is *Paramyxovirus;* only one serotype has been identified. Varicella zoster virus causes chickenpox, human herpes virus 6, roseola, parvovirus B19 erythema infectiosum, and rubella (German measles).

Rubeola has an incubation period of 8 to 12 days, during which there are no symptoms. Thereafter, patients present with a prodrome of malaise, high fever, cough, coryza, conjunctivitis, and photophobia. Within 2 to 3 days, Koplik spots develop, red spots with central white specks on the buccal mucosa. An erythematous maculopapular rash erupts after 5 days of symptomatic disease. The rash, lasting 4 to 5 days, begins on the head and spreads downward. A fourfold or greater increase in antibody titers in over 2 to 3 weeks confirms the diagnosis.

Treatment is primarily supportive. An association between vitamin A deficiency and measles does exist. Supplementation should be considered for patients 6 months to 2 years of age who are hospitalized or have complications, which include pneumonia, encephalitis, subacute sclerosing panencephalitis, pericarditis, and hepatitis. In malnourished children from developing nations, the mortality rate may approach 10%. Acyclovir or other antibiotics play no role. Immunoglobulin can be given prophylactically to a patient at high risk or to a patient with a severe complication. The measles–mumps–rubella (MMR) vaccine, a live attenuated vaccine, is highly effective and may provide some protection if given within 72 hours of measles exposure.

Recall that sensitivity equals true positives/(true positives + false negatives). Therefore, the new test has a sensitivity of 80%. The prevalence of disease is extraneous information but is useful in determination of the positive or negative predictive values.

62–66. The answers are: 62-D, 63-D, 64-E, 65-C, 66-E. (*Pediatrics*)

This young man has features of Klinefelter syndrome, which affects 1 of 800 newborns. Affected boys are usually taller than expected given their background, with an arm span greater than height. The testes remain small with infertility secondary to Leydig cell hyperplasia and seminiferous tubule dysgenesis. Serum testosterone levels are low; incomplete masculinization and female body habitus with decreased body hair are characteristic. Gynecomastia is a common feature, accounting for the increased risk for breast cancers when compared with 46,XY males. The mean IQ is 90, with an increased incidence of mental retardation. Patients do not have epicanthal folds or a flat nasal bridge, as seen in Down syndrome. Behavioral problems and immaturity are common with Klinefelter syndrome. Testosterone replacement therapy may result in improvement of many of the physical and social features associated with this 47,XXY karyotype defect.

The risk of conceiving another child with Klinefelter syndrome is not increased in a subsequent pregnancy. The likelihood would be the same as in the general population.

The majority of inherited diseases follow an autosomal recessive pattern of inheritance, which means that an abnormal allele must be inherited from both parents for the offspring to manifest the disease. If "A" is a normal gene and "a" is an abnormal gene for an autosomal recessive disease, only the offspring with two abnormal genes ("aa") will manifest the disease. For a male carrier ("Aa") who marries a woman with the disease ("aa"), 50% of their offspring will be carriers ("Aa") and 50% will have the disease ("aa"). This assumes 100% penetrance, which implies that all patients with the "aa" genotype will express the disease.

The X-linked disorders are slightly more complicated. It is necessary to know whether the disease is X-linked recessive or X-linked dominant, and this information has not been provided. With an X-linked dominant disease, 50% of all offspring, regardless of sex, would have the disorder. Even female offspring with one "bad" X chromosome will have the disease. Any question that relates to the percentage of offspring affected in an X-linked recessive trait must specifically ask about female versus male offspring. Again, this information was not provided. With an X-linked recessive disease, 50% of men would have the condition and 0% of women would have the condition. (However, 50% of these female individuals would be carriers.)

67–70. The answers are: 67-E, 68-E, 69-B, 70-C. (*Pediatrics*)

This patient has features suggestive of a neuroblastoma, which is a malignancy of neural crest cells—cells that give rise to the paraspinal sympathetic ganglia and the adrenal medulla. Neuroblastomas, the second most common solid tumor of childhood, second only to brain tumors, are slightly more predominant in boys and in whites. The mean age at diagnosis is 2 to 3 years of age; 50% of tumors are diagnosed by 2 years of age and 90% by 5 years of age. The Beckwith-Wiedemann syndrome may be associated with neuroblastoma and Wilms tumors. This syndrome is characterized by organ overgrowth with omphalocele, macroglossia, and mental retardation.

The most common location of neuroblastomas is the abdomen, where 50% occur from the adrenal medulla and 50% occur from extra-adrenal tissue. Findings include abdominal mass, abdominal pain, and systemic hypertension secondary to renovascular compression. The posterior mediastinal area is the second most common location; patients with these tumors present with respiratory distress or it is found as an incidental finding on chest radiograph. Head and neck locations can produce Horner syndrome with ptosis, miosis, and anhidrosis. Metastases are common at diagnosis and cause proptosis, periorbital ecchymoses ("raccoon eyes"), skull masses, subcutaneous nodules, lymphadenopathy, bone marrow failure, and hepatomegaly. Occasionally, patients present with diarrhea secondary to the secretion of vasoactive intestinal peptide by the tumor. Coloboma is part of the condition known as the CHARGE syndrome (**c**olobomas, **h**eart disease, choanal **a**tresia, **r**etardation, **g**enital abnormalities, and **e**ar abnormalities).

Amplification of the N-*myc* proto-oncogene is associated with this disease. The p53 suppressor gene is associated with numerous malignancies, including lung and colon cancer; the RB gene is mutated in retinoblastoma; the BRCA1 mutation is associated with a high risk of breast and ovarian cancer; and the WT-1 gene is mutated in Wilms tumor.

Because catecholamines are elaborated by most tumors, the measurement of urinary vanillylmandelic acid and homovanillic acid is useful. Both the urinary free cortisol and dexamethasone suppression tests are used to diagnose Cushing syndrome. The aldosterone and plasma renin levels are useful in diagnosing aldosteronism.

71–72. The answers are: 71-B, 72-E. (*Internal medicine*)
Broadly, syncope is divided into cardiac and noncardiac causes. The distinction is important because the cardiac causes of syncope have a much higher mortality. Cardiac causes can be divided into two groups: arrhythmogenic and low cardiac output–related. In this case, the patient is taking quinidine for atrial fibrillation. This drug is known to prolong the QT interval and promote torsades de pointes, a ventricular tachycardia. Hypoglycemia would be another potential cause of the syncope, but it is not commonly associated with metformin.

When this woman presented with an upper respiratory infection, she was likely treated with a macrolide antibiotic, such as clarithromycin or azithromycin, which can further prolong the QT interval and promote the development of ventricular tachycardia. The other antibiotics listed in question 72 are not common causes of QT prolongation. Atrial fibrillation should not cause syncope without a concomitant adverse effect.

73–75. The answers are: 73-D, 74-C, 75-D. (*Neurology, surgery*)
This patient has likely suffered a transient ischemic attack, a neurologic deficit that usually lasts 5 to 20 minutes—less than 24 hours. This event is unlikely to be a seizure because the probable location is subcortical, with involvement of both the Broca area and the left-sided internal capsule, causing right-sided weakness. This combination is not uncommon; the superior division of the middle cerebral artery feeds both these structures, which are in close proximity. Transient ischemic attacks usually do not precede embolic events in the brain, whereas they do occur before thrombotic strokes at least 20% of the time. Patients with subarachnoid hemorrhage most commonly present with headache and vomiting with or without cranial nerve findings, and occasionally, the bleeding can spread or cause a hematoma with enough mass effect to cause hemiparesis, aphasia, or abulia. But no spontaneous improvement occurs within 1 hour, as in this patient.

In the evaluation of patients with a history of transient ischemic attacks, Duplex ultrasound is a useful study to look for carotid artery stenoses. An echocardiogram is useful in the evaluation of embolic events to rule out a patent foramen ovale. An angiogram is useful as well but is much more invasive. A CT scan of the head is useful in cases with persistent neurologic findings.

Many studies have evaluated the efficacy of endarterectomy in patients with carotid artery stenoses. In patients *without* a history of symptoms such as transient ischemic attack, the Asymptomatic Carotid Atherosclerosis Study (ACAS) trial found that patients with stenoses of 60% to 99% had a 53% relative risk reduction at 5 years (from 11% to 5.1%) in ipsilateral stroke, perioperative stroke, or death; this benefit pertained to men only. The absolute risk reduction was 5.9% with a number-needed-to-treat of 17. It should be noted that a rate of surgical complications greater than 5% would negate any benefit. Some hospitals likely approach this complication rate.

In patients with a history of symptoms such as transient ischemic attack, the North American Symptomatic Carotid Endarterectomy Trial (NASCET) found that patients with stenoses of 70% to 99% had an overall relative risk reduction for stroke or death of 51% at 2 years (from 32.3% to 15.8%). For a stenosis of 50% to 69%, the results are less clear. For the patient in this case, an 80% stenosis of the carotid artery would be the clearest indication for endarterectomy. Patients with 100% stenosis are usually not considered candidates for surgery.

76–78. The answers are: 76-E, 77-E, 78-C. (*Internal medicine, obstetrics/gynecology*)
Menopause is defined as the cessation of menstruation due to failure of ovarian follicular development in a woman who previously had normal cycles. The average age of menopause in the United States is 51 years. Symptoms of menopause may be debilitating and include hot flashes, night sweats, insomnia, and vaginal dryness. Lack of estrogen protects against endometrial cancer. Long-term changes secondary to the lack of estrogen include osteoporosis and increased risk of cardiovascular disease.

In counseling women about estrogen replacement therapy (ERT), it is important to understand the risks associated with this treatment. Adverse effects include a doubling of the risk of gallbladder disease, a dose-dependent increase in thromboembolic disease, an increased risk of breast cancer, and an increased risk of endometrial cancer. It should be pointed out that the increased risk of breast cancer with ERT is probably small; the existence of such a risk is controversial. ERT is associated with no increased risk of pancreatitis.

Regimens for ERT involve either conjugated estrogens or micronized estrogens at a dose that prevents osteoporosis and minimizes postmenopausal symptoms (e.g., vaginal dryness, hot flashes). For most women, 0.625 mg of conjugated estrogen or 1 mg of micronized estrogen is sufficient. Alternative forms of estrogen therapy include transdermal administration and transvaginal delivery.

In women who have an intact uterus, it is important to add progestin to counteract the effects of unopposed estrogen. Because unopposed estrogen can lead to endometrial hyperplasia and an increased risk of adenocarcinoma, various regimens of combined estrogen–progestin therapy have been advocated. Continuous combined therapy is generally the best choice.

79–81. The answers are: 79-D, 80-B, 81-A. *(Neurology, psychiatry)*

This patient presents with the combination of deteriorating cognitive function and a movement disorder. His reported movement problems fit the description of chorea, which denotes rapid, irregular muscle jerks that occur involuntarily and unpredictably. Initial presenting features may include restlessness and clumsiness, and eventually, the patient has a lurching, dipping gait.

The particular combination of dementia and chorea limits the differential diagnosis to either Huntington disease or Wilson disease. Both of these conditions are inherited, and, therefore, a detailed and accurate family history is essential and can lead to the correct diagnosis. Wilson disease, an autosomal recessive disorder of copper metabolism, leads to cirrhosis, dementia, and chorea. Huntington disease, an autosomal dominant condition, leads to progressive dementia and worsening chorea. Given the patient's normal liver examination and absence of Kayser-Fleischer rings (copper deposits in the eyes), the most likely cause of the patient's symptoms is Huntington disease. Unfortunately, there is no cure for this disease, which follows a relentless course, culminating in death approximately 10 to 20 years after diagnosis.

82–85. The answers are: 82-E, 83-B, 84-C, 85-C. *(Obstetrics/gynecology)*

Hydramnios, or polyhydramnios, refers to an excessive volume of amniotic fluid (>2000 mL). The condition is generally suspected whenever the uterus is larger than expected for gestational age or whenever fetal parts cannot be easily palpated. Whenever hydramnios is suspected, the next step should be a detailed fetal ultrasound. Ultrasonography affords a detailed examination of the amount of amniotic fluid present (and, thus, makes the diagnosis of hydramnios) and also allows for a detailed anatomic examination of the fetus for possible underlying conditions that could lead to excessive amniotic fluid. None of the other answer choices in question 82 obviate the need for an ultrasound.

Hydramnios can be secondary to numerous conditions, although idiopathic causes are the most common (35%). Other possible causes include (1) central nervous system (CNS) abnormalities (e.g., anencephaly); (2) cardiovascular disorders (e.g., coarctation, arrhythmias, hydrops); (3) gastrointestinal (GI) disorders (e.g., abdominal wall defects); (4) respiratory disorders (e.g., pulmonary sequestration); (5) musculoskeletal disorders; (6) genitourinary disorders (e.g., uteropelvic junction obstruction); (7) diabetes mellitus; and (8) multiple gestations. Renal obstruction or agenesis, ruptured membranes, and intrauterine growth retardation generally lead to oligohydramnios. Toxoplasmosis usually has little effect on the amount of amniotic fluid.

Hydramnios can lead to many complications. The most common are preterm labor, premature ruptured membranes, maternal discomfort, and respiratory compromise. Uteroplacental insufficiency is not caused by hydramnios.

In some cases, the amount of amniotic fluid buildup is so great or so rapid that treatment must be instituted to avoid complications. It is always best to treat any underlying conditions (e.g., diabetes mellitus) that have a contributory role; however, no such condition exists in many cases. Medical treatment may involve indomethacin, which decreases fetal urine output and, as a result, decreases amniotic fluid output. However, no woman beyond 34 weeks' gestation should take indomethacin because of the risk of resulting fetal ductal closure. Ultrasonographic monitoring must be frequent during treatment to assess changes in amniotic fluid volume. Surgical treatment involves amniocentesis.

86–89. The answers are: 86-D, 87-D, 88-C, 89-C. (*Internal medicine*)
This patient suffers from chronic obstructive pulmonary disease (COPD). The history is suggestive; however, the differential diagnosis of dyspnea is broad and includes such disorders as cardiac problems; deconditioning; anemia; and pulmonary diseases, including COPD, asthma, interstitial lung disease, pulmonary embolism, and pulmonary hypertension. Pulmonary function testing can be invaluable in determining the cause. In this patient, the pulmonary function tests reveal a clear obstructive pattern with decreased expiratory flow and increased lung volume. This pattern may be consistent with either COPD or asthma; however, the significantly reduced diffusion capacity indicates disease of the alveolar membrane. This is seen only in COPD, which is characterized by progressive destruction of the elastic tissue of the lung as well as the alveolar membrane.

Arterial blood gases can also help guide therapy. In this case, hypercapnia and hypoxemia are evident. Controlled studies have shown that the only therapy that leads to an improvement in survival is supplemental oxygen to achieve an oxygen saturation of at least 90%. Although the other therapies listed in question 87 may afford symptomatic relief, they have little effect on overall survival.

With severe COPD and hypoxemia, pulmonary hypertension slowly develops secondary to hypoxic vasoconstriction, as well as destruction of the pulmonary capillary network by the disease process. It is not uncommon to see right heart strain, hypertrophy, and eventual development of right heart failure on echocardiography. Left heart failure may also occur, but it is not due to pulmonary disease. Aortic stenosis and mitral regurgitation have no relation to COPD.

Later, this patient presents with an exacerbation of COPD, which may be caused by viral or bacterial infections, arrhythmias, side effects of a sedating drug, pulmonary embolism, pneumothorax, or numerous other conditions. When increased shortness of breath occurs with increased and purulent sputum production, trials have shown that antibiotic therapy is beneficial. Albuterol nebulizer treatments and corticosteroids also have a positive effect. Patients with COPD are more likely to suffer from gram-negative infections, specifically from those caused by *Haemophilus influenzae*. Therefore, any antibiotic regimen must cover gram-negative organisms. The best choice is azithromycin.

90–91. The answers are: 90-D, 91-B. (*Emergency medicine, surgery*)
This patient most likely has a tear of the anterior cruciate ligament. The description of the injury can be helpful in determining the exact injury, but many patients cannot recall the exact mechanism (i.e., inversion, eversion). However, in more than 80% of cases, the documentation of a patient hearing a "pop" or "snap" is associated with a tear of the anterior cruciate ligament. The rapid appearance of bloody joint effusion is much more likely with injuries to the anterior cruciate ligament. The finding of anterior displacement of the knee confirms this suspicion. Unfortunately, in the acute setting with severe pain and guarding, it is difficult, if not impossible, to perform physical examination maneuvers, such as the Lachman test, that would aid in the exact diagnosis.

The initial treatment of injuries to the anterior cruciate ligament includes knee immobilization, crutches, ice, elevation and nonsteroidal anti-inflammatory drugs (NSAIDs). Aspiration of the knee effusion is not to be initially recommended because it would rapidly reappear. Reexamination by an orthopedic surgeon in the next 24 to 48 hours is recommended.

92–93. The answers are: 92-C, 93-D. (*Pediatrics, psychiatry*)
Attention deficit hyperactivity disorder is a condition that is characterized by an ever-changing definition and diagnostic criteria. It is typified by an inadequate attention span, impulsiveness, and hyperactivity. The disorder spans a spectrum, with three distinct types recognized by the *Diagnostic and Statistical Manual of Men-*

tal Disorders, fourth edition (DSM-IV): attention deficit hyperactivity disorder, predominantly inattentive type; attention deficit hyperactivity disorder, predominantly hyperactive-impulsive type; and mixed attention deficit hyperactivity disorder.

In many cases, it is the child's teacher who notes disruptive behavior in school on the part of the child and first makes others aware of the hyperactivity problem. It can be difficult to determine if there is an underlying learning disability (especially a speech–language problem) or an underlying neurologic problem. Furthermore, the symptoms may reflect social problems, such as parental neglect. Several minor physical anomalies seem to correlate with attention deficit hyperactivity disorder. These include epicanthal folds, hypertelorism of the eyes, low-set or malformed ears, clinodactyly (inward curvature) of the fifth finger, and high arched palate.

Medications may prove useful in increasing the child's attention span. However, to achieve maximal effectiveness, it is essential that these agents be used in conjunction with behavioral therapies. The mainstays of treatment are stimulants such as methylphenidate dextroamphetamine. Second-line agents include tricyclic antidepressants and selective serotonin reuptake inhibitors. Benzodiazepines, such as lorazepam, play no role in the treatment of attention deficit hyperactivity disorder.

94–95. The answers are: 94-E, 95-A. (*Pediatrics, surgery, emergency medicine*)
This patient presents with head trauma and cerebral edema with increased intracranial pressure. Proper management of this condition includes supportive care as well as maneuvers to decrease the intracranial pressure, which include mannitol, hyperventilation (leading to cerebral vasoconstriction), corticosteroids, and elevation of the head. In cases in which the increased intracranial pressure is a result of enlarged ventricles and increased cerebrospinal fluid (CSF), ventriculostomy and CSF removal can be useful. However, in this particular case, the pathogenesis of the increased intracranial pressure results from parenchymal injury, and it would not respond to removal of CSF.

The evaluation of brain death can be difficult. The assessment must be performed when the body temperature is higher than 35°C and when the blood pressure is within normal limits; pressor agents may even be necessary. Furthermore, agents such as barbiturates that may produce reversible coma-like states should not be present. A typical examination assesses pain response, muscle tone, voluntary movement, midbrain functions (oculocephalic and oculovestibular reflexes), and cranial nerve functions. The discovery of any level of brain function is incompatible with the diagnosis of brain death.

Assessment of respiratory drive occurs through an "apnea test." During this test, the patient is preoxygenated using 100% oxygen and ventilated to achieve a normal P_{CO_2}. Then the ventilator rate is turned to zero while the patient is monitored for any respiratory efforts until the heart rate, blood pressure, and oxygen saturation reach unacceptable levels. An arterial blood gas is often drawn at the end of the test before ventilation is resumed. If the P_{CO_2} rises by more than 20 mm Hg and no spontaneous ventilation occurs, the test is consistent with the diagnosis of brain death.

Other ancillary testing includes isoelectric electroencephalogram (EEG), negative brain-evoked potential, and a four-vessel cerebral angiogram that demonstrates no cerebral perfusion. The Glasgow Coma Score, a prognostic scoring system, has no role in the diagnosis of brain death.

96–98. The answers are: 96-A, 97-B, 98-C. (*Internal medicine*)
This history is classic for syndrome of inappropriate secretion of antidiuretic hormone (SIADH). This syndrome appears to be particularly common in women following gynecologic surgery. In this case, the combination of postoperative pain, nausea, and administration of hypotonic fluids at a rapid rate have led to the rapid development of hyponatremia. SIADH is characterized by hyponatremia and hypoosmolality; inappropriately high urine osmolality (>100 mOsm/L); urine sodium concentration greater than 40 mEq/L; normovolemia; and normal renal, adrenal, and thyroid functions. Hypothyroidism, Addison disease, and heart failure would be associated with other symptoms and are therefore unlikely.

The mainstay of SIADH treatment is fluid restriction. In severe circumstances, such as when the patient is seizing, hypertonic saline and diuretics may help afford a more rapid correction of the serum sodium. In cases of acute hyponatremia, it is generally safe to correct the serum sodium relatively quickly. Demeclocycline leads to a nephrogenic diabetes insipidus; this agent may be useful in cases of SIADH in which the underlying disorder cannot be corrected (such as in metastatic malignancies).

99–100. The answers are: 99-E, 100-D. (*Internal medicine*)
The most likely cause of intravascular catheter-related infections is either *Staphylococcus epidermidis* or *Staphylococcus aureus. Candida, Klebsiella,* and other gram-negative bacteria can be seen but are less common. While identification of the organism is pending, the most appropriate therapy is intravenous vancomycin. Patients who are frequently hospitalized have a high rate of resistance to methicillin and their infection is serious, with high fever, rigors, and hypotension. Vancomycin also has the advantage of a long half-life in this patient population, affording convenient dosing. The agents listed in question 100 do not provide adequate coverage of methicillin-resistant staphylococcal infections.

101–105. The answers are: 101-D, 102-E, 103-D, 104-A, 105-B. (*Internal medicine*)
Blood transfusions are often lifesaving and have become commonplace in the practice of medicine. However, this mundane procedure may be associated with several life-threatening reactions. It is essential that all physicians be familiar with the various transfusion reactions and their treatment.

Febrile reactions are the most common and generally are due to the presence of donor white blood cells (WBCs) in the unit of packed red blood cells (RBCs). These WBCs release pyrogens that lead to fever. In most cases, the use of selective filters that limit the transfusion of WBCs can prevent this reaction. However, it is important to realize that febrile reactions may signify more ominous disorders. For instance, febrile reactions can occur with bacterial contamination of the unit of RBCs. Thus, the proper treatment of any febrile reaction includes acetaminophen, as well as stopping the transfusion with reexamination of the cross matching and, perhaps, even culture of the unit of blood.

Anaphylactic reactions to blood transfusions are generally because of host responses to plasma proteins in the donor unit. Some of the most severe reactions are seen in recipients who suffer from a congenital absence of immunoglobulin A (IgA). In these situations, transfusions expose patients to foreign proteins, prompting the production of IgE and anaphylaxis on reexposure. Proper treatment involves the use of epinephrine (immediate effects), as well as corticosteroids and antihistamines (to prevent delayed responses).

The most serious transfusion reactions, which are associated with intravascular hemolysis of transfused cells and may be lethal, are a result of incompatibility. Acute onset of backache, malaise, fever, and hypotension develop. Soon thereafter, the urine may turn red secondary to filtering of the free hemoglobin; this may result in acute renal failure. Almost all hemolytic transfusion reactions are secondary to clerical errors with mislabeling of the blood. A rapid way to diagnose a hemolytic reaction is to centrifuge a sample of whole blood from the recipient. The presence of a red supernatant indicates free hemoglobin and, thus, hemolysis. Treatment of this reaction involves immediate cessation of the transfusion, intravenous hydration, and supportive care.

106–110. The answers are: 106-A, 107-D, 108-C, 109-D, 110-A. (*Emergency medicine, internal medicine*)
This patient presents with a combination of vague constitutional complaints (fatigue, malaise, constipation, and polyuria/polydipsia) along with findings on pulmonary examination that suggest a pleural effusion. Integrating this information with the patient's history of tobacco abuse, malignancy should be a concern. The initial workup should consist of those tests that would provide the information needed to support the suspected diagnosis without incurring excessive cost or morbidity to the patient. In this case, it is reasonable to obtain a complete blood count (CBC) to assess for anemia and an elevated white blood cell (WBC) count. A chemistry panel is appropriate to assess renal function and to check for hypokalemia and hypercalcemia. Liver function

tests should be checked given the patient's history of alcohol use. Finally, a chest radiograph is indicated based on the physical examination findings. Thyroid function tests are unlikely to yield useful information. Serum protein electrophoresis would take several days and is unlikely to yield useful information.

Like malignancy, hypercalcemia may result in all of these complaints. Furthermore, it may be secondary to malignancy (e.g., squamous cell carcinoma of the lung). Other possibilities include liver disease and tuberculosis. Major depression is unlikely to yield the constellation of symptoms reported by this patient. Although depression may lead to malaise and fatigue, it does not explain the other findings.

Several mechanisms may result in hypercalcemia. In this case, the most likely cause is production of parathyroid-related hormone by a squamous cell carcinoma of the lung. Other mechanisms include vitamin D production (e.g., lymphoma, granulomatous disease) and skeletal invasion by tumors (e.g., myeloma, prostate and breast cancers). Renal insufficiency is not associated with hypercalcemia and, in most cases, leads to lower levels of calcium secondary to decreased 1,25-dihydroxyvitamin D levels and elevated phosphate levels.

The pulmonary examination reveals dullness to percussion and decreased breath sounds at the right lung base. These findings are consistent with a pleural effusion. Given the concern for malignancy-induced hypercalcemia, hilar adenopathy may be expected. The other chest radiograph findings listed in question 109 are not consistent with the physical examination. Patients with bullous emphysema tend to have decreased breath sounds and increased resonance to percussion.

All of the therapies listed as possible answers for question 110 may be useful in the treatment of hypercalcemia. However, the most important initial maneuver is intravenous hydration with normal saline. Secondary to the calcium-induced polyuria, patients are volume-depleted at presentation, and volume-depletion further worsens the hypercalcemia. Volume expansion leads to calciuria, and once adequate hydration is achieved, calciuresis can be further increased with a loop diuretic. Glucocorticoids are effective in treatment of hypercalcemia secondary to lymphoma, myeloma, and vitamin D intoxication states. Bisphosphonates, such as pamidronate, which inhibits calcium release from bone, may be useful in patients with severe hypercalcemia or in those whose calcium remains elevated after hydration. Plicamycin, another antiresorptive agent, may be effective in patients unresponsive to pamidronate. Calcitonin is fast acting but weak.

111–113. The answers are: 111-E, 112-A, 113-D. (*Emergency medicine, neurology, internal medicine*)
This patient, who has advanced AIDS, presents with clinical signs of meningitis, including fever, headache, nausea, and vomiting. The profound immunosuppression leaves him susceptible to both common pathogens and unusual organisms, including fungi. A careful physical examination is critical in such a patient, who could have meningitis. The presence of skin findings, such as petechiae, could signify infection with *Neisseria meningitidis*.

The funduscopic examination is severely abnormal. Normally, the margins of the optic disc are sharp, and the retinal vasculature can be seen to cross over the margin of the disc. In this patient, the optic disc is bulging forward and the margins are obscured and the retinal vasculature is protruded forward. These findings are indicative of papilledema. Advanced diabetic retinopathy presents with hard and soft exudates, neovascularization, and vitreal hemorrhage. Optic neuritis demonstrates a pale optic disc. Retinal detachments are notable for a tear in the retina and a wrinkled appearance, and often there is associated hemorrhage.

Papilledema is a sign of increased intracranial pressure secondary to numerous causes, which may include meningitis, intracerebral hemorrhage, and mass lesions. The first step in management is an emergent head CT scan. It is essential to investigate the possibility of an intracranial mass that requires neurosurgery. In the absence of a mass lesion, it is safe to perform a low-volume lumbar puncture to obtain diagnostic information. Lumbar puncture should *never* occur in the setting of papilledema without a prior imaging study because, in the presence of a mass lesion, herniation and death can result. The use of intravenous mannitol and dexamethasone may decrease intracranial pressure; however, there is no urgent need for their use at this time, and diagnostic workup may swiftly continue. Furthermore, intravenous ceftriaxone alone would not be appropriate treatment in an immunocompromised patient if bacterial meningitis was being considered as a possible diagnosis. Appropriate antibiotic treatment should include vancomycin (for resistant *Streptococcus*) and ampicillin (for *Listeria*), as well as ceftriaxone.

The most likely diagnosis in this patient is cryptococcal meningitis. The subacute course, fever, and presence of papilledema are common and characteristic of this disease. Toxoplasmosis generally presents with fever, a mass lesion, and seizures. Lymphoma in the setting of fever is less common. Kaposi sarcoma rarely spreads to the central nervous system (CNS).

114–115. The answers are: 114-E, 115-D. (*Emergency medicine, obstetrics/gynecology*)
This patient clearly presents with symptoms consistent with pyelonephritis. Her urine displays white blood cell (WBC) casts, which confirm the diagnosis. Like all pregnant women, this patient is more prone to urinary tract infections and pyelonephritis; in part, this tendency is secondary to the effects of progesterone on the urinary system, leading to ureteral dilation and urine stasis. Nephrolithiasis could be a possible explanation for her symptoms; however, the urinalysis is diagnostic. Abruptio placentae results in severe uterine pain and vaginal bleeding in the third trimester. No evidence for glomerulonephritis (no red blood cell [RBC] casts) is present. Preeclampsia leads to hypertension, edema, and proteinuria.

Appropriate treatment must include hospital admission. Given the nausea, there is no assurance that the patient will tolerate oral antibiotics. Furthermore, dehydration is likely and requires intravenous hydration. Therefore, hospital admission and intravenous ceftriaxone is an appropriate choice. Nitrofurantoin is an effective agent for treatment of cystitis; however, it is not appropriate for the treatment of pyelonephritis, which requires an antibiotic that can produce high tissue concentrations.

116–117. The answers are: 116-C, 117-B. (*Emergency medicine, pediatrics, surgery*)
This patient presents with an intussusception, which occurs when there is invagination of one part of the intestine into another, resulting in abdominal pain, obstruction, and vomiting. It most commonly occurs before the age of 2 years, and the recurrence rate may be as high as 15%. Specific lead points for invagination, which include Meckel diverticulum, lymphoma, foreign bodies, and polyps, are found in only 5% of children. In many children, hypertrophy of Peyer patches secondary to a viral infection may ultimately serve as a lead point.

An intussusception may be serious if it is not rapidly identified; impaired arterial inflow and venous outflow to the involved bowel occur as a result, and necrosis and perforation may develop. An abdominal mass is felt in approximately 50% of cases and, with the proper clinical history, can point to the diagnosis.

It is important to obtain plain films first. Abdominal radiographs demonstrate a paucity of gas downstream from the obstruction and signs of obstruction proximally. Although ultrasound and CT would also be diagnostic, a plain radiograph is easier to obtain and results in a more rapid diagnosis.

If these films indicate obstruction, a barium enema is then warranted. In 75% of cases, this procedure is both diagnostic and therapeutic. The hydrostatic pressure reduces the obstruction. An appendectomy is inappropriate unless there is inflammation of the appendix, which is not present in this case.

118–120. The answers are: 118-D, 119-C, 120-D. (*Emergency medicine, surgery*)
Caustic injuries to the esophagus lead to serious short- and long-term morbidity and mortality. In adults, the majority of caustic ingestions occur as a result of suicide attempts. The initial treatment of these ingestions involves general supportive care with pain control, intravenous hydration, and careful monitoring. Early upper endoscopy is critical; it allows the grading of the injury and helps determine prognosis and treatment. For the majority of serious injuries, with mucosal ulcerations, severe edema, and eschar formation, treatment involves parenteral nutrition and no oral intake until healing occurs. Nasogastric tube placement is contraindicated because the tube may lead to perforation of the friable, injured mucosa. Induction of vomiting is also contraindicated because it may reexpose the esophagus to caustic injury.

Unfortunately, complications secondary to caustic injuries of the esophagus are common and include esophageal perforation, esophageal strictures, esophageal carcinoma, and aortoesophageal fistula. In this patient, the massive upper gastrointestinal (GI) tract bleeding was secondary to an aortoesophageal fistula. Cirrhosis is not a consideration in this case, and esophageal carcinoma takes years to develop.

121–123. The answers are: 121-C, 122-C, 123-D. (*Psychiatry, internal medicine*)
Alcohol abuse is prevalent in society. It is estimated that up to 23% of men may have a problem with alcohol sometime during their lives. The pathogenesis of alcoholism is complex and involves genetic predisposition, as well as physiologic and psychologic factors. Many patients who are interested in stopping their alcohol use present to their primary care physician. Unfortunately, for the majority of individuals, realizing that they need to stop consuming alcohol comes only after a serious event, such as job loss, a marital problem, or an arrest for alcohol-related behavior.

Disulfiram (Antabuse), an alcohol deterrent, works through the blockade of aldehyde dehydrogenase. If patients consume alcohol while taking disulfiram, acetaldehyde levels increase. Within 30 minutes of drinking, nausea, flushing, anxiety, tachycardia, and headache occur. In some patients, the reaction may be more severe, resulting in convulsions and myocardial infarction (MI). Because disulfiram is eliminated slowly from the body, patients who stop using the drug may still have reactions for up to 1 to 2 weeks. Patients also should understand that while they are taking disulfiram, any alcohol-containing medications may also elicit a reaction. In addition, they should not take disulfiram for more than 3 to 6 months because side effects (e.g., drowsiness, lethargy, transaminitis) worsen with time. Therefore, the drug is only effective as a short-term deterrent.

In the acute phase of alcohol cessation, withdrawal symptoms are common and may include tachycardia, fever, hallucinations, paranoia, and seizures. Rhinorrhea is not seen; it is characteristic of opioid withdrawal.

Many individuals who abuse alcohol are under the assumption that they can control their alcohol consumption; they may opt to pursue "controlled consumption." Various studies have repeatedly shown that this approach is doomed to fail. Inherently, alcoholics have lost the ability to control their alcohol intake, and there is no reason to believe that they can regain it. All of the answer choices in question 123 are true. The most successful programs rely on total abstinence as the cornerstone of therapy.

124–125. The answers are: 124-C, 125-D. (*Psychiatry*)
Electroconvulsive therapy is used as first-line therapy for patients with severe, life-threatening depression, bipolar illness, or catatonic schizophrenia. For patients with major depression accompanied by psychotic features, such as the one in this case, electroconvulsive therapy is more effective than antidepressants alone, with success rates approaching 90%. Symptom improvement also tends to be more rapid.

Unfortunately, electroconvulsive therapy is associated with severe side effects. Most patients experience memory loss, possibly long-term; after treatment, patients commonly do not remember the hospitalization. Fewer than 1% of patients complain of amnesia 6 months after the procedure. Seizures occur in essentially all patients; this is the nature of the treatment. A short-acting barbiturate is commonly given to mask and lessen the symptoms of the convulsions. Patients are also typically paralyzed with an agent such as succinylcholine. Other side effects include myalgia, headache, arrhythmia, myocardial infarction (MI), and broken teeth. Mania is not a side effect.

126–127. The answers are: 126-C, 127-D. (*Internal medicine*)
Traveler's diarrhea has several causes, including infection with strains of *Escherichia coli*. Although the condition is rarely life-threatening, as it can significantly impair enjoyment of a vacation, many patients are interested in prophylactic therapy. Several options exist, including: (1) ciprofloxacin or trimethoprim-sulfamethoxazole, given at the first sign of diarrhea; and (2) bismuth subsalicylate (Pepto-Bismol), taken daily during the trip. Unfortunately, exclusively using bottled water will not prevent all cases of diarrhea; a significant portion occur secondary to contaminated food.

It is important to realize that the use of Pepto-Bismol can be associated with side effects such as bleeding and salicylate toxicity. In this patient, the increased bleeding is secondary to the effect of the salicylate in the

Pepto-Bismol on platelet function. In combination with the anticoagulation properties of warfarin, this leads to prolonged bleeding.

128–130. The answers are: 128-D, 129-A, 130-D. (*Internal medicine*)
This patient presents with blood pressure measurements that clearly point to the diagnosis of hypertension and warrant treatment. However, blood pressures obtained away from the office are within normal limits, which suggests possible "white coat hypertension." A useful tool for confirming this diagnosis is the use of 24-hour ambulatory blood pressure monitoring. This can document the amount of time during a day that a patient meets the criteria for hypertension and can then guide the decision about starting antihypertensive therapy. It is premature to start antihypertensives or withhold oral contraceptives. A patient with this form of hypertension is likely part of a subgroup that is more likely to develop frank hypertension in the ensuing years.

Hypokalemia and hypertension occur in many disorders, including primary aldosteronism, Cushing disease, renal artery stenosis, and several other rare conditions. The first step in the diagnosis of these conditions is confirmation that the hypokalemia is due to enhanced renal losses of potassium. If this is true, a simultaneously obtained serum renin and aldosterone level may help. Three results are possible:

High renin/ high aldosterone	Occurs in renal artery stenosis, in which decreased renal perfusion leads to renin release and high levels of circulating aldosterone
Low renin/ high aldosterone	As a result of primary hyperaldosteronism
	Increase in circulating volume as a result of high levels of aldosterone leads to suppression of renin release
Low renin/ low aldosterone	Occurs in Cushing disease, in which high levels of corticosteroid lead to activation of the aldosterone receptor

Immediate MRI or CT scanning to look for adrenal masses is not a recommended choice because there is a high incidence of nonfunctioning incidental masses. It is critical to have biochemical evidence of oversecretion of hormone before embarking on imaging studies.

131–134. The answers are: 131-D, 132-B, 133-E, 134-B. (*Surgery, neurology*)
Incontinence is a common problem in older persons and in those with neurologic diseases. Behaviorial therapies tend to be more successful than medical treatment, and they avoid the side effects that are common with medications. Stress incontinence responds well to pelvic muscle exercises. Urge incontinence responds well to scheduled toileting, which involves the gradual increase of the interval between voiding while maintaining continence. Prompted voiding, in which the patient is asked to void, has been used to prevent incontinence in nursing home patients with dementia. Patients with overflow incontinence usually require medications, bladder drainage, or surgical correction.

Multiple sclerosis leads to incontinence through its effects on the central nervous system (CNS). Patients usually present with a combination of urge incontinence (overactivity of the detrusor muscle secondary to loss of inhibitory signals from the brain) and overflow incontinence from an adynamic bladder. Given the low postvoid residual urine volume in this patient, the most likely cause is urge incontinence. Typically, large volumes of urine are lost. The simplest and safest treatment is scheduled voiding, which avoids stretching the bladder walls and activating the reflex to void.

The second patient suffers from overflow incontinence as typified by her cystocele and large residual urine volume. She may ultimately require surgical repair but can also be treated with intermittent Foley catheterization.

The third patient, who suffers from dementia, is incapacitated. Therefore, she may not have the urge to void and may not be able to physically get to the toilet. The best therapy for this woman is prompted voiding.

The last patient has prostatic hypertrophy, which leads to overflow incontinence, as well as urge incontinence from overactivity of the detrusor muscle. Medications (α-blockers) may be helpful but are associated with orthostatic hypotension. Surgical procedures to improve the prostatic hypertrophy are also available. However, a simple solution involves the use of scheduled toileting. This allows the bladder volume to remain low and avoids bladder stretching with resulting detrusor hyperactivity or urinary overflow.

135–136. The answers are: 135-B, 136-A. (*Statistics*)

Positive predictive value is defined as the probability that a disease is present when a test or procedure is positive. This value is significantly influenced by the prevalence of disease and the sensitivity and specificity of the test or procedure. A clinically important variable, the positive predictive value allows practitioners to evaluate the importance of a positive test in any given patient. After all, clinicians want to know how well a certain test predicts the presence of disease in a given patient. The prevalence data along with the sensitivity and specificity data can be displayed in a 2 × 2 table as:

		DISEASE	
		Present	**Absent**
TEST	**Positive**	(a)	270 (b)
	Negative	43 (c)	630 (d)
	TOTALS	100	900

The positive predictive value is equal to a/(a + b); this is 57/(57 + 270), or approximately 17%.

137–138. The answers are: 137-B, 138-D. (*Internal medicine, neurology*)

This patient has clinical symptoms consistent with involvement of cranial nerve (CN) III with sparing of the pupillary fibers. The finding of ptosis and an eye deviated down and out should point to this diagnosis. Individuals with diabetes are prone to ischemic infarcts of CN III; the pupillary fibers tend to be spared because they are well vascularized, while the motor fibers are affected. Pain with the infarct is typical. The other answers listed in question 137 would not account for the patient's symptoms. CN VI lesions affect visual acuity, and they would not allow gaze to the left in the left eye. Occipital lobe strokes and retinal detachment would also affect visual acuity.

The most likely cause of this condition is an ischemic infarct of the cranial nerve secondary to poorly controlled diabetes mellitus. A common occurrence in diabetic patients, this is a result of small vessel atherosclerosis that develops when glycemic control is poor. Myasthenia gravis leads to global eye muscle weakness. Horner syndrome (often secondary to a Pancoast lung tumor) results in miosis, ptosis, and anhidrosis secondary to involvement of the sympathetic nerve chain. Multiple sclerosis most often affects the optic nerve, not the extraocular muscle. A stroke does not account for a single cranial nerve lesion.

139–142. The answers are: 139-D, 140-C, 141-A, 142-A. (*Internal medicine, obstetrics/gynecology*)

Both patients have various forms of vaginitis. In examining patients with vaginitis, the pH of the vaginal discharge can be diagnostic. In cases of *Candida* vaginitis, the pH is less than 4.5; in bacterial vaginosis, the pH is greater than 4.5.

In the first patient, the presence of a strong, foul odor when potassium hydroxide (KOH) is applied to the discharge is further evidence of bacterial vaginosis, the most common cause of vaginitis. A wet mount would reveal clue cells, which are bacteria-studded epithelial cells. The treatment of choice is either a 7-day course of metronidazole or a 2-g single dose of metronidazole. The 7-day course has a success rate of 95% versus 85% for the single dose course. Neither *Trichomonas* nor *Candida* is associated with a foul odor on addition of KOH.

The second patient suffers from severe *Candida* vaginitis. Budding yeast would be seen on a wet mount. Immunosuppression (HIV infection) and a recent course of antibiotics are two predisposing factors. Given the immunosuppression and failure of topical agents, the best treatment option would be a prolonged course of an oral azole, such as fluconazole. Metronidazole, estrogen, and ceftriaxone are not antifungal treatments.

Trichomonas infections also lead to vaginal discharge, which is less often accompanied by vulvovaginal irritation. A characteristic finding on examination is the presence of petechial hemorrhages on the cervix ("strawberry cervix"). The treatment of choice is metronidazole. Treatment of sexual partners is recommended.

143–145. The answers are: 143-D, 144-E, 145-B. (*Internal medicine, critical care medicine*)
The first patient presents with neutropenia and fever. The concerns for a possible pseudomonal infection are high, and coverage must include this organism. Many clinicians would also include vancomycin for patients who have a central line until culture results are available. If the fever continues despite antibiotic therapies and negative cultures, it may be necessary to add amphotericin B.

The second patient presents with a severe community-acquired pneumonia. Possible causes include *Streptococcus pneumoniae* and atypical organisms such as *Legionella*. Appropriate coverage would include ceftriaxone and azithromycin.

The third patient presents with signs of pelvic inflammatory disease (PID), which may be caused by *Neisseria gonorrhoeae*, *Chlamydia trachomatis,* or a mixture of aerobic and anaerobic organisms. The best treatment choice would be cefoxitin combined with doxycycline. None of the other answer choices in question 145 would provide adequate coverage of anaerobic and intracellular pathogens.

146–147. The answers are: 146-D, 147-B. (*Emergency medicine, surgery, internal medicine*)
During the surgery, this patient's terminal ileum was removed, and several months later, her symptoms of anemia developed. This portion of the ileum plays a critical role in numerous absorptive functions, including absorption of vitamin B_{12} and bile salts. The absence of significant disease of the terminal ileum may lead to serious conditions, which are likely due to vitamin B_{12} deficiency. The intrinsic factor–B_{12} complex cannot be absorbed and is lost in the stool. Over time, vitamin B_{12} stores are diminished until clinical deficiency results. This is pernicious anemia, which is typified by a maturation defect in all blood cell lines. Anemia characterized by macrocytosis is seen along with hypersegmented neutrophils. Iron deficiency, characterized by microcytosis, does not occur; iron is absorbed in the proximal bowel. Schistocytes are the result of microangiopathic hemolytic anemia. Thrombocytopenia, not thrombocytosis, may occur.

The terminal ileum is also responsible for the absorption of bile salts. Chronic loss of bile salts leads to body depletion and, eventually, steatorrhea because fats are not solubilized for absorption by the bile salts. The presence of free fatty acids in the bowel lumen allows calcium to bind to these acids, forming calcium salts (saponification), so the normally insoluble calcium oxalate present in the diet is absorbed as oxalate ions. This ultimately leads to the formation of calcium oxalate stones in the kidney as the concentration of calcium oxalate exceeds its solubility product.

148. The answer is B. (*Obstetrics/gynecology*)
This patient presents with infectious mastitis, which typically occurs when a milk duct becomes infected with a skin organism such as *Staphylococcus aureus* or *Streptococcus epidermidis*. Breast-feeding significantly increases the risk of this condition. Proper treatment certainly includes pain control but also uses antibiotics, such as cephalexin, to eradicate the infection. It is critical to rule out an abscess on examination; if infectious mastitis is not treated early, an abscess that requires drainage may develop. There is no reason to discontinue breast-feeding as long as an antibiotic is chosen that is safe for the infant. Suppression of lactation is not in-

dicated. Nonsteroidal anti-inflammatory drugs (NSAIDs), such as ibuprofen, are Class B in pregnancy and can be used for pain and inflammation.

149. The answer is E. (*Internal medicine, critical care medicine*)
Physicians often use a technique termed rapid-sequence induction for intubations that must be performed rapidly. This procedure involves using a rapid-onset induction agent (e.g., etomidate) along with a fast-acting paralytic agent. However, the use of a paralytic agent requires that either intubation is successful or that mask ventilation is convenient.

Neither of these conditions applies in this patient. In addition, in the setting of hypotension, most induction agents, such as propofol, further lower blood pressure. Thus, the safest airway management strategy involves the use of topical anesthesia with lidocaine followed by intubation.

150. The answer is D. (*Internal medicine*)
The inappropriate use of vancomycin has led to the increasing emergence of bacteria strains resistant to this antibiotic, especially vancomycin-resistant enterococci. Therefore, vancomycin should only be used in situations in which it is clearly efficacious and another antibiotic would not be effective. This requirement essentially limits use of vancomycin to the treatment of individuals with serious infections secondary to β-lactam–resistant gram-positive infections or with allergies to β-lactam antibiotics. Empirically, use of the antibiotic should be limited to those situations in which the suspicion of a resistant organism is high or the patient is critically ill.

Treatment of *Clostridium difficile* colitis should begin with metronidazole. Treatment of infective endocarditis, although it is guided by the results of blood culture, generally involves the use of a cephalosporin, ampicillin, or semisynthetic penicillin (e.g., nafcillin) with or without an aminoglycoside. Treatment of peritonitis in a patient with peritoneal dialysis also depends on culture results but begins with a cephalosporin and aminoglycoside.

Test V

QUESTIONS

DIRECTIONS: For each question, select the letter corresponding to the best answer. All questions have only one correct answer.

Setting: Emergency Department

Questions 1–3

A 29-year-old female nurse is brought in by the rescue squad after being found unconscious by a family member. After receiving 1 mg of glucagon, she becomes responsive and reacts appropriately. She takes no medications, is not a smoker, and drinks one or two glasses of wine with dinner. Several laboratory tests are obtained in the emergency department (ED).

1. Which of the following abnormalities is likely?

(A) Hyponatremia
(B) Hypercalcemia
(C) Hyperkalemia
(D) Hypernatremia
(E) Hypoglycemia

2. Which of the following conditions is NOT associated with this metabolic problem?

(A) Adrenal insufficiency
(B) Primary aldosteronism
(C) Liver failure
(D) Renal failure
(E) Pituitary failure

3. Which of the following laboratory tests is most likely to yield a diagnosis?

(A) Thyroid-stimulating hormone (TSH)
(B) Cortisol
(C) Alanine aminotransferase (ALT)
(D) C-peptide
(E) Chemistries

Setting: Satellite Clinic

Questions 4–5

A 24-year-old woman presents with complaints of dull, left lower quadrant abdominal pain of 48 hours' duration. She is sexually active, and her menstrual period is 1 week late. She takes no medications. Ipsilateral adnexal enlargement is apparent on pelvic examination. The woman claims to have monthly mittelschmerz; what she experienced 3 weeks ago was different from this pain.

4. Which of the following measures is the most appropriate next step?

(A) Cultures for chlamydia and gonorrhea
(B) β-Human chorionic gonadotropin (β-hCG)
(C) Abdominal ultrasound
(D) CT of the abdomen
(E) Complete blood count (CBC)

5. On further questioning, you learn that the woman has not had sexual intercourse in more than 8 weeks. Which of the following conditions is the likely cause of her pain?

(A) Ovarian adenocarcinoma
(B) Germ cell tumor
(C) Follicular cyst
(D) Corpus luteal cyst
(E) Choriocarcinoma

Setting: Emergency Department

Questions 6–11

A 34-year-old man with schizophrenia is brought in by his parents because they are concerned about his inability to communicate with them. They claim he has been drowsy and very rigid for the past 24 hours. His psychiatrist recently increased his dose of haloperidol.

6. Which of the following physical findings is most likely to be present?

(A) Hypotension
(B) Fever
(C) Bradycardia
(D) Hypothermia
(E) Apnea

7. Which of the following neurotransmitters is intimately associated with this phenomenon?

(A) Dopamine hydrochloride
(B) Serotonin
(C) Acetylcholine chloride
(D) γ-Aminobutyric acid
(E) Norepinephrine

8. The result of which of the following laboratory tests is most likely to yield a diagnosis?

(A) Potassium
(B) Creatinine
(C) Calcium
(D) Phosphate
(E) Creatine kinase

9. Which of the following agents do you recommend?

(A) Haloperidol
(B) Dantrolene sodium
(C) Trazodone hydrochloride
(D) Risperidone
(E) Clozapine

10. Twenty-four hours later, the man is still rigid and continues to exhibit an altered level of consciousness. Laboratory tests reveal:

Potassium	4.9 mEq/L
Phosphorus	4.2 mg/dL
Calcium	7.6 mg/dL

Which of the following conditions is the primary cause of the metabolic disarray?

(A) Hemolysis
(B) Hypoparathyroidism
(C) Rhabdomyolysis
(D) Hyperthyroidism
(E) Renal failure

11. An electrocardiogram (ECG) is within normal limits. Which of the following measures do you recommend?

(A) Aggressive hydration
(B) Dialysis
(C) Phosphate binders
(D) Calcium infusion
(E) Bicarbonate

Setting: Office

Questions 12–15

A 54-year-old woman presents with chronic abdominal pain. An extensive history and physical examination is unrevealing. A CT scan of the abdomen is normal except for a 4-cm density in the left adrenal gland.

12. The most important next step is

(A) 24-hour urine-free cortisol
(B) 24-hour urine metanephrines and catecholamines
(C) dehydroepiandrosterone sulfate (DHEAS)
(D) aldosterone
(E) plasma renin activity

13. Which of the following is the most sensitive test for the diagnosis of Cushing syndrome?

(A) Random cortisol
(B) Overnight 1-mg dexamethasone suppression test
(C) 24-hour urine-free cortisol
(D) Adrenocorticotropic hormone (ACTH) level
(E) High-dose dexamethasone suppression test

14. Which of the following groups of abnormalities are typical of primary aldosteronism?

(A) Hypertension, hypokalemia, high bicarbonate, and high plasma renin activity
(B) Hypertension, hyperkalemia, high bicarbonate, and increased aldosterone
(C) Hypotension, hypokalemia, low bicarbonate, and increased aldosterone
(D) Hypotension, hyperkalemia, low bicarbonate, and high plasma renin activity
(E) Hypertension, hypokalemia, high bicarbonate, and low plasma renin activity

15. No diagnosis is made, although several laboratory tests are obtained. On reviewing the CT scan, you learn that the mass has a high Hounsfield unit (>20). Which of the following procedures do you recommend?

(A) Biopsy
(B) Magnetic resonance imaging (MRI)
(C) CT repeated in 3 months
(D) Mammogram
(E) CT of the chest

Setting: Office

Questions 16–20

A 25-year-old man is referred to your office for evaluation of kidney stones. He has had three episodes of colicky, right-sided flank pain that radiates toward the groin. An abdominal plain film, taken in the ED, shows a ½-cm hyperdensity in the region of the left ureter.

16. The stone is least likely to have the following composition?

(A) Calcium oxalate
(B) Calcium phosphate
(C) Triple phosphate
(D) Uric acid
(E) Cystine

17. On further questioning, you learn that the man's mother and sister have a history of kidney stones; his sister has prolactinoma as well. His other three siblings have no medical problems. Which of the following conditions is NOT associated with the man's suspected disease?

(A) Parathyroid hyperplasia
(B) Pheochromocytoma
(C) Vasoactive intestinal polypeptide-secreting tumor
(D) Insulinoma
(E) Carcinoid tumor

18. This disease usually has which of the following patterns of inheritance?

(A) Autosomal dominant
(B) Autosomal recessive
(C) X-linked dominant
(D) X-linked recessive
(E) Cannot be determined

19. What gene is associated with this disease?

(A) *RET*
(B) *BCL-2*
(C) *TP53*
(D) *MENIN*
(E) *RB*

20. Which of the following laboratory tests is most likely to support a diagnosis?

(A) Calcitonin
(B) Calcium
(C) Prolactin
(D) Gastrin
(E) C-peptide

Setting: Emergency Department

Questions 21–24

A 32-year-old man is brought in after a motor vehicle crash. He was traveling at 50 mph when his vehicle hit the rear of another vehicle. He did not hit his head or lose consciousness; instead, he suffered blunt abdominal trauma. His blood pressure is 110/60 mm Hg, and his heart rate is 110 beats/minute. On physical examination, there is pain in the left upper quadrant on palpation. Breath sounds throughout his lung fields are good, but there is dullness to percussion of the left flank. Neurologic examination is within normal limits.

21. Which of the following procedures is the most appropriate next step?

(A) Head CT
(B) Abdominal radiography
(C) Abdominal CT
(D) Chest CT
(E) Chest radiography

22. Two hours later, the man's blood pressure drops acutely. Which of the following conditions is the most likely cause?

(A) Bowel perforation
(B) Adrenal insufficiency
(C) Liver laceration
(D) Aortic dissection
(E) Splenic rupture

23. Which of the following findings on peripheral blood smear is NOT associated with splenectomy?

(A) Howell-Jolly bodies
(B) Heinz bodies
(C) Pappenheimer bodies
(D) Target cells
(E) Nuclear remnant bodies within red blood cells (RBCs)

24. Which of the following pathogens is the most common cause of overwhelming sepsis in the splenectomized patient?

(A) *Streptococcus pneumoniae*
(B) *Haemophilus influenzae*
(C) *Pseudomonas aeruginosa*
(D) *Neisseria meningitidis*
(E) *Staphylococcus aureus*

Setting: Satellite Clinic

Questions 25–28

A 19-year-old African American man, who is sexually active, complains of pain on urination. He reports increased frequency and urgency but has no nausea, vomiting, abdominal pain, back pain, or fever. No abnormal penile discharge or odor is present. A urinalysis is ordered.

25. Which of the following results is least expected?

(A) More than 10 white blood cells (WBCs)/ high-power field (HPF)
(B) 1+ protein
(C) WBC casts
(D) Hyaline casts
(E) More than 10 red blood cells (RBCs)/HPF

26. The man receives an antibiotic and returns 48 hours later with weakness and yellow skin. Which of the following agents did he most likely take?

(A) Trimethoprim-sulfamethoxazole
(B) Amoxicillin
(C) Ciprofloxacin
(D) Doxycycline
(E) Pyridium

27. The man's disease involves the

(A) glycolytic pathway
(B) hexose monophosphate pathway
(C) Krebs cycle
(D) urea cycle
(E) electron transport chain

28. The man's peripheral smear shows

(A) target cells
(B) Howell-Jolly bodies
(C) sickle cells
(D) Heinz bodies
(E) Pappenheimer bodies

Setting: Office

Questions 29–31

A 42-year-old woman is referred to you for evaluation of a liver mass that was found on a CT scan ordered as part of a nephrolithiasis workup. The 3-cm mass has a central hypodense region with progressive peripheral-to-central enhancement. Her medical history includes only nephrolithiasis, and her medications include oral contraceptive pills and multivitamins.

29. Which of the following measures is the most appropriate next step?

(A) Fine needle aspiration
(B) CT-guided biopsy
(C) Observation with a follow-up CT scan
(D) Hepatic artery ligation
(E) Surgical removal

30. Which of the following diagnoses is the most likely?

(A) Adenoma
(B) Focal nodular hyperplasia
(C) Hepatocellular carcinoma
(D) Cholangiocarcinoma
(E) Hemangioma

31. Which of the following events occurs in the natural history of this disease?

(A) Metastasis to the liver via the bile ducts
(B) Little change in the mass
(C) Spontaneous rupture
(D) Local invasion
(E) Metastasis to the lung and bone

Setting: Satellite Clinic

Questions 32–37

A 20-year-old male college student presents to the university clinic with periumbilical pain that developed approximately 12 hours ago with fever, nausea, and vomiting. For 6 hours, the pain has been localized in the lower portion of his abdomen.

32. Which of the following physical findings is least likely to be present?

(A) Murphy sign
(B) Obturator sign
(C) McBurney sign
(D) Psoas sign
(E) Rovsing sign

33. The most common cause of periumbilical pain is

(A) parietal pleura inflammation
(B) foregut disease
(C) midgut disease
(D) hindgut disease
(E) retroperitoneal disease

34. Which of the following laboratory tests would be most helpful in making a diagnosis?

(A) Chemistries
(B) Complete blood count (CBC)
(C) Amylase
(D) Alanine aminotransferase (ALT)
(E) Urinalysis

35. Physicians most commonly establish a diagnosis by

(A) history and physical examination
(B) abdominal radiography
(C) abdominal CT
(D) abdominal ultrasound
(E) barium enema

36. The most common cause of this disease is

(A) foreign body obstruction
(B) fecalith obstruction
(C) torsion
(D) embolism
(E) lymphoid hyperplasia with obstruction

37. The blood supply of the involved organ is obtained from which of the following arteries?

(A) Gastroduodenal
(B) Superior mesenteric
(C) Inferior mesenteric
(D) Celiac
(E) Pudendal

Setting: Office

Questions 38–41

A 60-year-old man undergoes laboratory tests as part of a routine preoperative examination. His total hip replacement is scheduled for 1 week from today. Laboratory tests reveal:

Prothrombin time (PT)	14 seconds
Partial thromboplastin time (PTT)	44 seconds
Complete blood count (CBC)	Normal

38. All laboratory tests are repeated, and the results are unchanged. The most appropriate next step is

(A) bleeding time
(B) thrombin time
(C) mixing study
(D) lupus anticoagulant
(E) dilute Russell's viper venom clotting time

39. A bleeding time is a measure of

(A) liver function
(B) intrinsic clotting pathway function
(C) platelet function
(D) extrinsic clotting pathway function
(E) thromboplastin production

40. After the man's orthopedic surgery, which of the following methods of prophylaxis for deep venous thrombosis do you recommend?

(A) Unfractionated heparin
(B) Low-molecular-weight heparin
(C) Pneumatic compression devices
(D) Warfarin
(E) Hirudin

41. Which of the following procedures is associated with the greatest risk for deep venous thrombosis postoperatively?

(A) Elective hip arthroplasty
(B) Meniscectomy
(C) Pelvic fracture repair
(D) Elective knee arthroplasty
(E) Hip fracture repair

Setting: Hospital

Questions 42–48

A 56-year-old woman is admitted with complaints of fever, pleuritic chest pain, shortness of breath, and blood-streaked sputum. Her chest radiograph shows a new alveolar filling pattern in the left lower lobe.

42. Which of the following comorbidities would contribute most to your decision to treat this patient as an inpatient?

(A) Malignancy
(B) Congestive heart failure
(C) Chronic renal failure
(D) Liver disease
(E) Cerebrovascular disease

43. Which of the following organisms is most likely involved?

(A) *Staphylococcus aureus*
(B) *Haemophilus influenzae*
(C) *Streptococcus pneumoniae*
(D) *Moraxella catarrhalis*
(E) *Neisseria meningitidis*

44. Routine laboratory tests reveal hypokalemia. Which of the following agents is most likely to cause this abnormality?

(A) Captopril
(B) Propranolol hydrochloride
(C) Dapsone
(D) Trimethoprim
(E) Hydrocortisone

45. In hypokalemia, an ECG is likely to find

(A) flat P waves
(B) long PR interval
(C) large U waves
(D) wide QRS complex
(E) peaked T waves

46. As part of the workup for hypokalemia, you determine that the woman also has metabolic alkalosis. Which of the following tests is the most appropriate next step?

(A) Fractional excretion of sodium
(B) Urine sodium
(C) Fractional excretion of urea
(D) Urine potassium
(E) Urine chloride

47. The test referred to in question 46 results in a low value. In this setting, which of the following disorders is most likely?

(A) Cushing syndrome
(B) Primary aldosteronism
(C) Contraction alkalosis
(D) Prednisone therapy
(E) Licorice toxicity

48. Days later, you notice that the original sputum sample revealed gram-negative diplococci. Which of the following organisms has likely been isolated?

(A) *Klebsiella pneumoniae*
(B) *Haemophilus influenzae*
(C) *Streptococcus pneumoniae*
(D) *Moraxella catarrhalis*
(E) *Neisseria meningitidis*

Setting: Satellite Clinic

Questions 49–54

A 31-year-old Asian woman complains of diarrhea of 3 days' duration. It started 12 hours after she ate a ham sandwich with mayonnaise that she purchased at a local delicatessen. She has had fever (temperature to 39.4°C); more than 10 loose stools per day without blood; and mild pain in her right lower abdomen, which is no longer present. She has no significant medical history. On examination, vital signs are within normal limits, and the woman does not appear ill.

49. Which of the following tests is the most appropriate next step?

(A) Liver function tests
(B) Ova and parasites test on stool
(C) Abdominal radiograph
(D) Fecal leukocytes
(E) Chemistries

50. Which of the following laboratory results would you expect in the setting of intractable diarrhea?

(A) Hypokalemia, acidosis, and normal anion gap
(B) Hyperkalemia, alkalosis, and normal anion gap
(C) Hyperkalemia, acidosis, and high anion gap
(D) Hypokalemia, alkalosis, and normal anion gap
(E) Hypokalemia, acidosis, and high anion gap

51. A calculated stool osmolality far greater than a measured osmolality based on stool potassium and sodium suggests which of the following causes?

(A) Carcinoid tumor
(B) Zollinger-Ellison syndrome
(C) Celiac sprue
(D) Vasoactive intestinal polypeptide-secreting tumor
(E) Mastocytosis

52. If fecal leukocytes return positive, it suggests that the causal agent is NOT

(A) *Salmonella*
(B) *Campylobacter*
(C) *Shigella*
(D) *Yersinia*
(E) *Clostridium perfringens*

53. If the stool study reveals weakly acid-fast organisms, it suggests

(A) *Cryptosporidium*
(B) *Mycobacterium tuberculosis*
(C) *Mycobacterium avium-intracellulare* complex (MAC)
(D) *Campylobacter*
(E) *Salmonella*

54. Which of the following pathogens is associated with "rose spots" rash on the chest and abdomen?

(A) *Shigella*
(B) *Salmonella*
(C) *Campylobacter*
(D) *Yersinia*
(E) *Vibrio*

Setting: Office

Questions 55–59

A 12-year-old girl complains of sore throat. Her mother reports that last evening her daughter had a temperature of 38.6°C. She has had no cough or rhinorrhea. On physical examination, she is still febrile, with cervical lymphadenopathy and tonsillar erythema with an overlying exudate.

55. Which of the following organisms is the most likely?

(A) *Streptococcus pneumoniae*
(B) *Streptococcus pyogenes*
(C) *Neisseria meningitidis*
(D) *Chlamydia pneumoniae*
(E) *Haemophilus influenzae*

56. Which of the following treatments do you recommend?

(A) Erythromycin
(B) Cefuroxime
(C) Ampicillin
(D) Penicillin V
(E) Levofloxacin

57. Your associate treats the girl, who returns 3 days later with persistent symptoms, including fatigue and a faint maculopapular rash. Which of the following antibiotics did she likely receive?

(A) Erythromycin
(B) Cefuroxime
(C) Ampicillin
(D) Penicillin V
(E) Levofloxacin

58. Which of the following laboratory tests most likely confirms a diagnosis?

(A) Complete blood count (CBC) with differential
(B) Liver function tests
(C) Prothrombin time (PT)
(D) Chemistries
(E) Urinalysis

59. You see advertisements for a new throat swab that detects group A streptococcus. The test has a sensitivity of 80% and a specificity of 90%. If the girl's test is positive, how likely is she to have group A streptococcus infection?

(A) 50%
(B) 80%
(C) 90%
(D) 100%
(E) Cannot be determined

Setting: Office

Questions 60–62

A 38-year-old man presents with persistent fever of 2 weeks' duration. The sore throat he had 2 weeks ago has resolved. On physical examination, he is febrile to 38°C, has no lymphadenopathy, no pharyngitis, and the lungs are clear. The abdominal examination, the cardiovascular system, and the skin all appear within normal limits. The white blood cell (WBC) count is 12,500 cells/mm^3, with 55% lymphocytes and 35% segmented neutrophils. The blood smear contains atypical lymphocytes.

60. The likely cause is

(A) malignancy
(B) cytomegalovirus
(C) Epstein-Barr virus
(D) Reiter syndrome
(E) *Mycoplasma pneumoniae*

61. Which of the following infections is NOT associated with atypical lymphocytes?

(A) Cytomegalovirus
(B) Hepatitis A
(C) Toxoplasmosis
(D) Epstein-Barr virus
(E) *Streptococcus pneumoniae*–caused illness

62. Which of the following statements is true?

(A) IgM antibodies to cytomegalovirus are uniformly negative within 3 months postinfection
(B) In the United States, more than 90% of individuals are seropositive for hepatitis A by 50 years of age
(C) The Monospot test for Epstein-Barr virus is often negative within 1 week of infection onset
(D) More than 50% of Americans have serologic evidence of exposure to *Toxoplasma* by 21 years of age
(E) Hepatitis A infection is obtained primarily by the parenteral route

Setting: Office

Questions 63–66

A 63-year-old African American man complains of difficulty urinating. His medical history is notable for hypertension and diabetes mellitus. His medications include metformin and propranolol. He smokes one pack of cigarettes per day and drinks alcohol occasionally. His prostate-specific antigen (PSA) is high at 25 ng/mL.

63. Which of the following statements regarding the PSA test is true?

(A) It has 95% sensitivity
(B) It has 90% specificity
(C) It is higher in Caucasian men with benign prostatic hypertrophy than in African American men with the same condition
(D) It is elevated only in cases of adenocarcinoma
(E) The rate of rise of PSA (PSA velocity) can be used to determine PSA significance

64. Which of the following measures do you recommend?

(A) PSA repeated now
(B) Observation with PSA repeated in 1 year
(C) Transrectal biopsy
(D) Antibiotics with PSA repeated in 1 month
(E) Terazosin for benign prostatic hypertrophy

65. Which of the following statements regarding prostate cancer is true?

(A) Transitional cell is the most common type
(B) Risk of lymphatic spread correlates with the PSA level
(C) A tumor with a high Gleason tumor grade is less worrisome for metastatic spread
(D) The lung is the most common site of metastasis
(E) A radionuclide bone scan is less sensitive than a skeletal survey for prostatic bone metastasis

66. All of the following measures are useful therapies in prostate cancer EXCEPT

(A) testosterone
(B) orchiectomy
(C) leuprolide acetate
(D) aminoglutethimide
(E) flutamide

Setting: Office

Questions 67–70

A 30-year-old man complains of a testicular mass, which he first noticed 1 week ago while showering. The mass is not painful. The patient denies dysuria, hematuria, back pain, dyspnea, or testicular pain. He does not use tobacco; however, he drinks two or three beers per day. His family history is significant for a brother with Hodgkin lymphoma and a mother with breast cancer.

67. Which of the following statements about epididymitis is true?

(A) *Neisseria gonorrhoeae* is the most common cause in this patient's age group (30 to 35 years)
(B) Coliform bacteria are the most common cause in patients older than 35 years
(C) The affected testis is typically pain-free
(D) *Chlamydia trachomatis* is an uncommon cause
(E) *Chlamydia* and *Neisseria* are the exclusive causes in homosexual men

68. Which of the following statements regarding testicular cancer is true?

(A) The average age at diagnosis is 50 years
(B) The mortality rate is 50%
(C) Lymphoma should be considered in patients older than 50 years
(D) Orchiopexy eliminates the risk of cancer in a cryptorchid testis
(E) Typically, testicular pain is an associated symptom

69. Which of the following measures is the most appropriate next step?

(A) Observation
(B) Antibiotics
(C) Ultrasound of testis
(D) Mumps antibody titers
(E) Transscrotal biopsy

70. Which of the following tumors is associated with elevations in both α-fetoprotein (AFP) and β-human chorionic gonadotropin (β-hCG)?

(A) Embryonal carcinoma
(B) Endodermal sinus tumor
(C) Seminoma
(D) Teratoma
(E) Choriocarcinoma

Setting: Hospital

71. A 23-year-old woman, who is G_1P_0, ruptures her membranes at 39 weeks of pregnancy. Her cervix dilates, but it arrests at 4 cm for 2½ hours. Her pregnancy has been without complication. You recommend

(A) immediate cesarean section
(B) amniotomy
(C) oxytocin
(D) prostaglandin E_2
(E) management for malposition, disproportion, or malpresentation

Setting: Office

72. A 25-year-old woman, who is G_2P_1, experiences frequent contractions accompanied by cervical effacement at 26 weeks of pregnancy. The cervix is not dilated. You have many concerns, including the lack of pulmonary development. Which of the following measures might hasten lung development?

(A) Ritodrine hydrochloride
(B) Betamethasone
(C) Terbutaline sulfate
(D) Indomethacin
(E) Magnesium sulfate

Setting: Emergency Department

Questions 73–75

A 49-year-old man presents to the ED with abdominal pain. After an extensive workup, he is admitted and diagnosed with gastric ulcer.

73. Which of the following statements about gastric ulcers is true?

(A) The ulcers are most commonly found on the lesser curvature of the stomach
(B) Most are greater than 1 cm from the transition zone between the antrum and body of the stomach
(C) Unlike duodenal ulcers, *Helicobacter pylori* is NOT important
(D) Classically, pain is relieved with eating
(E) The ulcers are associated with gastric acid hypersecretion

74. A test for *Helicobacter pylori* antibodies is positive. The man has never been tested for this bacteria in the past. You recommend

(A) no treatment
(B) *H. pylori* breath test
(C) proton pump inhibitor
(D) macrolide antibiotics
(E) macrolide antibiotics and a proton pump inhibitor

75. The man later undergoes a truncal vagotomy and antrectomy. One week later, he complains of anxiety, weakness, sweating, and palpitations 15 minutes after eating. Which of the following disorders is the cause of these symptoms?

(A) Afferent loop syndrome
(B) Blind loop syndrome
(C) Alkaline reflux gastritis
(D) Dumping syndrome
(E) Recurrent ulcer

Setting: Office

76. You are trying to determine whether proton pump inhibitors protect against nonsteroidal anti-inflammatory drug (NSAID)–induced gastric ulcers. You have gathered several reports that address this question but are unsure which of these studies provides the best evidence for or against this practice. In evaluating these studies, which of the following studies provides the strongest clinical evidence of a cause-and-effect relationship?

(A) Cross-sectional study
(B) Case-control study
(C) Cohort study
(D) Randomized controlled trial
(E) Case series

Setting: Hospital

Questions 77–79

You are asked to see a 18-month-old girl with fever (temperature to 40°C), irritability, and a peculiar rash. Her parents report that yesterday evening their daughter was playful and displayed no unusual symptoms. This morning, however, she has a rash involving her trunk and bilateral red eyes, with no discharge. Except for minor upper respiratory infections, the girl has been healthy. She takes no medications. During the day, she is at a day-care center, and the parents know of no other children who are ill.

On examination, the girl is irritable, and a bilateral, nonpurulent, conjunctival erythema, as well as a diffuse, truncal morbilliform rash are apparent. You also find a similar rash around the peri-anal region. Diffuse cervical lymphadenopathy is present. Last, you note that the girl's lips are bright red, and her tongue has a white coating with red papillae.

77. All of the following disorders should be included in the differential diagnosis of this girl's illness EXCEPT

(A) streptococcal toxic shock syndrome
(B) scarlet fever
(C) measles
(D) hand-foot-and-mouth disease
(E) hypersensitivity reaction

78. The most appropriate therapy should include all of the following measures EXCEPT

(A) intravenous antibiotics
(B) aspirin
(C) intravenous immunoglobulin
(D) intravenous hydration
(E) intravenous corticosteroids

79. A long-term sequela of this disease is

(A) mental retardation

(B) vision loss

(C) coronary artery aneurysms

(D) seizures

(E) recurrent upper respiratory tract infections

Setting: Hospital

Questions 80–82

A 39-year-old woman with a history of mitral valve prolapse and mitral regurgitation is admitted following 7 days of low-grade fever, malaise, fatigue, and headache. Ibuprofen has provided no symptom relief. She has not traveled recently. She has no other significant medical history and takes no medications regularly.

Physical examination reveals an ill-appearing woman with a temperature of 39°C. Funduscopic, chest, and neurologic examinations are within normal limits. Cardiac examination is significant for a 3/6 holosystolic murmur radiating to the apex.

Laboratory work reveals:

Chemistries	Normal
White blood cell (WBC) count	12,000/mm^3, with 90% neutrophils
Echocardiogram	Probable small vegetation on posterior leaf of mitral valve

80. Which of the following antibiotic regimens would be appropriate initial therapy?

(A) Vancomycin and gentamicin

(B) Imipenem

(C) Ampicillin, nafcillin sodium, and gentamicin

(D) Ampicillin and gentamicin

(E) Nafcillin and gentamicin

81. After 7 days of therapy, the woman feels significantly better. Blood cultures from admission grow *Streptococcus viridans,* which has a minimal inhibitory concentration of less than 0.1 μg/mL for penicillin. Which of the following antibiotic regimens is most appropriate for completion of her treatment (duration of therapy, 4 to 6 weeks)?

(A) Vancomycin intravenously

(B) Ampicillin intravenously

(C) Imipenem intravenously

(D) Ceftriaxone intravenously

(E) Levofloxacin orally

82. After 21 days of therapy, the woman returns complaining of severe headache and right arm numbness. She reports that the symptoms began acutely and that the headache is "10 out of 10" in severity. Mild nuchal rigidity and mild photophobia are present. Neurologic examination reveals normal cranial nerves, normal upper and lower extremity strength, and a mild decrease in sensation in the right upper extremity. You order a CT scan of the brain. Which of the following findings might you expect to see?

(A) Findings within normal limits

(B) Subarachnoid hemorrhage

(C) Subdural hemorrhage

(D) Intracranial mass lesion

(E) Epidural hemorrhage

Setting: Emergency Department

83. An 80-year-old woman is brought to the ED after suffering a fall at a grocery store. Apparently, she slipped on spilled salad dressing, and she broke her fall with her outstretched hand. She is now complaining of severe right wrist pain. Her medical history is significant for hypertension and osteoporosis. Her current medications include atenolol, lisinopril, and calcium carbonate. On physical examination, dorsal angulation of the distal forearm is evident, with swelling around the wrist. You order a radiograph.

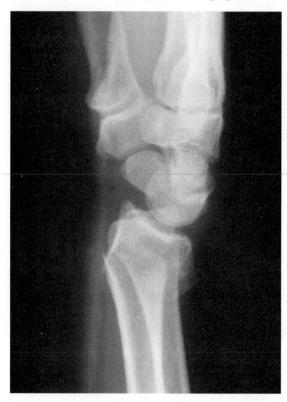

The proper treatment of this condition includes all of the following EXCEPT

(A) reduction of the fracture
(B) splinting of the forearm in a neutral position
(C) splinting of the forearm with the wrist in a flexed position
(D) nonsteroidal anti-inflammatory drugs (NSAIDs)
(E) splinting of the wrist for 2 weeks followed by 3 weeks of casting

Setting: Emergency Department

84. You are working as a physician in an ED in Vermont, during the ski season. A 22-year-old man is brought in by the ski patrol after a fall. His ski pole had jammed into the web space between his left thumb and index finger. He now has difficulty moving his thumb and complains of pain and swelling over the ulnar aspect of his metacarpophalangeal thumb joint. The abnormality is apparent on a radiograph.

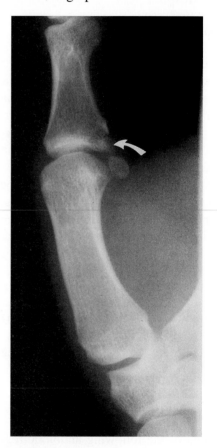

Which of the following injuries is associated with the radiograph and the clinical history?

(A) Radial collateral ligament injury
(B) Radial artery injury
(C) Ulnar collateral ligament injury
(D) Navicular fracture
(E) Fracture of the base of the thumb

Setting: Hospital

Questions 85–88

A 6-month-old female infant is admitted for evaluation of jaundice and anemia. Her mother has noted that the infant has become "more yellow" during the past 2 to 4 weeks. The infant's birth history and her mother's pregnancy were unremarkable. Family history is significant for a mild anemia of unknown etiology in the mother. Examination reveals a jaundiced infant who is only at the 20th percentile for height and weight. Several unusual findings, including frontal bossing, prominent cheekbones, and marked hepatosplenomegaly, are notable. Initial laboratory studies show a hematocrit of 15% with a reticulocyte count of 1%.

85. Which of the following laboratory results would you also expect?

(A) Serum creatinine, 2.5 mg/dL
(B) Platelet count, 10,000/mm^3
(C) Alanine aminotransferase (ALT), 10 U/L (normal, 6 to 62 U/L)
(D) Lactate dehydrogenase (LDH), 700 U/L (normal, 115 to 270 U/L)
(E) White blood cell (WBC) count, 1,000/mm^3

86. You obtain a peripheral blood smear. Which of the following would you expect to see?

(A) Schistocytes
(B) Microcytosis
(C) Macrocytosis
(D) Howell-Jolly bodies
(E) Spherocytes

87. You decide to order a hemoglobin electrophoresis. Which of the following findings is most likely?

(A) Normal hemoglobin pattern (Hgb A, 95%; Hgb A$_2$, 3%; and Hgb F, 2%)
(B) Hemoglobin Bart (four γ chains)
(C) Hemoglobin H (four β chains)
(D) Hemoglobin F, 90%
(E) Hemoglobin C, 30%; and hemoglobin A, 70%

88. Long-term management of this disease is associated with which of the following complications?

(A) Mental retardation
(B) Hemochromatosis
(C) Renal failure
(D) Myopathy
(E) Gastric cancer

Setting: Office

Questions 89–90

A 32-year-old woman is referred to you secondary to a recent diagnosis of bipolar disorder. For the past year, she describes both severe depression and episodes of manic behavior. She is interested in beginning lithium therapy but has several questions about its side effects.

89. Which of the following conditions is a common side effect of lithium use?

(A) Hypercholesterolemia
(B) Agranulocytosis
(C) Pancreatitis
(D) Gastritis
(E) Polyuria

90. The patient begins lithium therapy and initially does well, with improvement in her mood disorder. However, 15 months after starting treatment, she reports that she once again feels fatigued and depressed. Review of her chart reveals therapeutic lithium levels and no new medications. Which of the following measures should be your next step?

(A) Fluoxetine 20 mg daily
(B) Complete blood count (CBC)
(C) Thyroid panel
(D) Stopping the lithium
(E) Amitriptyline 25 mg daily

Setting: Hospital

Questions 91–93

An 18-year-old man is brought to the operating room for an emergent appendectomy. He receives succinylcholine chloride followed by inhalation anesthesia with a fluorocarbon. Soon after the operation begins, you note that the patient is tachycardic and has mottling of his skin and rigidity of his upper extremities and neck. Soon thereafter, his core temperature is recorded as 40.5°C and his blood pressure is 70/40 mm Hg.

91. The next step should involve intravenous

(A) fluid bolus and acetaminophen
(B) dopamine and fluid boluses
(C) esmolol
(D) dantrolene
(E) vancomycin and gentamicin

92. Which of the following complications is NOT associated with this man's condition?

(A) Hyperkalemia
(B) Metabolic alkalosis
(C) Elevated creatine kinase
(D) Hyperphosphatemia
(E) Lactic acidosis

93. The man is stabilized and discharged home. However, 25 years later, he is admitted to the hospital with acute cholecystitis. He recounts his medical history, including his hospital course and emergency appendectomy. To prevent a recurrence of the events in the operating room, which of the following measures is necessary?

(A) No specific action is needed; the past events represent an idiosyncratic reaction
(B) Avoidance of succinylcholine and use of nitrous oxide for anesthesia
(C) Avoidance of succinylcholine only
(D) Avoidance of all inhalation agents except nitrous oxide and use of succinylcholine
(E) Pretreatment with atenolol

Setting: Hospital

Questions 94–97

A 60-year-old man undergoes a routine screening flexible sigmoidoscopy. The findings include multiple sigmoid colon diverticula and one small polyp, which is removed. The patient, who is otherwise healthy, expresses concern about the presence of the diverticula.

94. Which of the following conditions is the most common complication of diverticulosis?

(A) Hemorrhage
(B) Malignancy
(C) Diverticulitis
(D) Rectal prolapse
(E) Sigmoid volvulus

95. Follow-up continues for the next 14 months, and the man does well. However, he is admitted to the ICU for profuse, bright-red, rectal bleeding. On admission, his hematocrit is 25% and his vital signs are notable only for tachycardia. He receives four units of packed red blood cells (RBCs) overnight before the bleeding stops. Which of the following statements regarding lower gastrointestinal (GI) bleeding secondary to diverticulosis is true?

(A) CT scans can localize the site of bleeding
(B) Resection of the involved segment of colon is usually required to stop the bleeding
(C) Spontaneous cessation of bleeding occurs in 85% of cases
(D) Antibiotics are necessary because there is a high probability of a subclinical bowel perforation
(E) Bleeding often signifies the presence of an enteric–vascular structure fistula

96. The man is stabilized and does well. However, he presents to the office 6 months later with fever, chills, and left lower quadrant pain of 3 days' duration. His white blood count (WBC) is 19,000 cells/mm^3. A CT scan reveals some inflammation around the sigmoid colon with no evidence of abscess. You decide to admit the patient to the hospital for therapy. Appropriate treatment should include

(A) emergent surgery with bowel resection
(B) barium enema
(C) colonoscopy
(D) ampicillin/sulbactam intravenously
(E) corticosteroids

97. The man is discharged from the hospital feeling significantly improved. However, 10 days later, he returns with a fever (temperature to 40°C), severe left lower quadrant pain with rebound and guarding, and nausea. A CT scan now shows a 5-cm abscess in the left lower quadrant, and an upright chest radiograph demonstrates free air in the peritoneum. Which of the following should be the next step?

(A) Emergent resection of the involved region of the colon with abscess drainage and intravenous antibiotics
(B) Total colectomy with abscess drainage and intravenous antibiotics
(C) CT-guided drainage of the abscess and intravenous antibiotics
(D) Operative drainage of the abscess and intravenous antibiotics
(E) Broad-spectrum antibiotics and elective colectomy

Setting: Emergency Department

Questions 98–99

A 62-year-old man with end-stage renal disease requiring hemodialysis has missed a dialysis session because he attended his daughter's wedding. He presents with nausea, vomiting, abdominal pain, and dyspnea. Physical examination is notable for a blood pressure of 210/100 mm Hg, heart rate of 60 beats/minute, and a respiratory rate of 30/minute. Chest examination demonstrates rales over the entire lung fields bilaterally. Cardiac examination is notable for a loud S_4 heart sound and a 2/6 holosystolic murmur radiating to the axilla. Abdominal examination is within normal limits. Laboratory work is performed, and a 12-lead ECG (*below*) is obtained.

98. The next step should be

(A) transcutaneous pacing
(B) thrombolysis
(C) intravenous bicarbonate (1 ampule)
(D) calling the cardiac catheterization laboratory
(E) intravenous calcium chloride (1 ampule)

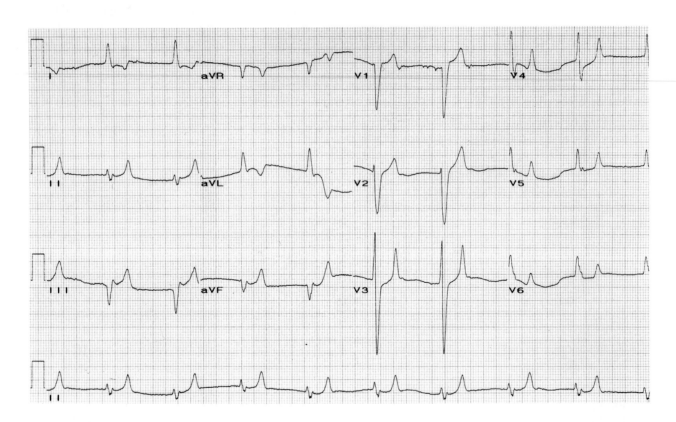

99. You call to arrange for emergent dialysis for the man; you are told that it will take approximately 90 minutes before this can occur. He is becoming more dyspneic and agitated, and a blood gas reveals a PO_2 of 50 mm on 100% nonrebreather face mask. He has minimal urine output. After intravenous labetalol, his blood pressure is now 160/100 mm Hg. You next step should be

(A) intravenous furosemide drip at 40 mg/hour
(B) nitroglycerin paste 1 inch applied to chest wall
(C) emergent intubation
(D) intravenous nitroprusside drip
(E) intravenous verapamil

Setting: Office

Questions 100–104

A 26-year-old woman comes to see you for several neurologic problems. During the past few months, she has had intermittent weakness in her arms, a loss of dexterity, and a tingling sensation in her right foot. In the past week, she has experienced blurred vision in her right eye, with pain that she describes as localized behind the eye. She has no medical history and takes only one multivitamin per day. She smokes one pack of cigarettes per day, drinks no alcohol, and uses no drugs. She is unmarried and has no children. She currently teaches first grade. Family history is significant for coronary artery disease in her father and diabetes mellitus type 2 in her mother.

Physical examination reveals an anxious woman with vital signs within normal limits. Neurologic examination is notable for:

Funduscopic examination	Possible swelling of right optic disc
Motor examination	Within normal limits
Sensory examination	Slightly decreased sensation in right foot
Deep tendon reflexes	Within normal limits
Cerebellar examination	Mild ataxia of right arm on finger-to-nose testing

100. Which of the following cranial nerve findings might you expect?

(A) Bell palsy
(B) Pupillary dilation in response to direct light in the right eye, following constriction in response to indirect light in the left eye
(C) Decreased sensation over the distribution of the right trigeminal nerve
(D) Normal examination
(E) Right CN VI lesion

101. You decide to obtain a MRI of the brain in search of which of the following findings?

(A) Mass lesion
(B) Vascular aneurysm
(C) White matter lesions
(D) Encephalomalacia
(E) Dilated cerebral ventricles

102. The MRI suggests the diagnosis you suspect. You recommend that the woman have a lumbar puncture, and she reluctantly agrees. Which of the following findings on examination of the cerebrospinal fluid (CSF) supports the suspected diagnosis?

(A) Normal CSF (normal protein, cell count, glucose)
(B) Elevated immunoglobulin G (IgG) level with oligoclonal bands
(C) Low glucose concentration
(D) Neutrophilic pleocytosis
(E) High protein content with normal IgG levels

103. A medication improves the woman's symptoms. However, in the next 6 months, she has two additional relapses, which are marked by lower extremity weakness and numbness with right hand ataxia. Treatment of these relapses is successful. She asks about the availability of a treatment that will decrease the frequency of relapses. Which of the following agents has been used successfully to decrease annual exacerbation rates?

(A) Interferon beta
(B) Amantadine hydrochloride
(C) Prednisone
(D) Low-dose cyclosporine
(E) Angiotensin-converting enzyme (ACE) inhibitors

104. The woman returns 1 year later complaining that she has to urinate every 5 to 10 minutes. Urine culture is negative. Urodynamic testing demonstrates a hyperreflexic bladder. Which of the following therapies is indicated for this condition?

(A) Intermittent self-catheterization
(B) Terazosin 5 mg every night
(C) Oxybutynin 5 mg 2 times a day
(D) Bethanechol 10 mg 4 times a day
(E) No treatment indicated

Setting: Hospital

105. A 56-year-old man is involved in a motor vehicle accident in which he suffers extensive injury to his abdomen, requiring splenectomy and small bowel resection. He is placed on total parenteral nutrition (TPN). During the next week, you note that he has lost 2 kg and wonder if he is receiving adequate caloric intake. The TPN formula is:

Weight	80 kg
Carbohydrates	5 g/kg per day
Protein	0.8 g/kg per day
Lipids	0.5 g/kg per day

What is the man's approximate total caloric intake from TPN per day (in kcal)?

(A) 1,500
(B) 1,750
(C) 2,000
(D) 2,200
(E) 2,400

Setting: Hospital

Questions 106–107

A 40-year-old man is admitted to the ICU with respiratory failure. Fever, chills, and shortness of breath developed 3 days ago; these symptoms have worsened during the past 48 hours. On initial evaluation in the ED, oxygen saturation on 100% oxygen was 75%, and he was in severe respiratory distress. After being emergently intubated, he is transferred to the ICU. Chest radiography shows severe bilateral pneumonia. Initial ventilator settings are synchronized intermittent mandatory ventilation at a rate of 12, fractional concentration of oxygen in inspired gas (FIO_2) of 65%, tidal volume of 850 mL, and a positive end-expiratory pressure (PEEP) of 2 cm H_2O. An arterial blood gas is performed; the pH is 7.39, the $PaCO_2$ is 42 mm Hg, and the PaO_2 is 55 mm Hg.

106. The man's oxygenation can be improved by

(A) decreasing the respiratory rate to 10/minute
(B) increasing the respiratory rate to 16/minute
(C) increasing the FIO_2 to 100%
(D) increasing the PEEP to 10 cm H_2O
(E) increasing the tidal volume to 1,100 mL

107. The man receives antibiotics and supportive care and, ultimately, is extubated on hospital day 5. However, the night after extubation, you are called because he is in severe respiratory distress with an oxygen saturation of 90% on 100% nonrebreather face mask. An emergent chest radiograph (*below*) is obtained.

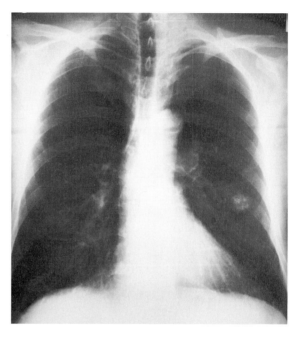

Which of the following conditions is the most likely diagnosis?

(A) Empyema
(B) Collapse of the left lung
(C) Hemothorax
(D) Pulmonary embolus
(E) Malignant pleural effusion

Setting: Emergency Department and Hospital

Questions 108–112

A 65-year-old man presents to the ED with severe, substernal chest pain radiating to the left jaw, with associated dyspnea, nausea, and diaphoresis of 4 hours' duration. Medical history is significant for obesity, hypertension, hyperlipidemia, and type 2 diabetes mellitus. His medications include insulin, benazepril hydrochloride, and simvastatin.

On physical examination, he appears in moderate distress with a blood pressure of 160/100 mm Hg, a heart rate of 60 beats/minute, and respiratory rate of 16/minute. Cardiac examination reveals a regular rate with an S_4 heart sound. Pulmonary examination finds few bibasilar rales. Abdominal examination is within normal limits, with no bruits.

At the time of admission, the man has an ECG (*below*).

108. The diagnosis is

(A) pericarditis
(B) hypokalemia
(C) hypercalcemia
(D) acute anterior myocardial infarction (MI)
(E) acute inferior MI

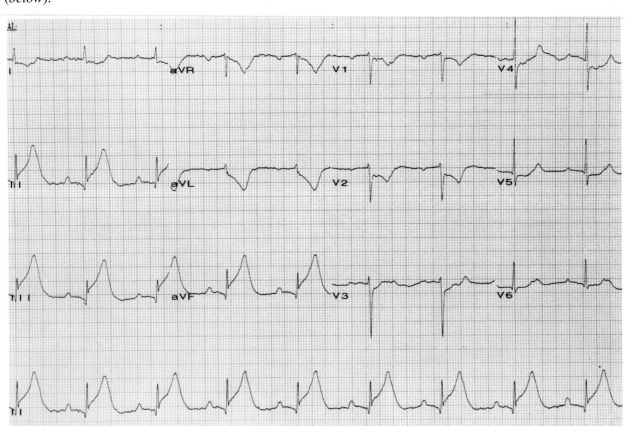

109. You treat the man with aspirin and intravenous metoprolol, and you decide to initiate thrombolysis with tissue plasminogen activator (tPA). Which of the following conditions is an absolute contraindication against giving tPA?

(A) Previous MI
(B) Diabetic retinopathy, with only hard exudates
(C) Peptic ulcer disease, with last upper gastrointestinal (GI) bleeding 1 year ago
(D) Laparoscopic cholecystectomy 1 week ago
(E) Age 65 years

110. The man initially does well with tPA, with resolution of the chest pain and evidence of reperfusion. However, Q waves develop in the inferior ECG leads. On hospital day 4, you are called to see him secondary to severe, acute onset of dyspnea. You arrive to find the patient sitting upright in moderate respiratory distress, with a respiratory rate of 30/minute and oxygen saturation of 92% on 100% face mask oxygen. You hear a new 3/6 holosystolic murmur radiating to the axilla. The diagnosis is

(A) pericarditis
(B) reinfarction
(C) free wall rupture
(D) papillary muscle rupture
(E) aspiration pneumonia

111. The best treatment for the man's current problem is

(A) antibiotics
(B) nonsteroidal anti-inflammatory drugs (NSAIDs)
(C) angiotensin-converting enzyme (ACE) inhibitors
(D) anticoagulation with heparin
(E) emergent surgery

112. It is useful to identify patients with acute MIs who are at high risk for poor outcomes. Numerous clinical trials have investigated this question, and several factors have been identified that put patients at high risk after an MI. These patients seem to benefit from a more invasive protocol utilizing cardiac catheterization rather than a noninvasive stress test. Which of the following features is NOT a high-risk characteristic?

(A) Congestive heart failure
(B) Ventricular tachycardia within the first 48 hours after MI
(C) Recurrent myocardial ischemia
(D) Diabetes mellitus
(E) Large infarction (more than four leads with ST-segment elevation)

Setting: Office

Questions 113–115

A 67-year-old man comes to the office because his wife is concerned about some recent changes in his appearance and behavior. During the past year, a resting tremor has developed, and he seems to move much more slowly. His medical history is significant for hypertension for which he takes verapamil. His family history is notable for colon cancer and breast cancer. On physical examination, significant findings include a masked facial appearance, a bilateral resting tremor of his hands, a flexed posture, and a shuffling gait.

113. Which of the following physical examination findings would you also expect to find?

(A) Decreased motor strength
(B) Hyperactive deep tendon reflexes
(C) Decreased peripheral sensation
(D) Hypersensitivity to touch
(E) Increased resistance to passive movement of the upper extremities

114. The man begins to take a combination of levodopa and carbidopa. The addition of carbidopa to the preparation

(A) provides another dopamine precursor
(B) reduces the side effects of levodopa
(C) inhibits peripheral dopa decarboxylase
(D) provides anticholinergic effects
(E) directly stimulates dopamine receptors

115. Common side effects of levodopa include all of the following EXCEPT

(A) postural hypotension
(B) nausea
(C) cardiac arrhythmias
(D) transient deterioration of symptoms prior to the next daily dose
(E) gastritis

Setting: Satellite Clinic

Questions 116–117

A 45-year-old man presents with severe diarrhea of 7 days' duration. He has five to six diarrheal stools per day with prominent nausea, occasional vomiting, diffuse abdominal pain, and the sensation of bloating. He has no medical history and takes no medications. He lives on a farm and works herding cattle. On physical examination, no signs of hypovolemia are apparent, and the abdominal examination is in normal limits. You decide to offer conservative treatment with continued hydration. However, 10 days later, the man returns with the same symptoms. You suspect a particular diagnosis and send stool samples for testing.

116. Which of the following agents should be used?

(A) Loperamide hydrochloride
(B) Metronidazole
(C) Ampicillin
(D) Amoxicillin
(E) No drug treatment

117. To prevent recurrence of this disease, you recommend

(A) boiling and filtering all water
(B) no special measures
(C) long-term therapy with antibiotics to treat persistent reservoirs of infection
(D) insect repellents
(E) weekly metronidazole

Setting: Office

Questions 118–119

A 28-year-old woman who is pregnant with her first child has been referred to you; on her first prenatal visit, her blood pressure was 140/85 mm Hg. Currently, she is at 18 weeks' gestation, and she has had no other problems during the pregnancy. She has no medical history; she has not seen a physician since she was 16 years of age. Her only medication is a multivitamin. She denies alcohol, tobacco, or drug abuse. Her family history is significant for hypertension in her mother and father. Except for a blood pressure of 137/86 mm Hg, physical examination is within normal limits. Urinalysis shows no proteinuria.

118. The most likely diagnosis is

(A) eclampsia
(B) pregnancy-induced hypertension
(C) essential hypertension
(D) glomerulonephritis
(E) cocaine abuse

119. On repeat examination 2 weeks later, the woman's blood pressure is 143/100 mm Hg. You decide to initiate antihypertensive therapy. Which of the following agents is contraindicated in pregnancy?

(A) Nifedipine
(B) Amlodipine
(C) Methyldopa
(D) Labetalol hydrochloride
(E) Enalapril

Setting: Office

Questions 120–122

A 20-year-old obese woman is 28 weeks into her first pregnancy. She had a blood pressure of 128/80 mm Hg at 10 weeks' gestation. Her blood pressure is now 150/98 mm Hg. Urinalysis shows 2+ protein, and a 24-hour urine shows 650 mg total urinary protein. Physical examination is notable only for trace peripheral edema, which the woman says is always present. She denies tobacco, alcohol or drug abuse.

120. The most likely diagnosis is

(A) eclampsia
(B) pregnancy-induced hypertension
(C) essential hypertension
(D) glomerulonephritis
(E) cocaine abuse

121. Appropriate treatment of this patient should include all of the following EXCEPT

(A) hospitalization and bed rest
(B) blood pressure control with antihypertensive agents
(C) serial fetal ultrasounds
(D) serial 24-hour urine protein measurements
(E) magnesium sulfate infusion

122. Which of the following statements about eclampsia is NOT true?

(A) Magnesium sulfate is the drug of choice for treating convulsions

(B) Eclampsia may occur in the immediate post-partum period

(C) The definitive cure for eclampsia is delivery of the infant

(D) In cases of respiratory depression secondary to magnesium sulfate infusion, calcium infusion is necessary

(E) It is important to give phenytoin with magnesium to prevent seizures

Setting: Office

123. A 6-year-old boy is brought into the office for evaluation of several skin lesions that have developed during the past few weeks. They are essentially asymptomatic and are mostly limited to the face. The child's mother has been treating them with topical hydrocortisone cream without effect. His medical history is benign, and the boy is well otherwise.

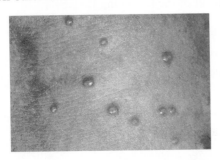

Treatment of these lesions should include

(A) intralesional corticosteroid injection

(B) high-dose topical corticosteroids

(C) topical clindamycin

(D) oral tetracycline

(E) no therapy

Setting: Hospital

Questions 124–126

A 23-year-old woman is admitted to the hospital with acute onset of left leg swelling and shortness of breath. A ventilation-perfusion scan ($\dot{V}/\dot{Q}$) is high-probability, and therapy with intravenous heparin begins. The patient's medical history is unremarkable. Her medications include multivitamins and oral contraceptive pills. Her family history is significant for a sister who had deep venous thrombosis 2 years ago. She also thinks that her grandmother may have had pulmonary embolus.

124. Which of the following conditions is the most likely cause of this woman's increased susceptibility to venous thrombosis?

(A) Protein C deficiency

(B) Protein S deficiency

(C) Antithrombin III deficiency

(D) Antiphospholipid antibody syndrome

(E) Factor V Leiden mutation

125. The anticoagulation regimen that should be given at discharge is

(A) warfarin titrated to an international normalized ratio (INR) of 3 to 4 for 3 to 6 months

(B) warfarin titrated to an INR of 2 to 3 for 3 to 6 months

(C) low-molecular-weight heparin

(D) no anticoagulation needed; stop the oral contraception

(E) warfarin titrated to an INR of 2 to 3 indefinitely

126. The woman follows your treatment recommendations. One month after discharge, however, she calls to tell you that she is pregnant. She asks what she should do about her anticoagulation. Your response is

(A) Continue the warfarin at the current dose.

(B) Stop the warfarin immediately because it is associated with a risk of congenital malformations. There is no need for continued anticoagulation.

(C) Stop the warfarin immediately because it is associated with a risk of congenital malformations. Initiation of subcutaneous heparin is necessary.

(D) Stop the warfarin immediately. An inferior vena cava filter is necessary.

(E) Continue the warfarin at the current dosage for now. It is likely that the warfarin dosage will need to be increased as the pregnancy progresses.

Setting: Emergency Department

Questions 127–128

A 34-year-old man with a history of cocaine abuse is brought to the ED after developing 10/10 substernal chest pain associated with diaphoresis and shortness of breath. On arrival at the scene, the rescue squad found signs that he had recently used cocaine. On physical examination, he is combative, and his blood pressure is 210/120 mm Hg with a pulse of 120/minute. His lungs are clear and cardiac examination is only notable for a loud S_4 heart sound. Intravenous access is obtained. An ECG shows an ST-segment elevation of 3 mm in leads V_2 to V_4. Initially, he receives treatment with aspirin, nitroglycerin, and lorazepam.

127. Which of the following therapies should be instituted next?

(A) Intravenous metoprolol

(B) Intravenous enalapril

(C) Emergent cardiac catheterization and percutaneous angioplasty

(D) Intravenous tissue plasminogen activator (tPA)

(E) Intravenous verapamil

128. You institute the appropriate treatment, and the man recovers. He wants to know if his cocaine use contributed to his myocardial infarction (MI). Cocaine has all of the following effects EXCEPT

(A) increased myocardial oxygen consumption

(B) enhanced platelet aggregation

(C) possible intense vasoconstriction

(D) possibly impaired fibrinolytic system activity

(E) increased afterload

Setting: Office

129. A 40-year-old woman presents for an initial visit with a chief complaint of fatigue of approximately 4 months' duration. She has no other problems. Physical examination is unrevealing. Which of the following tests is most likely to reveal the cause of her fatigue?

(A) Thyroid-stimulating hormone (TSH) level

(B) Multiscore Depression Inventory

(C) Epstein-Barr serology

(D) Complete blood count (CBC)

(E) Lyme titer

Setting: Office

Questions 130–133

The response options for the next four items are the same. You will be required to select one answer for each item in the set.

For each patient at risk for bacterial endocarditis, select the most appropriate antibiotic regimen.

(A) Amoxicillin 2 g orally 1 hour before the procedure

(B) Ampicillin 2 g either intravenously or intramuscularly 30 minutes before the procedure

(C) Clindamycin 600 mg orally 1 hour before the procedure

(D) Clindamycin 600 mg intravenously 30 minutes before the procedure

(E) No prophylaxis is necessary

130. A 67-year-old man who had successful, four-vessel, coronary artery bypass 4 months ago now requires oral surgery (root canal).

131. A 57-year-old woman who has had a dual-chamber pacemaker inserted for sick sinus syndrome is scheduled to undergo a colonoscopy next week.

132. A 32-year-old man with a history of intravenous drug abuse, cirrhosis, and bacterial endocarditis is admitted to the ICU with upper gastrointestinal (GI) bleed. He is to undergo upper endoscopy and likely sclerotherapy for bleeding esophageal varices.

133. A 26-year-old woman with mitral valve prolapse with mitral regurgitation is scheduled for a tonsillectomy. Two years ago she experienced hives and wheezing after receiving penicillin for streptococcal pharyngitis.

Setting: Hospital

Questions 134–135

The response options for the next two items are the same. You will be required to select one answer for each item in the set.

You are the intern on call in a busy obstetrical ward. At present, four women are in labor. During the night, you are called for several problems that occur during the labor of each of these women. For each patient, select the most likely cause of the prolonged labor.

(A) False labor

(B) Malposition

(C) Cephalopelvic disproportion

(D) Anesthesia

(E) Uteroplacental insufficiency

134. A 23-year-old primigravida is admitted after the onset of labor pain and rupture of the amniotic membranes. The pain is severe, and placement of an epidural catheter for anesthesia provides excellent pain relief. On initial examination, her cervix is dilated to 2.5 cm. Ten hours later, she remains at 2.5 cm; 20 hours later, she is at 3.5 cm.

135. A 32-year-old woman, who is G_3P_2, has been in labor for 6 hours. Her cervix is completely dilated. However, after 45 minutes of continued labor, there has been no progress. Uterine contractions are strong, and fetal monitoring shows no evidence of distress. She has not received any analgesia. An ultrasound performed 5 weeks ago was within normal limits. On questioning, you learn that the woman had similar problems with her second pregnancy; in that instance, a cesarean section was necessary.

Setting: Emergency Department

Questions 136–139

The response options for the next four items are the same. You will be required to select one answer for each item in the set.

For each patient who suffers from poisoning, select the most appropriate therapy.

(A) Alkalinization of urine and blood
(B) Hemodialysis
(C) *N*-Acetylcysteine
(D) Pralidoxime chloride
(E) Naloxone hydrochloride

136. A 26-year-old man who is found unconscious in his garage is brought to the ED, where initial blood gas reveals pH of 6.9, serum bicarbonate of 5 mmol/L, and anion gap of 40 mmol/L. Some crystals are apparent on analysis of the patient's urine.

137. An 18-year-old woman who is found stuporous and unresponsive at a local bus station is brought to the ED. Her respiratory rate is 4/minute. Physical examination is significant for a blood pressure of 70/40 mm Hg, constricted pupils, and needle marks on the left forearm.

138. A 6-year-old boy is brought to the ED by his parents, who note that he has become lethargic during the past 2 hours. They report two episodes of vomiting, a large amount of oral secretions, and tremors. On examination, you note the increase in oral secretions, as well as miosis, diffuse sweating, and muscle fasciculations.

139. A 75-year-old woman with chronic osteoarthritis is brought to the ED by her family, who report that she has become increasingly confused in the past 12 hours. She complains of "a funny sound" in her ears. On examination, she is confused, and vital signs are notable only for a respiratory rate of 30/minute. Arterial blood gas reveals a pH of 7.35, an HCO_3^- of 12 mmol/L, and a PCO_2 of 39 mm Hg.

Setting: Office

Questions 140–143

The response options for the next four items are the same. You will be required to select one answer for each item in the set.

For each patient with asthma, select the most appropriate therapy for asthma management in adults and children older than 5 years of age.

(A) Symptomatic use of albuterol by metered-dose inhaler

(B) Daily inhaled fluticasone and symptomatic use of albuterol by metered-dose inhaler

(C) Daily inhaled fluticasone, daily inhaled salmeterol, and symptomatic use of albuterol by metered-dose inhaler

(D) Daily inhaled fluticasone; oral prednisone; and daily inhaled salmeterol, with symptomatic use of albuterol by metered-dose inhaler

(E) No therapy is needed

140. A 21-year-old female college student complains of occasional, brief episodes of shortness of breath, wheezing, and cough. These episodes occur twice a month on average, never more than once a week. Office pulmonary function tests are within normal limits.

141. An 18-year-old woman with a history of severe eczema complains of continued wheezing, shortness of breath, and cough. Her symptoms are continuous in nature. During the past 2 weeks, she has visited the ED with these complaints 3 times. Last year, she was admitted to a hospital on four occasions with severe shortness of breath and wheezing. She has never been intubated. Office pulmonary function testing reveals a peak flow that is 40% of predicted.

142. A 25-year-old man is referred to you secondary to worsening complaints of wheezing and dyspnea. He says that he has symptoms every day despite using an albuterol inhaler 7 to 10 times a day. He reports that, perhaps once a week, the symptoms become so severe that he has to limit his activity. Office pulmonary function testing reveals a peak flow that is 65% of predicted.

143. A 30-year-old man complains of episodic wheezing and dyspnea, which occur 3 or 4 times per week. They rarely force him to limit his activity. Once a month, perhaps, he suffers from nighttime wheezing. Office pulmonary function testing reveals a peak flow that is 90% of predicted.

Setting: Office and Hospital

Questions 144–146

The response options for the next three items are the same. You will be required to select one answer for each item in the set.

For each patient with a possible thyroid condition, select the likely results of a thyroid profile, which includes triiodothyronine (T_3), T_3 resin uptake (T_3RU), thyroxine (T_4), and thyroid-stimulating hormone (TSH).

	Total T_4	T_3RU	Free T_4	TSH
(A)	Decreased	Decreased	Decreased	Increased
(B)	Increased	Increased	Increased	Decreased
(C)	Normal	Normal	Normal	Decreased
(D)	Decreased	Increased	Normal	Normal
(E)	Normal	Normal	Normal	Normal

144. A 45-year-old woman presents with sweating, palpitations, and weight loss. Physical examination is notable for a diffuse goiter and mild exophthalmos.

145. A 60-year-old patient has been admitted to the ICU for sepsis, pneumonia, and respiratory failure.

146. A 30-year-old woman begins lithium therapy. She experiences lethargy and fatigue.

Setting: Office

Questions 147–150

The response options for the next four items are the same. You will be required to select one answer for each item in the set.

For each patient with viral hepatitis, choose the serologic profile that best fits the clinical history.

	HBsAg	Anti-HBs	IgM Anti-HBc	Total Anti-HBc	HBeAg	Anti-HCV
(A)	+	−	−	+	+	+
(B)	−	+	−	−	−	−
(C)	−	+	−	−	−	+
(D)	+	−	−	+	−	−
(E)	−	−	−	−	−	−

Anti-HBs = antihepatitis B surface antigen antibody; anti-HCV = antibodies to the hepatitis C virus; HBeAg = hepatitis B e antigen; HBsAg = hepatitis B surface antigen; IgM and total anti-HBc = antibodies to the hepatitis B core antigen.

147. A previously healthy 30-year-old woman, who is a nun, goes to Thailand on a mission. She eats raw shellfish. Within 10 days, she experiences the acute onset of jaundice, malaise, and fatigue.

148. A 32-year-old surgical resident experiences a needlestick in the operating room. He is previously healthy and has received the hepatitis B vaccine. Recent liver function tests were within normal limits. Postexposure blood is sent for hepatitis serologies.

149. A 59-year-old salesman, who admits to experimenting with intravenous drugs in the 1960s, is referred to you after routine laboratory work shows an elevated aspartate aminotransferase (AST) and alanine aminotransferase (ALT). He has received the hepatitis B vaccine.

150. A 49-year-old man with chronically elevated liver function tests has chronic hepatitis B infection. It is believed that he acquired the infection as a result of intravenous drug abuse. He is interested in beginning therapy with interferon.

ANSWER KEY

1-E	31-B	61-E	91-D	121-E
2-B	32-A	62-C	92-B	122-E
3-D	33-C	63-E	93-B	123-E
4-B	34-B	64-C	94-A	124-E
5-C	35-A	65-B	95-C	125-B
6-B	36-E	66-A	96-D	126-C
7-A	37-B	67-B	97-A	127-C
8-E	38-C	68-C	98-E	128-D
9-B	39-C	69-C	99-C	129-B
10-C	40-B	70-A	100-B	130-E
11-A	41-D	71-E	101-C	131-E
12-B	42-A	72-B	102-B	132-B
13-C	43-C	73-A	103-A	133-D
14-E	44-E	74-E	104-C	134-D
15-A	45-C	75-D	105-D	135-C
16-D	46-E	76-D	106-D	136-B
17-B	47-C	77-D	107-B	137-E
18-A	48-D	78-E	108-E	138-D
19-D	49-D	79-C	109-D	139-A
20-B	50-A	80-C	110-D	140-A
21-C	51-C	81-D	111-E	141-D
22-E	52-E	82-B	112-B	142-C
23-D	53-A	83-C	113-E	143-B
24-A	54-B	84-C	114-C	144-B
25-C	55-B	85-D	115-E	145-D
26-A	56-D	86-B	116-B	146-A
27-B	57-C	87-D	117-A	147-E
28-D	58-A	88-B	118-C	148-B
29-C	59-E	89-E	119-E	149-C
30-E	60-B	90-C	120-B	150-D

ANSWERS AND EXPLANATIONS

1–3. The answers are: 1-E, 2-B, 3-D. (*Emergency medicine, internal medicine*)
This patient arrives at the emergency department (ED) with hypoglycemia. The clue is her response to a 1-mg injection of glucagon, which raises cAMP levels and increases glycogenolysis to elevate plasma glucose levels. Hypoglycemia is associated with many different diseases. The differential diagnosis includes **re**nal failure, **ex**ogenous insulin, **p**ituitary insufficiency, **l**iver failure, **a**drenal insufficiency, **i**nsulinoma, and **n**eoplasm (REEXPLAIN). Other causes include trimethoprim-sulfamethoxazole, pentamidine, and quinine sulfate. Primary aldosteronism is not classically associated with hypoglycemia.

Some individuals do not respond to glucagon because their glycogen stores are depleted (e.g., malnutrition). Patients who respond to glucagon have hypoglycemia that is mediated by insulin or an insulin-like factor. This young woman may have insulinoma, a rare condition, or she could be taking exogenous insulin. Her position as a health care worker should raise the suspicion for factitious exogenous insulin administration; somatoform disorders are more common in the health care profession. A C-peptide would distinguish between these two disorders; it would be low with exogenous insulin administration and high with an insulinoma. A thyroid-stimulating hormone (TSH) test is not as helpful because hypothyroidism is not associated with hypoglycemia, unless panhypopituitarism is present. A cortisol value and liver function tests are less helpful in the absence of other findings that suggest adrenal insufficiency or liver failure.

4–5. The answers are: 4-B, 5-C. (*Obstetrics/gynecology, surgery*)
In women of reproductive age, the normal ovary is palpable about 50% of the time. Important features on pelvic examination include ovarian size, shape, consistency, and mobility. In patients who take oral contraceptives, the ovaries are palpable with less frequency. This patient has an adnexal mass that could be an ovary. However, she is sexually active, and her menses are 1 week late. In addition, her mittelschmerz occurred 3 weeks ago, and she probably ovulated at that time. Although it would be early to palpate a tubal pregnancy, a β-human chorionic gonadotropin (β-hCG) is the most important first test. If it is negative, an ultrasound is warranted to evaluate the abnormality further. If the woman is pregnant, she is approximately 3 weeks from conception, and, therefore, a urine β-hCG would be adequate. (Recall that urinary pregnancy tests that detect β-hCG at levels of 50 mIU/mL can identify β-hCG as early as 14 days after conception. Serum β-hCG tests are even more sensitive.) If the serum β-hCG level is less that 5,000 mIU/mL, a transvaginal ultrasound is necessary to evaluate for intrauterine gestation.

Because this patient has not had sexual intercourse in more than 8 weeks, it less likely that she has an ectopic pregnancy. However, a negative β-hCG is important to corroborate this information. The most likely cause of the adnexal enlargement is a functional ovarian cyst. When an ovarian follicle fails to rupture completely during follicular maturation, ovulation does not occur, and a follicular cyst develops. Occasionally, this cyst can be painful and always results in a prolonged follicular phase with secondary amenorrhea. The estrogen-rich environment with the lack of ovulation overstimulates the endometrium, causing irregular bleeding. Unilateral tenderness with a palpable, mobile, cystic, adnexal mass is evident on pelvic examination. In most cases, the cyst resolves in 6 to 8 weeks. In this setting, a clinician might choose to follow-up with the patient for 6 to 8 weeks and repeat a pelvic examination. An alternative is to confirm diagnosis of a follicular cyst with ultrasound. If the cyst persists for more than 6 to 8 weeks, the physician should consider another diagnosis. (The occurrence of ovulation based on the patient's monthly mittelschmerz might not support this diagnosis.)

A corpus luteal cyst, the other common type of functional ovarian cyst, develops after ovulation when the corpus luteum produces progesterone for longer than the usual 14 days. The corpus luteum enlarges, menstruation is delayed, and associated dull, lower quadrant pain is present. Pelvic examination usually discloses an enlarged, tender, cystic, or solid adnexal mass. The triad of missed menstrual period, lower quadrant pain, and adnexal enlargement is seen with a corpus luteal cyst. However, these features also are seen in ectopic pregnancy. Therefore, it is necessary to rule out pregnancy before considering a corpus luteal cyst.

The most common benign germ cell tumor is the benign cystic teratoma. Patients are generally asymptomatic. Treatment is surgical. Malignancy is rare ($<1\%$).

A serous ovarian neoplasm (adenocarcinoma) may be benign or malignant. Although it is more common in a perimenopausal or postmenopausal woman, it can occur at any time. A neoplasm is larger than a functional ovarian cyst. Statistically, its occurrence is less likely.

Choriocarcinoma, a rare malignancy of gestational trophoblastic tissue, is associated with elevated hCG levels. This tumor has a propensity to bleed and to metastasize to the brain. It is highly sensitive to chemotherapy.

6–11. The answers are: 6-B, 7-A, 8-E, 9-B, 10-C, 11-A. (*Psychiatry, emergency medicine, internal medicine*)

This patient, who demonstrates rigidity and changes in mental status after taking an increased dose of a neuroleptic medication, has neuroleptic malignant syndrome. Definitions of this condition vary, but most experts consider fever a criterion of this disease. In 1985, a consensus panel proposed that the most commonly used diagnostic criteria be considered "major" (i.e., fever, rigidity, elevated creatine kinase) and "minor" (i.e., tachycardia, abnormal blood pressure, tachypnea, altered consciousness, diaphoresis, leukocytosis). Parkinsonism and hyperpyrexia are the cornerstone of the diagnosis. The primary cause of the disease is the administration of dopamine receptor antagonists or the withdrawal of dopamine agonists. The other answer choices listed in question 7 are other neurotransmitters that may play a role in various psychiatric disorders. For example, serotonin and norepinephrine are involved in the pathogenesis of depression. However, only dopamine is implicated in the pathogenesis of neuroleptic malignant syndrome.

Characteristic laboratory findings include elevated creatine kinase in approximately 40% to 50% of cases, which likely relates to the hyperpyrexia with extreme muscle rigidity. This may be a sign of rhabdomyolysis, a potential complication. Other typical features include leukocytosis, hypophosphatemia, elevated liver transaminases, and proteinuria. Hyperphosphatemia, hyperkalemia, and hypocalcemia may occur in the setting of rhabdomyolysis.

Treatment consists of intravenous hydration and cessation of the offending drugs. Sodium dantrolene, which stabilizes the sarcoplasmic reticulum and decreases rigidity, is useful, and bromocriptine mesylate, a centrally acting dopamine agonist, may also be effective. Electroconvulsive therapy has been successful in some cases. The dopamine antagonists would not be helpful.

After 24 hours, the patient is still rigid and has laboratory findings consistent with rhabdomyolysis. Hemolysis can cause similar results, but it is not as common in this setting. Hypoparathyroidism is uncommon and does not explain the hyperphosphatemia and hyperkalemia. Renal failure may occur, it is secondary to rhabdomyolysis.

The treatment for rhabdomyolysis is aggressive hydration to maintain the urine output above 200 mL/hour, if possible. Phosphate binders are not warranted unless the calcium-phosphorus product exceeds 70, the level at which calciphylaxis can occur. Calcium infusion should be avoided because the patient's calcium levels return to normal spontaneously as calcium phosphate breaks down; infusions of calcium may result in hypercalcemia. The use of bicarbonate, which may worsen the hypocalcemia of rhabdomyolysis, is controversial.

12–15. The answers are: 12-B, 13-C, 14-E, 15-A. (*Surgery, internal medicine*)

Adrenal incidentalomas are detected on 1% to 2% of all abdominal computed tomography (CT) scans. Benign adenomas account for 50% of these lesions. Pheochromocytomas, metastases, or primary cancers are other possibilities. A physician must answer two questions about these masses: (1) Are they malignant? and (2) Are they secretory?

All patients warrant evaluation for pheochromocytoma by a 24-hour urine test for metanephrines and catecholamines. If the history and physical examination suggest that other conditions may be present, the following screening tests are necessary: urine-free cortisol for Cushing syndrome, dehydroepiandrosterone sulfate

(DHEAS) for excess androgen production, and plasma renin activity or aldosterone for primary hyperaldosteronism.

A 24-hour urine-free cortisol is the most sensitive screening test for suspected Cushing syndrome. Because random cortisol measurements vacillate and exhibit diurnal variation, they are not useful in the diagnosis of Cushing syndrome. A overnight 1-mg dexamethasone suppression test is less sensitive. A high-dose dexamethasone suppression test, which is used after the initial screening test is positive, can help distinguish between a pituitary adenoma and other causes of Cushing syndrome.

Primary aldosteronism (Conn syndrome) is characterized by hypertension, hypokalemia, alkalosis, a high aldosterone level, and low plasma renin activity. These conditions are secondary to the effect of aldosterone on the collecting duct.

In this case, all of the patient's tests are in normal limits or negative. The next diagnostic consideration is the size of the lesion. Tumors greater than 4 cm in diameter should be more worrisome; adrenal carcinomas typically exceed 5 cm. Some clinicians recommend resection for any lesion greater than 4 cm. The next consideration is the amount of attenuation on CT. A mass with a high Hounsfield unit value (>20) is of concern for malignancy. In the setting of a 4-cm mass with greater than 20 Hounsfield units of attenuation, a biopsy or resection is recommended. A MRI scan will not affect the decision to proceed with a biopsy. A repeat CT scan in 3 months is too risky; this management step would be reasonable if the lesion were smaller.

16–20. The answers are: 16-D, 17-B, 18-A, 19-D, 20-B. (*Internal medicine, surgery*)
This patient appears to have recurrent kidney stones. This condition has many possible causes, including low urinary volumes (26%), hypercalciuria (14%), hypocitraturia (9%), hyperuricosuria (8%,) hyperoxaluria (8%), and hypomagnesemia (5%). Calcium phosphate and calcium oxalate stones are radiodense; struvite (triple phosphate) stones are usually radiodense; cystine stones are poorly visualized; and uric acid stones are completely radiolucent. This stone is evident on a plain radiograph, so a uric acid stone is least likely.

On learning about the family history of kidney stones and a prolactinoma, the clinician must consider a potential genetic syndrome that involves these two diseases. This condition affects two generations and afflicts both men and women; thus, it is likely to have an autosomal dominant inheritance pattern. Multiple endocrine neoplasia (MEN) satisfies these criteria. MEN type 1 (MEN1) includes parathyroid hyperplasia (causing hypercalciuria and stones) and anterior pituitary tumors (e.g., prolactinomas), as well as pancreatic islet cell tumors (e.g., gastrinomas, vasoactive intestinal polypeptide-secreting tumors, insulinomas), carcinoid tumors, and lipomas, but not pheochromocytomas, which occur in MEN2A and MEN2B. An autosomal dominant disorder, MEN1 has variable penetrance. The gene, referred to as the *MENIN* gene, has been mapped to the long arm of chromosome 11. The *RET* proto-oncogene is associated with MEN2A and MEN2B, which may involve medullary thyroid carcinoma and pheochromocytoma.

Primary hyperparathyroidism is the most common disorder in MEN1, so a calcium level is the laboratory test most likely to aid in making a diagnosis. A calcitonin value might be useful if MEN2 were the suspected diagnosis.

21–24. The answers are: 21-C, 22-E, 23-D, 24-A. (*Emergency medicine, surgery*)
The spleen is the organ most commonly injured as the result of blunt abdominal trauma. Signs of peritoneal irritation and splenic hemorrhage include left upper quadrant tenderness, referred pain at the left shoulder (Kehr sign), and dullness of the left flank to percussion (Ballance sign). It must be understood that isolated splenic injuries are rare; concomitant orthopedic or neurologic injuries are more common. Splenic rupture occurs in 30% of cases. However, the history and physical examination suggest a splenic injury, and the patient appears not to have suffered any neurologic injury. Evaluative options include abdominal CT, abdominal ultrasound, and diagnostic peritoneal lavage. In this case, lavage is not indicated because the patient appears stable. An abdominal CT scan is the option of choice because it provides information about organs other than the spleen.

At a later time, when the patient becomes hypotensive, splenic rupture is the major concern. Adrenal insufficiency should always be considered because it is treatable and because adrenal hemorrhage can occur in this setting. Aortic dissection should always be considered in deceleration injuries. A tear occurs where the aortic arch is tethered by the ligamentum arteriosum. A bowel perforation would lead to peritoneal signs. A liver laceration would result in right upper quadrant pain.

Splenectomy, the treatment of choice for this patient, is associated with numerous abnormalities on peripheral blood smear. The spleen acts as a filter of the blood and removes aged erythrocytes, damaged erythrocytes, nuclear remnants within erythrocytes (Howell-Jolly bodies), denatured hemoglobin within erythrocytes (Heinz bodies), and iron inclusions within erythrocytes (Pappenheimer bodies). Target cells are associated with thalassemia, liver disease, and any disease in which the surface-to-volume ratio of the erythrocyte is increased.

Because postsplenectomy sepsis is such a concern, many centers are developing strategies to preserve the spleen whenever possible. Encapsulated organisms cause the overwhelming infections. *Streptococcus pneumoniae* is the most common agent, followed by *Haemophilus influenzae, Neisseria meningitidis,* β-hemolytic streptococcus, *Escherichia coli,* and *Pseudomonas* species.

25–28. The answers are: 25-C, 26-A, 27-B, 28-D. (*Internal medicine*)

This patient has signs and symptoms of urinary tract infection. It is possible to make the diagnosis by examining unspun urine under the microscope. The presence of one or more pathogens correlates with a quantitative culture of 10^5 CFU/mm, which is sufficient for the diagnosis of a urinary tract infection. Pyuria, which is defined as more than 10 leukocytes/high-power field (HPF) in a centrifuged specimen, is also suggestive. The leukocyte esterase test on dipsticks correlates with greater than 10 leukocytes/HPF. Mild proteinuria is commonly seen in a urinary tract infection. Hyaline casts do not signify disorder because they consist of Tamm-Horsfall protein aggregates. They are most commonly in the setting of dehydration with prerenal azotemia but can be seen in this setting as well. The patient should not have white blood cell (WBC) casts in his urine. Nausea, vomiting, abdominal pain, fever, and flank pain are not present, which tends to rule out pyelonephritis.

After the patient receives an antibiotic, he returns with jaundice and weakness. The likely cause in this setting would be hemolysis secondary to glucose-6-phosphate dehydrogenase deficiency, which is the most common enzyme defect associated with hereditary hemolytic anemia. Because this defect is X-linked, it occurs phenotypically primarily in men. The most common abnormal variant, present in 10% of African Americans, is referred to as the A⁻ variant; it is associated with an isoenzyme that deteriorates rapidly (half-life, 13 days). The Mediterranean variant, found in individuals of Greek and Italian descent, is associated with almost complete absence of enzyme activity (half-life, only hours).

This enzyme is the first enzyme of the hexose monophosphate pathway, which produces (reduced) nicotinamide adenine dinucleotide phosphate (NADPH), which in turn provides glutathione reductase with hydrogen ions to generate reduced glutathione. This glutathione can respond to oxidizing agents and protect erythrocytes from destruction. In the absence of glucose-6-phosphate dehydrogenase, there is less NADPH and, thus, less reduced glutathione to handle an oxidizing agent, such as sulfonamides, salicylates, phenacetin, or an oxidizing event, such as infection.

Heme and globin moieties dissociate, and globin precipitates as Heinz bodies, which are removed by the spleen. Target cells are associated with thalassemia, liver disease, and any disease in which the surface-to-volume ratio of the erythrocyte is increased. Nuclear remnants within erythrocytes (Howell-Jolly bodies) and iron inclusions within erythrocytes (Pappenheimer bodies) are other erythrocyte abnormalities.

29–31. The answers are: 29-C, 30-E, 31-B. (*Surgery, internal medicine*)

With the increasing use of abdominal imaging, clinicians discover incidental liver abnormalities with greater frequency. Benign liver cysts and tumors are common; therefore, it is important to determine which lesions require further workup. Cavernous hemangiomas, which occur in 8% of patients, are the most common benign liver tumor. These tumors may enlarge over time; if greater than 4 cm in size, they are termed "giant" hemangiomas. In some cases, the tumors are hormone-responsive and, occasionally, undergo spontaneous thrombosis and lead to pain and elevated liver transaminases. However, most of these tumors are asymptomatic, and spontaneous rupture is rare. As in this case, contrasted CT usually shows a progressive peripheral-to-central prominent enhancement and a central hypodense region. Serial CT scans can be used to monitor patients. Surgical removal is recommended if they are associated with pain.

Hepatic adenomas are benign tumors that occur in women 30 to 50 years of age, most of whom have a history of estrogen use. These solitary, unencapsulated masses appear as sheets of hepatocytes without triads histologically. Because these tumors may grow and rupture in as many as 30% of cases, a surgical approach is recommended. Occasionally, larger lesions (>5 cm) may develop into hepatocellular carcinoma.

Focal nodular hyperplasia involves well-circumscribed benign lesions with a central fibrous scar and nodular hyperplasia. These lesions have no premalignant potential and rarely grow or rupture. Histologically, they have bile ducts throughout. Unfortunately, diagnosis without pathologic specimens is difficult, and, therefore, the masses are removed if the patient is a good surgical candidate.

Hepatocellular carcinoma is rare without underlying liver disease and hepatitis B or C. In the appropriate setting, it is important to consider metastasis.

Cholangiocarcinoma generally leads to jaundice because the bile ducts are obstructed. Outside of the United States, this condition is most commonly associated with a liver fluke (*Clonorchis sinensis*).

32–37. The answers are: 32-A, 33-C, 34-B, 35-A, 36-E, 37-B. (*Surgery*)

Appendicitis is the most common cause of an acute surgical abdomen, occurring in 4% to 6% of the population. Most patients are between the ages of 5 and 35 years, and they present within 1 to 2 days of the onset of pain. The appendix is 6 to 10 cm long. Usually located in the right lower quadrant at the apex of the cecum, it may lie inferior, medial, lateral, or retrocecal to the cecum. The location of the pain is a diagnostic clue.

The initial pain is periumbilical in nature—a nonspecific, referred "visceral" pain. Any organ of the midgut, from D2 of the duodenum to the splenic flexure, can refer pain to the periumbilical region when it is distended. As the peritoneum becomes involved, the pain then is located at the area of inflammation ("peritoneal pain"). In appendicitis, this pain is usually in the right lower quadrant. The McBurney point, which is located between the middle and outer third of a line drawn between the anterior superior iliac spine and the umbilicus, is often the site of this rebound tenderness. The obturator sign is elicited by passively rotating the flexed right thigh with the patient in the supine position. A positive obturator sign indicates local inflammation of the adjacent obturator internus muscle. The psoas sign, which is elicited on extension of the right hip, indicates inflammation of the psoas muscle by the adjacent appendix. The Rovsing sign is the sensation of right lower quadrant pain when palpating over the left lower quadrant. Inflammation of the iliopsoas muscle occurs more commonly with a retrocecal appendix. The Murphy sign, which is pain over the right upper quadrant with inspiration, is seen in cholecystitis, not with appendicitis.

Appendicitis is characterized by rebound tenderness to palpation. In addition, it is usually associated with fever, nausea and, occasionally, vomiting. Leukocytosis is usually present, which means that a complete blood count (CBC) is the most useful diagnostic laboratory test. No imaging study is part of the standard of care of appendicitis; history and physical examination are the basis of diagnosis. Occasionally, a plain film of the abdomen reveals a calcified fecalith. A CT scan may detect appendiceal inflammation, but it may miss the diagnosis. Similarly, ultrasound may be misleading.

Obstruction of the appendiceal lumen leads to inflammation of the organ. The columnar epithelium of the appendix contains several lymph follicles, which decrease after 20 years of age. Obstruction of the appendiceal lumen often occurs secondary to lymphoid hyperplasia caused by a viral or bacterial illness. This obstruction causes increased pressure, which reduces the blood supply to the appendix. Occasionally, the obstruction can be secondary to a foreign body or a fecalith. The superior mesenteric artery, which essentially supplies the midgut, supplies the ileocolic artery, which then feeds the appendicular artery in the mesoappendix.

38–41. The answers are: 38-C, 39-C, 40-B, 41-D. (*Internal medicine*)
In this case, the prothrombin time (PT) is normal and the partial thromboplastin time (PTT) is prolonged. The PT measures the integrity of the extrinsic and common pathways of the clotting cascade (factors II, VII, V, X, and fibrinogen), and the PTT measures the integrity of the intrinsic and common pathways of the clotting cascade (factors XII, XI, IX, VIII, X, V, II, fibrinogen, and high-molecular-weight kininogen). This patient probably has a factor deficiency or a factor inhibitor, and the first step is to repeat the PTT before embarking on a potentially expensive workup. A mixing study, which mixes equal parts of the patient's plasma and "normal" plasma, is the test of choice for distinguishing between these two conditions. If the PTT corrects itself, a factor deficiency is likely. If the PTT does not correct itself, a factor inhibitor, most commonly a factor VIII inhibitor or a lupus anticoagulant, is probable.

The bleeding time, a test of platelet–vessel wall interaction and function, measures the time to cessation of bleeding after a standard incision over the ventral aspect of the forearm. The bleeding time is prolonged in thrombocytopenia, qualitative platelet abnormalities, von Willebrand disease, and primary vascular disorders, not in factor deficiencies. The thrombin time, the time it takes for plasma to clot when adding thrombin, is prolonged in afibrinogenemia, dysfibrinogenemia, disseminated intravascular coagulation (DIC), and in the presence of heparin. Russell's viper venom is used to look for a lupus anticoagulant.

After the patient's elective total hip replacement, prophylaxis for deep venous thrombosis (DVT) is necessary because the frequency of DVT occurrence in unprotected patients is 70%. Of note, the risk of DVT complicating a total knee arthroplasty is even higher, approaching 85% in some studies. The approximate incidence of DVT is:

Elective knee arthroplasty	80%
Elective hip arthroplasty	70%
Hip fracture	60%
Meniscectomy	20%
Pelvic fracture	20%

In 1995, the Prevention of Thromboembolism Task Force of the American College of Chest Physicians reported that low-molecular-weight heparin is more effective in preventing DVT after total knee arthroplasty than warfarin, aspirin, or heparin. This is a controversial subject, but low-molecular-weight heparin is likely more effective than low-dose warfarin as prophylaxis for DVT after total knee and hip arthroplasties. Hirudin, a direct thrombin inhibitor, is approved for the treatment of DVT and pulmonary embolism in patients with a history of heparin-induced thrombocytopenia.

42–48. The answers are: 42-A, 43-C, 44-E, 45-C, 46-E, 47-C, 48-D. (*Internal medicine*)
This patient has signs and symptoms consistent with community-acquired pneumonia. The decision of hospital admission is difficult, and it is important to gather supportive data, if possible. A tool designed to assist physicians in making admission decisions is now part of the recent guidelines of the Infectious Disease Society of America for the care of patients with community-acquired pneumonia. Patients receive points for age and comorbid conditions. Neoplastic disease receives the highest, with 30 points; liver disease, 20 points; and most other diseases (e.g., renal disease, congestive heart failure, cerebrovascular disease), 10 points. The scores help predict patients' 30-day mortality. It may be more harmful to admit low-risk patients to the hospital.

Streptococcus pneumoniae is the most common bacterial cause of community-acquired pneumonia. *Haemophilus influenzae, Moraxella catarrhalis,* and *Legionella* are more likely to colonize those who smoke.

Routine laboratory studies determine that the patient has hypokalemia. Medications are an important cause of hypokalemia. Hydrocortisone, which has some mineralocorticoid activity, may cause hypokalemia by increasing the excretion of potassium at the distal segments of the kidney. The other agents listed in question 44 cause hyperkalemia, not hypokalemia. Captopril decreases aldosterone and its effect on both the distal convoluted tubule and the collecting duct. Propranolol and all β-blockers affect transcellular transport of potassium and alter renin release at the juxtaglomerular apparatus. Both dapsone and trimethoprim affect sodium reabsorption in the distal segments of the kidney, altering the ability to excrete potassium.

In the setting of hypokalemia, an ECG reflects the repolarization abnormalities. Sagging of the ST segment, T-wave depression, and U-wave elevation are evident. In the setting of hyperkalemia, flat P waves, lengthened PR intervals, a wide QRS, and peaked T waves are apparent.

Metabolic alkalosis is commonly associated with hypokalemia. Causes may be either saline-responsive or saline-resistant. The saline-responsive causes are primarily characterized by vomiting and dehydration. The saline-resistant causes are associated with conditions of mineralocorticoid excess, such as Cushing syndrome and hyperaldosteronism. To help distinguish between these two types of metabolic alkalosis, a urine chloride is most useful. A low urine chloride suggests a volume-depleted state, or contraction alkalosis, as in this patient. The high urine chloride suggests mineralocorticoid excess. Licorice excess causes an increase in mineralocorticoids as well.

M. catarrhalis is a gram-negative diplococcus that grew later in this patient's culture. *Klebsiella pneumoniae* and *Haemophilus influenzae,* which are also gram-negative organisms, are not diplococci; instead, they are rods. *S. pneumoniae* is gram-positive. *Neisseria meningitidis* does not cause pneumonia.

49–54. The answers are: 49-D, 50-A, 51-C, 52-E, 53-A, 54-B. (*Internal medicine*)

This patient has acute diarrhea. She has had a significant fever for several days, and she also has abdominal pain. Her history makes an invasive pathogen a concern. Because her vital signs are within normal limits, the next important step is to look for fecal leukocytes to distinguish between invasive and noninvasive pathogens. Liver function studies would be particularly important if jaundice were present or if viral hepatitis were suspected. Although ova and parasite tests are rarely useful, they warrant checking if there is a history of recent travel. Chemistries would be important if dehydration were present. With weakness, hypokalemia with a non–anion gap acidosis is possible; the cause of this finding is the loss of potassium and bicarbonate in the secretory diarrhea.

The primary differential diagnosis of diarrhea involves viral, bacterial, or parasitic agents. Among the bacterial causes of acute diarrhea are toxin-related foodborne illness (*Clostridium perfringens, Staphylococcus aureus*) and foodborne invasive bacteria (*Campylobacter, Shigella, Salmonella, Yersinia*). *C. perfringens* and *S. aureus,* which cause diarrhea within 6 to 12 hours after ingestion, are not associated with fecal leukocytes. *Yersinia enterocolitica* can mimic appendicitis, causing a mesenteric lymphadenitis. In the setting of recent antibiotics or surgery, it is important to check for *C. difficile* toxin. In travelers, it is necessary to consider *Entamoeba histolytica, Giardia lamblia,* and *Cryptosporidium. Giardia,* associated with well water, can cause chronic diarrhea. *Cryptosporidium,* a weakly acid-fast organism, may cause diarrhea in HIV and other immunocompromised states. The invasive pathogens are associated with fever, abdominal pain, bloody stools, and fecal leukocytes. In viral gastroenteritis, the presenting features are nausea, vomiting, headache, diarrhea, and low-grade fever. Rarely does the stool contain leukocytes.

A stool osmolality is calculated ($2 \times$ [$Na^+ + K^+$]) and compared with the measured osmolality. If the difference between them, the osmotic gap, is greater than 50 mOsm/kg, it suggests the presence of osmotically active substances in the stool as the cause of the diarrhea. Celiac sprue is a cause of osmotic diarrhea; the small intestine is unable to absorb nutrients secondary to an immune destruction of the villi. Carcinoid tumors, Zollinger-Ellison syndrome, vasoactive intestinal polypeptide-secreting tumors, and mastocytosis are all associated with a secretory diarrhea and, therefore, a normal osmotic gap.

Salmonella typhi causes typhoid fever, which may be foodborne or waterborne. It is associated with a "pea soup" diarrhea that develops in the third week of illness. Fever, a relative bradycardia, a "rose spots" rash on the trunk, splenomegaly, cough, and headache are also evident.

55–59. The answers are: 55-B, 56-D, 57-C, 58-A, 59-E. (*Pediatrics, statistics*)
This patient appears to have pharyngitis. The extensive differential diagnoses of this condition includes group A β-hemolytic streptococci (*Streptococcus pyogenes*), other streptococci, *Chlamydia trachomatis*, Epstein-Barr virus (mononucleosis), adenovirus, mycoplasma, and influenza. It is important but difficult to distinguish between group A streptococcus pharyngitis and other causes. Certain features are predictors of group A streptococcus pharyngitis, including fever, cervical lymphadenopathy, exudative tonsillitis, and lack of cough or rhinorrhea. This patient requires treatment with penicillin V, the treatment of choice for group A streptococcus. No penicillin-resistant group A streptococcus is yet known.

However, a patient with Epstein-Barr virus–related mononucleosis or adenovirus could present in the same manner. In fact, this patient returned with the fine maculopapular rash suggestive of ampicillin treatment of a patient with mononucleosis. Up to 70% of mononucleosis patients treated with ampicillin develop this rash. Patients with mononucleosis commonly present with a persistent or recurrent sore throat, posterior (or anterior) cervical lymphadenopathy, malaise, fever, tonsillar exudate and, occasionally, splenomegaly. A complete blood count (CBC), which shows lymphocytosis with atypical lymphs, or a Monospot test is used to make the diagnosis. Note that the Monospot test can be negative early in infection and that it can remain positive for many months to a year. Of note, atypical lymphocytes are also seen in cytomegalovirus, acute viral hepatitis, toxoplasmosis, syphilis, leukemia, or lymphoma.

When evaluating the performance characteristics of the new swab, it is important to recall that sensitivity is a measure of the likelihood of a positive test in a patient with disease. Clinically, the likelihood of disease in a patient with a positive test is interesting to physicians. This is the positive predictive value and is dependent on the prevalence of disease in the patient population under study. This information is missing, which means that the positive predictive value cannot be determined.

60–62. The answers are: 60-B, 61-E, 62-C. (*Internal medicine*)
This patient is approaching the time consistent with a fever of unknown origin (defined variably as 2 to 4 weeks). He is febrile and had a sore throat weeks ago. Low-grade fever is present, with atypical lymphocytes, but no lymphadenopathy and splenomegaly. These findings are consistent with cytomegalovirus. Although symptomatic cytomegalovirus is rare in immunocompetent hosts, an infectious mononucleosis–like syndrome may be evident. Cytomegalovirus causes approximately 8% of cases of infectious mononucleosis; these viral infections are indistinguishable from Epstein-Barr virus infections except that the cytomegalovirus-caused disorders are Monospot-negative. In addition, affected patients often present with less severe pharyngitis, no lymphadenopathy, and no splenomegaly, as in this case. Reiter syndrome is characterized by the triad of arthritis, urethritis, and conjunctivitis; this "classic" triad is seen in one third of patients. The incidence of this condition peaks during the third decade. Post–sexually transmitted disease syndrome is more common in men, but postdysentery syndrome affects both sexes equally. Sacroiliitis, enthesitis, keratoderma blennorrhagicum, and other extra-articular manifestations may also occur.

The appearance of atypical lymphocytes is nonspecific. This finding is seen in association with Epstein-Barr virus infection, cytomegalovirus infection, viral hepatitis, toxoplasmosis, syphilis, rubella, drug reactions, leukemia, and lymphoma.

The Monospot test for Epstein-Barr virus is positive in only 40% to 50% of acute infections; however, during the third week of illness, it is positive in more than 80% of cases. The immunoglobulin M (IgM) antibodies to cytomegalovirus may be present for months to years after infection. Therefore, the presence of IgM does not strictly imply acute infection. Hepatitis A, an RNA virus of the picornavirus family, is transmitted almost exclusively by the fecal–oral route. In the United States in the 1970s, serologic evidence of infection was present in 40% of adults from urban populations. Subsequent studies have found a decreasing prevalence of hepatitis A infection. In the United States, 5% to 30% of individuals 10 to 19 years of age have serologic evidence of *Toxoplasma* exposure; this increases to 10% to 67% by age 50. In France and Central America, the seroprevalence approaches 90% by age 40.

63–66. The answers are: 63-E, 64-C, 65-B, 66-A. (*Internal medicine, surgery*)
A high prostate-specific antigen (PSA) value is a nonspecific finding that may be elevated in prostate cancer, prostatitis, benign prostatic hypertrophy, and prostatic infarction. An imperfect tumor marker, PSA is positive in only 65% of cases; therefore, its sensitivity is 65%. Its specificity is less than 50%. PSA values tend to be higher in African American men with or without benign prostatic hypertrophy. In borderline cases of PSA elevation (4.1 to 10 ng/mL), several factors may be useful in determining risk of cancer: the rate of PSA rise (PSA velocity), PSA density (prostate mass/volume), age-specific reference ranges, and quantification of free PSA.

The high PSA value in this case warrants further evaluation. Prostate cancer is rare before the age of 50 years and is more common in African Americans, so the patient has an increased risk of prostate cancer. If an annual digital rectal examination is abnormal or if the PSA is greater than 10 ng/mL, a transrectal biopsy under sonography is necessary. Adenocarcinoma of the prostate should not be missed. Observation would be unreasonable in this setting. Antibiotics would not be reasonable because there is little suspicion for prostatitis. Terazosin would be useful if the patient had symptoms suggestive of benign prostatic hypertrophy that was confirmed by transrectal biopsy.

Prostate cancer is the most common malignancy that affects men in the United States. More than 90% of tumors are adenocarcinomas that occur in the acini, which have a predilection for the periphery of the prostate gland. The Gleason tumor grade is used to determine biologic behavior; it is calculated by grading the two most dominant histologic patterns and assigning a number (1 to 5) based on differentiation. The higher the Gleason score, the less differentiated the tumor and, therefore, the worse the prognosis. Spread of prostatic adenocarcinoma occurs via three routes: direct extension, the lymphatic system, and the bloodstream. Lymphatic spread occurs in the obturator, internal iliac, common iliac, presacral, and para-aortic nodes (in decreasing order). The risk of lymphatic spread correlates with the size and grade of the tumor as well as the PSA level. Hematogenous metastasis occurs most commonly to bone (pelvis > vertebrae), followed by the lung, liver, and adrenal glands in decreasing frequency. Direct extension can occur to surrounding tissues, such as the rectum.

One of the important therapies for prostate cancer is androgen deprivation because the tumors are often androgen-responsive. Methods of androgen-deprivation include orchiectomy, leuprolide (luteinizing releasing-hormone analog), flutamide (androgen receptor antagonist), and aminoglutethimide (inhibits androgen synthesis by testes and adrenals). Testosterone could accelerate tumor growth.

67–70. The answers are: 67-B, 68-C, 69-C, 70-A. (*Internal medicine, surgery*)
The differential diagnosis of testicular mass in a young man is extensive. It is essential to assume that this mass is malignant until proven otherwise. Conditions to rule out include varicocele, epididymal cyst, hydrocele, spermatocele, epididymitis, and testicular torsion. A varicocele is a dilated plexus of scrotal veins that is usually asymptomatic and more prominent when standing. A hydrocele is a cystic accumulation of clear fluid within the tunica vaginalis that is usually painless. A spermatocele is a sperm-containing cyst that is painless and benign. Epididymitis refers to inflammation of the epididymis, most commonly due to trauma or bacterial infection. Chlamydia and gonorrhea are common causes in patients younger than 35 years, and coliform bacteria (e.g., *Escherichia coli*) are more common in patients older than 35 years. The testicle is very tender, and the patient is occasionally febrile. Testicular torsion, a medical emergency, is characterized by the acute onset of severe testicular pain. The condition occurs most often at approximately 16 years of age. On examination, the testicle is enlarged and exquisitely tender. The window for saving of the testicle is approximately 6 hours.

In this case, the mass is painless, which makes torsion and epididymitis unlikely. Testicular cancer in this young man is a concern, and an ultrasound is of critical importance. Neither observation nor antibiotics will help rule out a malignancy. A transscrotal biopsy should never occur in the event that the mass is malignant because it can cause scrotal spread of the tumor.

Recall that testicular tumors are either germ cell tumors (95%) or non–germ cell tumors (5%; Leydig and Sertoli cell tumors). Germ cell tumors, which can occasionally arise from extragonadal tissue in the mediastinum and retroperitoneum, are split into two groups: seminomatous (50%) and nonseminomatous (50%). Seminomatous tumors occur most frequently between the ages of 20 and 40 years, with a mean age of approximately 30 years. The classic presentation is a painless mass. Any mass in a patient older than 50 years is presumed to be lymphoma until proven otherwise. About 50% of tumors in young men are seminomas. Most patients present with stage I disease limited to the testis, epididymitis, and spermatic cord. The cure rate is more than 90% for patients with seminomatous disease; it is highest when diagnosis occurs at stages I or II. Men with an undescended testis (cryptorchid) are at greater risk of later development of germ cell tumors; orchiopexy (surgical descent) reduces, but does not entirely eliminate, this risk.

Nonseminomatous tumors are more aggressive and metastasize earlier. The four subtypes are embryonal carcinoma, teratoma, choriocarcinoma, and endodermal sinus tumor. α-Fetoprotein (AFP) is elevated in patients with nonseminomatous disease only. β-Human chorionic gonadotropin (β-hCG) is elevated in both seminomatous and nonseminomatous disease. (If a biopsy finds seminomatous tissue but the patient has an increased AFP, treatment for nonseminomatous disease is necessary.) Classically, a choriocarcinoma is associated with elevated β-hCG, endodermal sinus tumor with elevated AFP, and embryonal carcinoma with both AFP and β-hCG elevation.

71. The answer is E. (*Obstetrics/gynecology*)
Labor has been divided into three stages, with a fourth stage occurring during the postpartum period. The four phases of labor are:

1. Latent phase: cervical effacement through dilation to 3 cm
   Active phase: 3–10 cm (complete dilation)
2. Complete cervical dilation through delivery of infant
3. After delivery of the infant through delivery of placenta
4. Immediate postpartum through 2 hours' postpartum

Abnormal labor patterns include a prolonged latent phase, a prolonged active phase, an arrest of dilation, and an arrest of descent. This patient, who began to dilate but then stopped for more than 2 hours, has arrest of dilation. Dilation ceases either because uterine contractions are inadequate to maintain labor or an aspect of fetal size, lie, or position causes problems.

Before giving oxytocin to augment uterine contractions or performing an immediate cesarean section, it is important to rule out fetal malposition, fetopelvic disproportion, and malpresentation. In these circumstances, a cesarean section is indicated. Anatomy is usually considered for a prolonged latent phase, but membrane rupture and dilation to 4 cm have already occurred. Prostaglandin E₂ gel is also used during the first stage of labor, and this patient is past this point.

72. The answer is B. (*Obstetrics/gynecology*)
At 26 weeks' gestation, the fetal lungs are poorly developed. Even at 32 weeks' gestation, the production of surfactant is still poor. This patient is in preterm labor, defined as regular uterine contractions with cervical change between 20 and 36 weeks of pregnancy. The administration of a steroid, such as betamethasone, hastens pulmonary maturity and reduces the incidence and mortality from respiratory distress syndrome. The β₂-agonists ritodrine and terbutaline are used to inhibit uterine contractions in preterm labor. Indomethacin is used occasionally in preterm labor because it inhibits prostaglandin production, which causes uterine contractions. If indomethacin is used after 34 weeks, it can cause premature closure of the ductus arteriosus. Magnesium sulfate competes with calcium at the neuromuscular junction to inhibit uterine contractions as well.

73–75. The answer is: 73-A, 74-E, 75-D. (*Emergency medicine, surgery, internal medicine*)
Gastric ulcers are usually located on the lesser curvature of the stomach within 1 cm of the gastric antrum. The pain caused by gastric ulcers classically occurs at the epigastrium and may radiate through to the back; it worsens with the ingestion of food. Classically, duodenal ulcer pain is relieved with the ingestion of food. Clinically, this finding is rarely useful. *Helicobacter pylori* clearly plays an important role in the pathogenesis of gastric ulcers, although the exact cause of these ulcers is unclear. Most patients have a pattern of normal or low gastric acid secretion; therefore, the underlying cause of the ulcers is probably not acid hypersecretion. Many studies that suggest that *H. pylori* is important in the pathogenesis of ulcers also promote the treatment of *H. pylori*.

Several studies are useful in the detection of *H. pylori*. The CLO test takes advantage of the urea-splitting ability of the bacterium. During an esophagogastroduodenoscopy, a biopsy of the ulcer is obtained. Ammonia forms on exposure to urea if *H. pylori* is present. The enzyme-linked immunosorbent assay (ELISA) test for the existence of *H. pylori* antibodies in plasma also may be useful. However, if a patient has a history of *H. pylori,* the ELISA is likely to remain positive, and it cannot detect relapses. If circumstances prevent the use of ELISA, the ^{14}C-urea breath test may eliminate the need for another esophagogastroduodenoscopy. The patient ingests a ^{14}C-urea load. A short time later, the expired air tests for ^{14}C because if *H. pylori* is present, it splits the ^{14}C-urea bond.

In this case, the patient has a gastric ulcer and a positive test for *H. pylori* antibodies. The most effective treatment for *H. pylori* is a macrolide antibiotic (clarithromycin); a proton pump inhibitor (omeprazole); and a second antibiotic (metronidazole or amoxicillin). This regimen is approximately 90% effective in eliminating *H. pylori*.

Evidently, medical therapy fails, and the patient requires a vagotomy and antrectomy. Removal of the pyloric mechanism results in the loss of the tight control of gastric emptying. This problem accounts for many of the postgastrectomy syndromes. In this case, the patient has early dumping syndrome, which results in anxiety, weakness, tachycardia, diaphoresis, and palpitations 15 minutes after a high osmolar load. Uncontrolled emptying of hypertonic fluid into the small intestine draws intravascular fluid into the small intestines, causing acute intravascular volume depletion. Apparently, the release of serotonin, histamine, glucagon, and vasoactive intestinal peptides also accounts for the symptoms. Patients should eat smaller meals with some fat in each meal to help slow gastric emptying.

Late dumping syndrome is characterized by similar symptoms to those of early dumping syndrome, but they do not occur until 3 hours after ingestion of a meal. The condition is thought to be related primarily to glucose and insulin changes.

Afferent loop syndrome occurs only after Billroth II reconstruction. In this procedure, the body of the stomach is anastomosed with a proximal loop of jejunum, and the remaining loop of duodenum is left as a "blind" loop proximal to the flow of gastric contents. This "afferent limb" can become kinked, causing the collection of pancreatic and biliary secretions. This, in turn, causes cramping abdominal pain after the ingestion of a meal. Patients often vomit dark brown material 45 minutes after a meal. Treatment consists of a Billroth I conversion or a Roux-en-Y gastrojejunostomy.

Blind loop syndrome is associated with bacterial overgrowth in the afferent limb of a Billroth II procedure, as previously described. These bacteria interfere with the metabolism of vitamin B_{12} and folate. In addition, they can deconjugate bile acids, causing steatorrhea. Therefore, these patients have diarrhea, weight loss and, occasionally, anemia. Treatment consists of antibiotics with a conversion to Billroth I if the syndrome recurs.

Alkaline reflux gastritis occurs when duodenal, pancreatic, and biliary fluid refluxes back into the denervated stomach. On esophagogastroduodenoscopy, the gastric mucosa is inflamed, edematous, and bile-stained. Patients suffer from weakness, nausea, epigastric pain that radiates to the back and, occasionally, anemia. Treatment is a Roux-en-Y conversion with a long (40 cm) limb to prevent reflux.

Recurrent ulcer disease most commonly results from an incomplete vagotomy, often of the right posterior vagal branch. Truncal vagotomy and antrectomy is associated with the lowest recurrence rate.

76. The answer is D. (*Statistics*)

Increasingly, physicians are attempting to practice "evidence-based" medicine in which practice patterns and decisions are based on clinical studies. In judging the literature, it is important to be able to evaluate the evidence presented in a study. Randomized controlled trials provide the best evidence of a cause-and-effect relationship. These trials involve the comparison of a drug with placebo (or two different drugs) over time in a large population randomly assigned to different treatment arms. Randomized controlled trials have the lowest risk of bias and confounding factors.

Cross-sectional studies provide only weak evidence of a causal relationship. In these types of studies, investigators focus on a portion (cross section) of a population and quantify various characteristics. Case-control series compare a population with an exposure to a population selected to match the exposed group. Cohort studies follow populations with varying exposures over time. Case series studies, which merely describe several cases, supply the weakest evidence of a cause-and-effect relationship. Thus, they are prone to reporting bias and offer no comparisons of different treatment. However, they are useful in describing rare conditions and novel approaches.

77–79. The answers are: 77-D, 78-E, 79-C. (*Pediatrics*)

This child presents with clinical signs and symptoms suggestive of Kawasaki syndrome (mucocutaneous lymph node syndrome). This acute, febrile, multisystem disease affects children, most often between the ages of 1 and 2 years. Diagnostic features include:

Fever > 5 days
Rash (may be morbilliform, scarlatiniform, or target-like)
Bilateral conjunctival erythema
Cervical lymphadenopathy
Bright red erythema of lips and tongue ("strawberry tongue")
Erythema of the palms and soles with later desquamation

In the early stages of the disease, it is important to consider several possible causes. The nonspecific appearance of the rash along with fever should suggest conditions such as streptococcal toxic shock syndrome, scarlet fever, measles, and hypersensitivity rash. Hand-foot-and-mouth-disease, an acute viral infection, manifests as painful vesicular eruptions on the tongue, buccal mucosa, hands, and feet.

Initial therapy should address all the important possibilities. For Kawasaki syndrome, it is necessary to administer aspirin and intravenous antibiotics; for possible streptococcal infection, intravenous antibiotics; and for the high fever and oral lesions, intravenous hydration. Corticosteroids have no role in the initial treatment of this patient.

The most feared complications of Kawasaki syndrome are cardiac in nature. They include:

Pericardial effusion
Tachyarrhythmia
Tricuspid or mitral regurgitation
Coronary artery aneurysm, with resulting thrombosis and infarction

The other choices in question 79 are not complications of Kawasaki syndrome.

80–82. The answers are: 80-C, 81-D, 82-B. (*Internal medicine, neurology*)

This patient has infective endocarditis. The empiric treatment of this condition must cover the most common bacterial causes [viridans streptococci; enterococci; *Staphylococcus aureus;* and ***Haemophilus, Actinobacillus, Cardiobacterium, Eikenella corrodens,*** and ***Kingella*** (HACEK group of bacteria)]. A common regimen consists of nafcillin (*S. aureus* and viridans streptococci) and ampicillin (enterococci and HACEK group bacteria) combined with gentamicin for bacteriocidal synergy. In most regimens, gentamicin can be discontinued after 2 weeks of therapy, with the exception of therapy for enterococcus, in which prolonged gentamicin therapy is indicated.

Once the microorganism is isolated, antimicrobial therapy can be adjusted accordingly. The discovery of viridans streptococci that is susceptible to penicillin allows for various choices, including penicillin G, ceftriaxone, and cefazolin. Vancomycin is appropriate only in cases of penicillin allergy or resistance.

One of the feared complications of infective endocarditis is mycotic aneurysm, which occurs as the result of an embolus of bacteria to a vessel in the brain, resulting in vascular infection and weakening of the vessel wall. These aneurysms are at risk for rupture, causing subarachnoid hemorrhage; this is what happened to the patient in this case. Epidural or subdural hemorrhages are more often associated with trauma. An intracranial mass lesion is not associated with endocarditis unless a brain abscess develops. Affected patients often present with seizures and a focal neurologic deficit.

83. The answer is C. (*Emergency medicine, surgery*)

This patient has a Colles fracture, one of the most common fractures of the forearm. This type of fracture often follows a fall on an outstretched arm. Colles fractures involve the distal radius and often the ulnar styloid process, with dorsal displacement of the distal radius fragment. This results in the characteristic dorsal angulation of the wrist ("silver fork" deformity) seen on physical examination. Older individuals are particularly prone to Colles fractures secondary to age-associated osteoporosis.

Treatment involves reduction of the fracture followed by splinting of the arm in a neutral position. Following splinting, up to 3 weeks of casting may be necessary. It is important to obtain follow-up radiographs to ensure that there is no loss of reduction. Nonsteroidal anti-inflammatory drugs (NSAIDs) may be used to treat the associated pain and inflammation. Splinting with wrist flexion, which may compromise the median nerve, should be avoided when treating Colles fractures.

84. The answer is C. (*Emergency medicine, surgery*)

This patient has suffered an acute injury to the ulnar collateral ligament, which occurs with forced radial abduction of the thumb. A small avulsion injury on the ulnar aspect of the first metacarpophalangeal joint, the location of insertion of the ulnar collateral ligament, is an associated radiographic finding (arrow on the radiograph). Historically, this injury is often referred to as "gamekeeper's thumb." This refers to the chronic sprain of the ulnar collateral ligament suffered by English game wardens, who sacrificed rabbits by breaking their necks between the thumb and index finger.

Such injuries to the ulnar collateral ligament are common in skiers. Complete tears of this ligament require surgical intervention; an orthopedic surgeon should evaluate all suspected cases.

85–88. The answers are: 85-D, 86-B, 87-D, 88-B. (*Pediatrics*)

This infant has β-thalassemia major (Cooley anemia). The molecular defect responsible for this condition is the absence of β-globin synthesis, which results in the complete absence of Hgb A_1 and the resulting increase in the synthesis of Hgb F and smaller amount of Hgb A_2 (two α and two δ chains). Clinically, affected children suffer from a severe hemolytic anemia that is manifested within the first 6 to 8 months of life. Marked bone marrow hyperplasia is present secondary to increased erythropoiesis, leading to frontal bossing, prominent cheek bones, and hepatosplenomegaly. Laboratory clues include severe anemia with reticulocytopenia and evidence of hemolysis (elevated lactate dehydrogenase [LDH]). Liver enzymes (except alanine aminotransferase [AST]), renal function, and other cell lines on the complete blood count (CBC) are normal.

A peripheral smear is likely to show microcytosis, hypochromia, and anisocytosis. Schistocytes are seen in microangiopathic hemolytic anemia (usually associated with thrombocytopenia). Macrocytes are seen in folate and vitamin B_{12} deficiency. Howell-Jolly bodies are seen in asplenic states. Spherocytes can be seen in hereditary spherocytosis, another cause of a congenital hemolytic anemia. In hereditary spherocytosis, however, the reticulocyte count is often normal.

Hemoglobin electrophoresis is diagnostic. In this case, there would be a large increase in hemoglobin F and a lesser increase in hemoglobin A_2. Hemoglobin Bart (four γ chains) is seen in hydrops fetalis or α-thalassemia major. Hemoglobin H (four β chains) is seen in variants of α-thalassemia in which three α-globin genes are deleted. Hemoglobin C is seen in hemoglobin C disease in which a lysine substitutes for a normally occurring glutamine at position 6 of the hemoglobin molecule.

Long-term sequelae of β-thalassemia include hemochromatosis secondary to the massive transfusion requirements that are often necessary. The transfused iron accumulates in the liver, skin, heart, pancreas, and gonads. Treatment with an iron chelator (deferoxamine) is effective in preventing this disease. The other choices in question 88 are not possible outcomes of β-thalassemia.

89–90. The answers are: 89-E, 90-C. (*Psychiatry*)

Lithium is an effective agent in the treatment of bipolar disorder. However, it has significant side effects and a narrow therapeutic index. Patients on chronic lithium must be educated about the side effects of the medication and carefully followed-up. The two most common side effects are polyuria and hypothyroidism. Polyuria, which occurs in up to 40% to 50% of patients on chronic lithium therapy, may be quite severe (up to 11 L/day of urine) and irreversible. Other long-term renal side effects include interstitial fibrosis and decreased renal function. The other listed choices are not seen with lithium use. In fact, a benign, reversible leukocytosis is commonly seen after initiation of lithium therapy.

Hypothyroidism, which occurs in up to 15% of patients on chronic lithium therapy, is more common in women with symptoms that may mimic depression. A serum thyroid-stimulating hormone (TSH) level is warranted.

91–93. The answers are: 91-D, 92-B, 93-B. (*Surgery, internal medicine*)

Malignant hyperthermia has developed in this patient. In this poorly understood genetic disorder, inhalational anesthetic agents (except nitrous oxide) and succinylcholine lead to the intracellular accumulation of toxic amounts of calcium. Presenting features include a host of clinical findings, which may develop during anesthesia induction or at any subsequent time in a patient undergoing surgery. Clinical findings include unexplained tachycardia, dysrhythmia, skin mottling, skeletal muscle rigidity, acidosis, cyanosis, hyperthermia, hemodynamic instability, and rhabdomyolysis. Intravenous dantrolene, the treatment of choice, may be lifesaving. Dantrolene, a muscle relaxant, inhibits calcium release from the sarcoplasmic reticulum. Of course, intravenous fluids and pressor agents may be required. Esmolol (a short-acting β-blocker), antibiotics, and acetaminophen have no role in the treatment of malignant hyperthermia.

Several metabolic complications may develop as a result of malignant hyperthermia, including hyperkalemia, hyperphosphatemia (from rhabdomyolysis), lactic acidosis, and elevated creatine kinase. However, metabolic alkalosis does not occur.

Prevention centers on avoidance of causal agents—inhalational anesthetics and succinylcholine. There is little evidence that prophylactic dantrolene is efficacious.

94–97. The answers are: 94-A, 95-C, 96-D, 97-A. (*Surgery, internal medicine*)

Diverticulosis involves the formation of diverticula in the colon. Diverticula are herniations of the mucosa through the muscularis that usually occur at points at which a nutrient artery penetrates the muscularis, occurring most commonly in the sigmoid colon. One theory postulates that high intraluminal pressures (secondary to constipation and a low-fiber diet) predispose to diverticula formation. Diverticula, which increase in frequency with age, most often are asymptomatic and found on routine endoscopy. However, diverticula can lead to serious complications; the most common is hemorrhage. Less common complications include diverticulitis, abscess formation, bowel perforation, and fistula formation. Malignancy, rectal prolapse, and sigmoid volvulus are not consequences of diverticulosis.

Approximately 85% of diverticular hemorrhages stop spontaneously, so watchful waiting is safe if the patient is hemodynamically stable. If bleeding continues, endoscopy, nuclear medicine scans, or angiography may be used to localize the bleeding. CT scans are not helpful. Only if all conservative measures fail or the patient is unstable should partial colectomy be considered as a treatment option. Antibiotics are not necessary in this setting. Enteric–vascular fistulas are rare and usually present with catastrophic hemorrhage.

Treatment of the patient's diverticulitis should include bowel rest and intravenous broad-spectrum antibiotics. Both barium enema and colonoscopy should be avoided because of the associated high risk of perforating the inflamed bowel. Neither emergent surgery nor corticosteroids are warranted.

Signs of colonic diverticula rupture, with abscess formation and peritonitis, are now apparent. Because of the presence of free peritoneal air, emergent surgery is required. The surgery should include resection of the involved colonic segment, end colostomy, and formation of a Hartmann pouch (oversewing of the uninvolved segment of the rectosigmoid, creating a segment that drains through the anus). Drainage of the abscess and antibiotics are also necessary. Total colectomy is not necessary, and abscess drainage alone is not appropriate because of the presence of a bowel perforation.

98–99. The answers are: 98-E, 99-C. (*Internal medicine, critical care medicine*)
Patients with end-stage renal disease are prone to electrolyte abnormalities and volume overload, especially if they miss scheduled dialysis sessions. In this case, the ECG shows classic changes consistent with hyperkalemia: peaked, symmetrical T waves; absent P waves; and accelerated ventricular or junctional rhythm, which may degenerate into ventricular fibrillation. As a result of hyperkalemia, the earliest change on the ECG is peaking of T waves, followed by widening of the QRS complex and, eventually, impairment of atrioventricular conduction. Intravenous calcium, which will stabilize the myocardium, is the necessary emergent treatment. It is also necessary to provide definitive treatment, which may include insulin/dextrose, sodium polystyrene sulfonate (Kayexalate), or hemodialysis. Intravenous bicarbonate plays little, if any, role in the treatment of hyperkalemia in a patient with end-stage renal disease. Coronary revascularization is not indicated in this case.

Emergent intubation is later necessary. The patient is rapidly deteriorating, and dialysis cannot be started in time to affect significant volume removal. Intubation allows for the improvement of oxygenation, a reduction in cardiac stress, and sedation of the agitated patient. It is unlikely that this patient will significantly respond to diuretics; in any case, his blood pressure has already been controlled. In the meantime, dialysis can be arranged and performed safely. After volume removal with dialysis, extubation may safely proceed.

100–104. The answers are: 100-B, 101-C, 102-B, 103-A, 104-C. (*Neurology*)
This patient has multiple sclerosis, a chronic demyelinating disease with lesions that are disseminated in time and space. It commonly affects young women (older than 35 years of age). Multiple sclerosis appears to be an autoimmune disease mediated by T lymphocytes with the initiating factors not clearly understood. Diagnostic criteria for multiple sclerosis include:

Examination revealing objective abnormalities of CNS
Involvement predominantly affecting white matter tracts of nervous system (e.g., pyramidal, cerebellar pathways, optic nerves, posterior columns)
Examination or history that MUST implicate involvement of two or more areas of CNS
Clinical pattern that MUST consist of two or more separate episodes of CNS involvement (each lasting >24 hours and separated by at least 1 month) or gradual, stepwise progression for 6 months with finding of either increased CSF IgG or CSF oligoclonal bands
Age of onset: 15 to 60 years
Exclusion of other diseases (e.g., Lyme disease, systemic lupus erythematosus, sarcoidosis)

CSF = cerebrospinal fluid; CNS = central nervous system.

Presenting signs suggest optic neuritis. Involvement of the optic nerve leads to an afferent pupillary defect. In this case, direct light on the involved eye results in pupillary dilation. However, indirect light on the uninvolved eye (left) leads to normal constriction of the pupil of the involved eye (right), because the optic nerve of the uninvolved eye is normal. The other answer choices in question 100 may occasionally occur in multiple sclerosis; however, as the patient's history is not suggestive, these findings would be less likely.

MRI of the brain is extremely useful in showing the characteristic changes in white matter. (On T1-weighted images, these lesions appear hypointense; on T2-weighted images, they appear hyperintense.) Lesions are most often seen in the brainstem, cerebellum, and spinal cord. The findings listed as other possible answers to question 101 are not characteristic of multiple sclerosis.

The presence of oligoclonal immunoglobulin G (IgG) bands and increased amounts of IgG on cerebrospinal fluid (CSF) examination is characteristic. Cell counts are usually normal but may demonstrate a monocyte pleocytosis. Glucose concentrations are within normal range.

A major advance in the treatment of multiple sclerosis has been interferon beta. Clinical trials have shown that this agent decreases annual exacerbation rates by one third and reduces the number of new, white matter lesions visible on monthly MRI scans. Thus, interferon beta should be used as prophylaxis against relapses. Corticosteroids are warranted for treatment of acute exacerbations. Methotrexate, azathioprine, and cyclophosphamide are useful for multiple sclerosis that progresses despite therapy with interferon beta. Cyclosporine and angiotensin-converting enzyme (ACE) inhibitors have no role in multiple sclerosis management.

Bladder problems eventually occur in nearly all individuals with multiple sclerosis. Because symptoms of bladder dysfunction correlate poorly with physiologic dysfunction, it is recommended that all patients undergo urodynamic testing. This testing allows classification of bladder problems into three categories: hyperreflexia; hyporeflexia; and dyssynergy, in which the detrusor muscle and external urinary sphincter muscle do not operate in concert. Treatment of bladder hyperreflexia involves anticholinergic agents, such as oxybutynin or propantheline; treatment of bladder hyporeflexia involves cholinergic agents, such as bethanechol; and treatment of dyssynergy involves a combination of intermittent self-catheterization and anticholinergic agents.

105. The answer is D. (*Surgery*)
To determine the total amount of calories delivered by total parenteral nutrition (TPN), it is necessary to know the caloric values of carbohydrates, lipids, and proteins. These values are carbohydrates, 4 kcal/g; lipids, 9 kcal/g; and proteins, 4 kcal/g. Thus, the total caloric intake from TPN is:

Carbohydrate	4 kcal/g $\times$ 80 kg $\times$ 5 g/kg per day = 1,600 kcal
Protein	4 kcal/g $\times$ 80 kg $\times$ 0.8 g/kg per day = 256 kcal
Lipids	9 kcal/g $\times$ 80 kg $\times$ 0.5 g/kg per day = 360 kcal
TOTAL	2,216

106–107. The answers are: 106-D, 107-B. (*Internal medicine, critical care medicine*)
This patient presents with respiratory failure secondary to severe pneumonia. Despite intubation and ventilation, his oxygenation remains suboptimal. The next step should be to increase positive end-expiratory pressure (PEEP) to 10 cm H_2O. This enhances oxygenation by increasing the mean airway pressure, improving ventilation of collapsed alveoli. It is important to realize that increasing PEEP may have detrimental effects; (1) it may lead to airway and alveoli injury (pneumothorax), and (2) it can impede venous return of blood, decreasing cardiac output. Therefore, changes in PEEP must be monitored closely.

Decreasing the respiratory rate worsens ventilation and does not improve oxygenation. Increasing the tidal volume or respiratory rate decreases the carbon dioxide level (by improving ventilation) but has little effect on oxygenation. Although raising the fractional concentration of oxygen in inspired gas (FIO_2) increases the oxygenation of the patient, the price is high; it results in an increased direct oxygen toxicity on the lung.

The chest radiograph shows complete collapse of the left lung likely secondary to a mucus plug. The clues to lung collapse are the shift of the mediastinum to the left, the opaque appearance of the left hemithorax, and the tracheal shift. Pleural effusions, whether malignant, bloody, or purulent, would not lead to shift of the mediastinum toward the side of the effusion.

108–112. The answers are: 108-E, 109-D, 110-D, 111-E, 112-B. (*Emergency medicine, internal medicine*) The ECG displays findings consistent of acute inferior myocardial infarction (MI). ST-segment elevation is evident in leads II, III, and aVF, with reciprocal depression in leads I and aVL. The prominent ST-segment depression in the right precordial leads, which may represent posterior wall infarction, is also noteworthy. Interestingly, this patient also has a sinus rhythm with a 2:1 atrioventricular block, which is best seen in leads V_5 and V_6.

Because of the early presentation, ST-segment elevation MI, and the patient's age (younger than 75 years), he is a candidate for reperfusion therapy with tissue plasminogen activator (tPA). It is important to determine whether the patient has any contraindications to thrombolytic therapy. In general, these contraindications fall under the category of conditions in which the risk of bleeding is too high to justify the risk of using tPA. Common contraindications include:

High blood pressure
Systolic >200 mm Hg or
Diastolic >120 mm Hg
Acute pancreatitis
Cerebral aneurysm or recent stroke
Suspected aortic dissection
Prolonged cardiopulmonary resuscitation (CPR)
Diabetic retinopathy with hemorrhage
Recent head trauma
Hemoptysis
Active hematuria
Surgery within past 2 weeks
Gastrointestinal bleeding within past 2 months

Because there are many other potential contraindications, tPA therapy must be individualized to minimize complications. The recent laparoscopic surgery mentioned in question 109 precludes the use of tPA, and percutaneous interventions are favored.

The patient in questions 110 and 111 has acute, severe mitral regurgitation secondary to papillary muscle rupture. This complication, which is seen in 1% of MIs, occurs most often with inferior infarcts; involving ischemia to the posteromedial papillary muscle, which is supplied by only one blood vessel. The development of acute pulmonary edema 2 to 7 days postinfarct should lead to suspicion of papillary muscle rupture. Echocardiography is usually diagnostic. Pericarditis, which occurs in up to 10% of Q-wave infarcts, is usually benign; however, tamponade may occur, especially if the patient is receiving anticoagulants. Free wall rupture is a catastrophic event that occurs after large anterior MIs.

Although medical therapy with vasodilators may temporarily improve symptoms, surgery is the definitive therapy. Except for emergent surgery, none of the other answer choices in question 111 fit the clinical scenario.

It is important to be able to risk stratify patients with MI because not all patients benefit from the most aggressive approach (such as percutaneous revascularization). High-risk characteristics postinfarction include:

Large infarcts (more than four leads with ST-segment elevation)
Recurrent ischemia
Poor ejection fraction (<40%)
Diabetes mellitus
Ventricular tachycardia 48 hours after MI
Congestive heart failure
Suspected mechanical defect

Ventricular tachycardia occurring within the first 48 hours after an MI has no prognostic significance.

113–115. The answers are: 113-E, 114-C, 115-E. (*Internal medicine, neurology*)

This patient is suffering from Parkinson disease, which is typified by tremor, rigidity, bradykinesia, and unstable gait and posture. The condition is most common in patients who are older than 65 years. It is believed that symptoms are caused by the loss of neurons in the substantia nigra and the locus ceruleus in the brainstem. This process leads to loss of dopaminergic cells and striatal dopamine depletion, as well as loss of thalamic excitation of the cerebral cortex with the characteristic symptoms. Physical examination almost certainly finds increased rigidity of the extremities. Deep tendon reflexes, motor strength, and sensation should all be preserved.

Levodopa, the metabolic precursor of dopamine, is the mainstay treatment of Parkinson disease. However, oral administration of the drug exposes levodopa to peripheral (mainly intestinal) dopa decarboxylase, which converts levodopa to dopamine outside of the central nervous system (CNS), making the drug less effective. Therefore, levodopa is given in conjunction with carbidopa, a peripheral dopa decarboxylase inhibitor that allows a larger amount of levodopa to enter the CNS and be converted to dopamine. The other answer choices in question 114 are not mechanisms of action for carbidopa.

Although levodopa is an effective therapy for Parkinson disease, it has significant side effects, including nausea and vomiting, postural hypotension, nightmares, and cardiac arrhythmias. Another important side effect is the "wearing-off" phenomenon, in which patients experience transient deteriorations in symptoms just before their next dose. This can be managed easily by decreasing the time interval between doses. A more difficult problem is the "on–off" phenomenon, in which patients experience abrupt, transient deteriorations without warning and without relationship to the dosing interval. The exact mechanisms associated with this phenomenon are not known but may involve progressive deterioration of presynaptic dopaminergic nerve terminals.

116–117. The answers are: 116-B, 117-A. (*Internal medicine*)

The most likely cause of this patient's diarrhea is *Giardia lamblia*. Not only does the patient live in a rural setting, but his diarrhea is associated with prominent upper gastrointestinal (GI) symptoms. However, these findings are suggestive, not diagnostic. It is necessary to send a stool sample to look for either cysts or trophozoites. Alternatively, a test that checks for *Giardia* antigens in the stool, which is easier to perform and as sensitive and specific as microscopic examination, has recently become available. Treatment should commence with metronidazole 250 mg 3 times a day for 5 days. This therapy offers cure rates as high as 80%.

To prevent further recurrences, the most likely source of infection must be identified. In most cases, this is well water. Boiling or filtering contaminated water prevents most further outbreaks.

118–119. The answers are: 118-C, 119-E. (*Obstetrics/gynecology*)

This patient has essential hypertension. Often, it can be very difficult to determine whether a patient has preexisting hypertension or pregnancy-induced hypertension. Of course, if prepregnancy blood pressures are available, and they become elevated, the diagnosis is easier. But remember, even if this is the case, pregnancy-induced hypertension can be superimposed on existing hypertension. Because blood pressure normally falls during the second trimester, the diagnosis of essential hypertension is confirmed if elevated blood pressures are present before the 20th week of gestation. It is also important to look for other underlying diseases that may be associated with preexisting hypertension (diabetes, vascular disease, renal disease). In this case, the presence of hypertension early in pregnancy, the absence of proteinuria, and the strong family history point to the diagnosis of essential hypertension.

The treatment of essential hypertension during pregnancy is difficult and controversial. Because placental perfusion is critically dependent on blood pressure, overtreatment of hypertension can be dangerous. For this reason, many obstetricians opt for treatment only when the diastolic pressure is above 100 mm Hg. Of the agents listed in question 119, only enalapril (and all angiotensin-converting enzyme [ACE] inhibitors) is contraindicated. These agents have been associated with fetal renal failure and death.

120–122. The answers are: 120-B, 121-E, 122-E. (*Obstetrics/gynecology*)
This patient has pregnancy-induced hypertension, which is primarily a disease of first pregnancy that is more common in younger and older mothers. The finding of new-onset hypertension late in pregnancy along with edema and proteinuria is consistent with the diagnosis.

Treatment depends somewhat on the severity of the condition and gestational age. Severe pregnancy-induced hypertension is defined as blood pressure higher than 160/110 mm Hg, proteinuria greater than 5 g/day, oliguria, visual blurring, and pulmonary edema or cyanosis. In severe pregnancy-induced hypertension or late in gestation, delivery of the infant is necessary. However, with mild pregnancy-induced hypertension or early in gestation, a conservative approach is warranted. This includes bed rest, frequent fetal ultrasounds, antihypertensive therapy as needed, and monitoring of renal function and proteinuria. Magnesium infusions should be reserved for severe pregnancy-induced hypertension and eclampsia.

Eclampsia is the extension of pregnancy-induced hypertension to include seizures, coma, or both. It is associated with a significant maternal and fetal mortality rate, and prevention is possible, with early recognition and treatment. Although most cases of eclampsia occur before birth of the infant, up to 25% can occur after delivery. Magnesium sulfate is the agent of choice to both treat and prevent convulsions. Because magnesium can lead to respiratory depression and cardiac arrest, close monitoring of levels and clinical signs is critical. Loss of the patellar reflex is one of the earliest signs of magnesium toxicity and should guide titration of the infusion. Calcium, which antagonizes the neuromuscular blockade of magnesium, serves as the antidote for toxicity. The addition of phenytoin to magnesium can lead to serious sedation and high risk for pulmonary aspiration, and it should be avoided. Definitive treatment is delivery of the infant.

123. The answer is E. (*Pediatrics*)
The lesions of molluscum contagiosum result from an infection of the superficial layers of the epidermis by a pox family virus. The lesions are seen in three clinical contexts:

Young, healthy children
HIV-positive individuals
Sexually active young adults, who can spread the virus by contact

The lesions are painless and flesh-colored, with a central umbilication. They commonly appear together on the face but can be found anywhere; this distribution may be secondary to autoinoculation.

In healthy children, such as the patient in this case, the course is self-limited, and no treatment is required. In immunocompromised patients, the diagnosis should be confirmed with skin biopsy; several conditions (disseminated fungal infections) can have a similar appearance.

124–126. The answers are: 124-E, 125-B, 126-C. (*Internal medicine, obstetrics/gynecology*)
Increasingly, it is recognized that a significant portion of suspected idiopathic venous thromboses are due to an underlying hypercoagulable state. Some of these hypercoagulable states include protein C and S deficiencies, factor V Leiden, and antiphospholipid antibody syndrome. By far, the most common inherited hypercoagulable disorder is factor V Leiden, in which a substitution of a glutamine for an arginine at amino acid position 506 alters the ability of protein C to degrade the activated factor. The combination of factor V Leiden and the use of oral contraception increase the risk of venous thrombosis up to 50-fold. The other inherited hypercoagulable states are much rarer and less likely.

The discharge anticoagulation regimen should include warfarin titrated to an international normalized ratio (INR) of 2 to 3. The length of warfarin therapy is a subject of controversy. For a first episode of venous thrombosis, most clinicians select a 3 to 6-month course of therapy and reserve indefinite therapy for patients with recurrent episodes. Even in the presence of factor V Leiden, most clinicians choose limited-duration therapy with warfarin. Low-molecular-weight heparin is an option for patients who do not tolerate warfarin, but the expense of this therapy makes it a second-line treatment. In this case, it is also important that the use of oral contraceptives stop.

The management of anticoagulation in pregnancy is difficult. A small molecule, warfarin easily crosses the placenta and leads to birth defects such as limb hypoplasia. This agent is contraindicated in pregnancy. During pregnancy, a switch to subcutaneous heparin is appropriate, with close monitoring of the partial thromboplastin (PTT) time. An inferior vena cava filter is unnecessary unless the patient cannot take heparin or has recurrent episodes of pulmonary emboli despite anticoagulation.

127–128. The answers are: 127-C, 128-D. (*Emergency medicine, internal medicine*)
This patient presents with an acute anterior myocardial infarction (MI) in the setting of recent cocaine use. Coronary angiography with possible angioplasty is the best option. Many cocaine-associated MIs are due to vasospasm, but a significant number are secondary to rupture of coronary artery plaque and thrombosis. Clinically, it is difficult to distinguish these possibilities; therefore, angiography is the best option for both diagnosis and treatment. β-Blockage may make cocaine-associated vasoconstriction worse, because α-receptor effects are unopposed. Neither intravenous enalapril nor verapamil plays a role in this setting. The rationale for calcium-channel blockade is to reduce vasospasm, but this has not been clinically proven.

Cocaine has several effects on the cardiovascular system, which include increasing systemic afterload; increasing myocardial workload and oxygen consumption (both by increasing heart rate and afterload); enhancing platelet aggregation; intensifying vasoconstriction; increasing heart rate and blood pressure; and increasing shear stress on the vascular wall, possibly increasing the risk for plaque rupture. However, cocaine has no effect on the fibrinolytic system.

129. The answer is B. (*Internal medicine*)
Fatigue, which accounts for approximately 7 million office visits per year in the United States, ranks seventh among initial complaints. Psychiatric problems account for 45% to 80% of the diagnoses that result in fatigue. The most common disorders are major depression, panic disorder, and somatization disorder.

An organic etiology is found in 2% to 13% of cases. The most common organic causes are anemia, hypothyroidism, occult malignancy, diabetes mellitus, and obstructive sleep anemia. When the history and physical examination are unrevealing, laboratory tests are rarely fruitful. A formal depression screening test and alcohol screening test are essential.

Chronic fatigue syndrome is rare, and its diagnosis requires satisfying the published criteria. Epstein-Barr virus is not likely to be related to chronic fatigue syndrome. Lyme disease as a cause of chronic fatigue is unclear as well. Unless the diagnosis is considered for objective reasons, Lyme serologies should not be drawn.

130–133. The answers are: 130-E, 131-E, 132-B, 133-D. (*Internal medicine*)
Antibiotic prophylaxis for procedure-related endocarditis is indicated in several clinical circumstances in which the risk of bacterial seeding and infection of a heart valve is high. Such situations include:

High-risk conditions	Prosthetic heart valves
	Previous endocarditis
	Cyanotic congenital heart disease
	Surgically corrected systemic–pulmonary shunts and conduits
Moderate-risk conditions	Acquired valvular dysfunction (rheumatic heart disease)
	Hypertrophic cardiomyopathy
	Mitral valve prolapse with mitral regurgitation
Other conditions	Invasive dental, respiratory, and esophageal procedures

Prophylaxis is not recommended in conditions associated with negligible risk, which include isolated secundum atrial septal defects (ASDs), surgical repair of ASDs or ventricular septal defects (VSDs), previous coronary artery bypass graft, mitral valve prolapse without regurgitation, functional heart murmurs, and cardiac pacemakers or defibrillators.

In questions 130 and 131, no antibiotic prophylaxis is warranted because the clinical situations are low risk. The patient in question 132 presents with a high-risk predisposing factor and a high-risk procedure. In this case, the recommended prophylaxis is intravenous ampicillin. In question 133, antibiotic prophylaxis is necessary, but given the patient's allergic response to penicillin, ampicillin is contraindicated. Furthermore, because the patient will have nothing-by-mouth (be NPO) before surgery, intravenous clindamycin is the best choice.

134–135. The answers are: 134-D, 135-C. (*Obstetrics/gynecology*)
Labor has been conveniently divided into three stages. The first stage, which is further divided into latent (slow dilation) and active phases, consists of the onset of labor to complete cervical dilation. On average, the duration of the first stage is approximately 20 to 24 hours in nulliparas and an average of 14 to 16 hours in multiparas. By definition, latent phase disorders, which occur before the cervix reaches 4 cm of dilation, are longer than 20 hours in nulliparas and 14 hours in multiparas. Causes include unripe cervix, false labor, uterine inertia, sedation, anesthesia, and idiopathic and unknown factors. Active phase disorders, also termed "primary dysfunctional labor," are defined as cervical dilations of less than 1.2 cm/hour in nulliparas and less than 1.5 cm/hour in multiparas. Causes of these disorders include cephalopelvic disproportion, malposition, sedation, and anesthesia.

In the case described in question 134, the prolonged first stage of labor is likely due to anesthesia. There is no evidence of malposition. False labor is unlikely given the history of ruptured membranes. Cephalopelvic disproportion, a rare cause of a prolonged latent phase, is less likely than anesthesia. Uteroplacental insufficiency does not lead to prolonged labor.

In the case described in question 135, the most likely explanation is cephalopelvic disproportion. The cesarean section is suggestive. The woman has received no anesthesia, and the other selections are not common causes of prolonged labor in this setting.

136–139. The answers are: 136-B, 137-E, 138-D, 139-A. (*Emergency medicine, critical care medicine*)
Antidotes and specific therapies exist for a number of important poisonings. It is imperative that both the clinical signs and symptoms, as well as specific therapies, are known for the clinically important toxins.

In the case described in question 136, the presence of metabolic acidosis with a large anion gap has a limited differential diagnosis. The causes of anion gap acidosis include methanol, uremia, diabetic ketoacidosis, paraldehyde, iron intoxication, lactic acidosis, ethanol, and salicylates. The occurrence of crystals strongly suggests ethylene glycol poisoning. Oxalate is a metabolite of ethylene glycol; therefore, urine oxalate crystals are a common and often diagnostic finding. Hemodialysis warrants strong consideration as first-line treatment for ethylene glycol poisoning, especially if the pH is less than 7.15 or the ethylene glycol levels are greater than 60 mmol/L. Ethanol and fomepizole also inhibit the metabolism of ethylene glycol into its toxic metabolites and should be used as specific antidotes.

In the case described in question 137, narcotic overdose should be the primary concern. The combination of stupor, constricted pupils, hypopnea, and needle tracks on the arm should lead to rapid treatment of the patient with naloxone (Narcan), an opioid antagonist.

In the case described in question 138, the patient is suffering from organophosphate intoxication or cholinergic poisoning. Organophosphates such as malathion are commonly found in insecticides. The mnemonic DUMBELS describes the signs of cholinergic excess: **d**iarrhea, **u**rination, **m**iosis, **b**ronchospasm, **e**mesis, **l**acrimation, and **s**alivation. Nicotinic effects lead to increased muscular twitching, fasciculations, and cramps. Pralidoxime is the specific antidote in this case.

In the case described in question 139, the presence of combined respiratory alkalosis and metabolic acidosis should strongly lead to the suspicion of salicylate overdose. Furthermore, the complaint of "a funny sound" in her ears should suggest tinnitus. Because salicylate is a weak acid, alkalinization of the urine traps salicylate in its anion form and leads to increased excretion in the urine. In the setting of high salicylate levels, severe acidosis, or severe mental status changes, hemodialysis may also be used.

140–143. The answers are: 140-A, 141-D, 142-C, 143-B. (*Pediatrics, internal medicine*)
The National Asthma Education and Prevention Program has published expert guidelines for the classification and stepwise approach for managing patients with asthma. Determination of asthma severity is the first step in the evaluation process. Asthma is classified into the following four types:

Step	Symptoms	Nocturnal Symptoms	Lung Function
1 Mild Intermittent	<2 times/week, with brief exacerbations and normality in between episodes	≤2 times/month	FEV_1 or peak flow >80% of predicted
2 Mild Persistent	>2 times/week, but <1 time/day	>2 times/month	FEV_1 or peak flow >80% of predicted
3 Moderate Persistent	Daily with limiting of activity, exacerbations >2 times/week	>1 time/month	FEV_1 or peak flow 60%–80% of predicted
4 Severe Persistent	Continual, limited activity with frequent exacerbations	Frequent	FEV_1 or peak flow <60% of predicted

FEV_1 = forced expiratory volume in 1 second.

Therapy for asthma is then tailored to the patient's particular step, using an approach designed to achieve long-term control.

Step	Long-term Control	Quick Relief
1	None needed	Inhaled β-agonist for symptom relief
2	**Daily medication (ONE)**	Inhaled β-agonist for symptom relief
	Inhaled corticosteroid (low-dose) OR	
	Cromolyn/nedocromil OR	
	Theophylline OR	
	Leukotriene modulator	
3	**Daily medications**	Inhaled β-agonist for symptom relief
	Inhaled steroid (medium-dose)	
	OR	
	Inhaled steroid and long-acting bronchodilator or theophylline	
4	**Daily medications**	Inhaled β-agonist for symptom relief
	High-dose inhaled steroids	
	AND	
	Long-acting bronchodilator or theophylline	
	AND	
	Oral corticosteroids	

In question 140, the patient has symptoms consistent with step 1 asthma. Symptomatic treatment with albuterol is indicated.

In question 141, the patient has severe, persistent symptoms. Aggressive treatment with oral steroids, inhaled steroids, and a long-acting bronchodilator is warranted at this time.

In question 142, the patient has step 3 asthma. He should receive an inhaled steroid with a long-acting bronchodilator.

In question 143, the patient has step 2 asthma. He should receive inhaled steroids.

144–146. The answers are: 144-B, 145-D, 146-A. (*Internal medicine*)
Thyroid disorders are extremely common. Distinct clinical syndromes allow for the recognition of the different thyroid conditions.

The patient in question 144 has Graves disease, in which thyroid-stimulating antibodies cause the increased formation and secretion of thyroid hormone, as well as exophthalmos. The thyroxine (T_4) level is elevated. Triiodothyronine resin uptake (T_3RU) is a measure of thyroid-binding globulin. Radioactive triiodothyronine

(T_3) competes with the T_4 in the serum for the binding sites on thyroid-binding globulin, and the excess T_3 is then bound to a resin and quantitated. Thus, the value of the T_3RU is inversely proportional to the number of available thyroxine binding sites. In cases of T_4 excess, most of the binding sites on thyroid-binding globulin are occupied, so the binding resin takes up the added T_3, resulting in an elevated T_3RU. The high levels of T_4 inhibit secretion of thyroid-stimulating hormone (TSH).

The patient in question 145 has "sick euthyroid syndrome." In critical illness, the total T_4 level decreases, possibly secondary to changes in the amount of thyroid-binding globulin. The increase in T_3RU reflects this; there are fewer free sites available on thyroid-binding globulin. The important measure is the TSH value, which remains in the normal range. In most cases, follow-up thyroid function testing is normal after the patient's condition has improved. Other clues to sick thyroid syndrome are a low T_3 and an increased reverse T_3 because of impaired peripheral conversion of T_4 to T_3. Essentially, critically ill patients can have abnormal thyroid studies without having significant thyroid disease.

The patient in question 146 has lithium-induced hypothyroidism. This is reflected in the low T_4; low T_3RU, with more free binding sites on thyroid-binding globulin and less radioactive T_3 available to bind to the resin; and elevated TSH.

147–150. The answers are: 147-E, 148-B, 149-C, 150-D. (*Internal medicine*)
The patient in question 147 likely has acute hepatitis A infection acquired by eating raw shellfish. She is at low risk for hepatitis B and C; serologies should be negative. An immunoglobulin M (IgM) antihepatitis A virus titer may be positive. The patient should improve with supportive care.

The patient in question 148 has received the hepatitis B vaccine, and, therefore, anti-HBs should be positive. He has no risk factors for hepatitis C. If he were exposed to hepatitis C, it would take time for seroconversion (up to 6 months), and this would not be apparent on immediate postexposure blood work.

The patient in question 149 represents a common scenario. Increasingly, clinicians are using elevated liver function tests to identify certain individuals who engaged in high-risk activities in the 1960s; these patients have hepatitis C. In this patient, vaccination with the HBsAg vaccine would also lead to the positive result for anti-HBc.

The patient in question 150 has chronic hepatitis, which is manifested by persistent HBsAg, no anti-HBs and, often, elevated liver function tests. Antibodies to HBc are also present but are usually the IgG isoform and not IgM (reflecting past infection). Patients with chronic disease may also have HBeAg, which reflects active viral replication and high risk of infectivity. However, this patient has no evidence of concomitant hepatitis C infection.

References

American Psychiatric Association. *Diagnostic and Statistical Manual of Mental Disorders.* 4th ed. Washington, DC: American Psychiatric Association, 1994.

Becker KL, ed. *Principles and Practice of Endocrinology and Metabolism.* 3rd ed. Philadelphia: Lippincott Williams & Wilkins, 2001.

Benson MD. *Obstetrical Pearls: A Practical Guide for the Efficient Resident.* Philadelphia: FA Davis, 1984.

Brant WE, Helms CA. *Fundamentals of Diagnostic Radiology.* 2nd ed. Philadelphia: Lippincott Williams & Wilkins, 1999.

Collins J, Stern EJ. *Chest Radiology: The Essentials.* Philadelphia: Lippincott Williams & Wilkins, 1999.

Ellenhorn MJ. *Ellenhorn's Medical Toxicology: Diagnosis and Treatment of Human Poisoning.* Baltimore: Williams & Wilkins, 1997.

Fowler NO. *Clinical Electrocardiographic Diagnosis: A Problem-Based Approach.* Philadelphia: Lippincott Williams & Wilkins, 2000.

Frankel DH. *Field Guide to Clinical Dermatology.* Philadelphia: Lippincott Williams & Wilkins, 1999.

Goodheart HP. *A Photoguide of Common Skin Disorders: Diagnosis and Management.* Baltimore: Williams & Wilkins, 1999.

Humes DH, ed. *Kelley's Textbook of Internal Medicine.* Philadelphia: Lippincott Williams & Wilkins, 2000.

Irwin RS, Cerra FB, Rippe JM. *Intensive Care Medicine.* 4th ed. Philadelphia: Lippincott-Raven, 1999.

Kaplan HI, Sadock BJ. *Synopsis of Psychiatry.* 8th ed. Baltimore: Williams & Wilkins, 1998.

Masear VR. *Primary Care Orthopedics.* Philadelphia: WB Saunders, 1997.

O'Connor BH. *A Color Atlas and Instruction Manual of Peripheral Blood Cell Morphology.* Baltimore: Williams & Wilkins, 1984.

Schwartz GR, ed. *Principles and Practice of Emergency Medicine.* 4th ed. Philadelphia: Lippincott Williams & Wilkins, 1999.

Scully JH. *National Medical Series for Independent Study: Psychiatry.* 4th ed. Philadelphia: Lippincott Williams & Wilkins, 2001.

Wright KW, ed. *Textbook of Ophthalmology.* Baltimore: Williams & Wilkins, 1997.

Review for USMLE Step 3 Answer Sheet

TEST I

1 A B C D E	51 A B C D E	101 A B C D E
2 A B C D E	52 A B C D E	102 A B C D E
3 A B C D E	53 A B C D E	103 A B C D E
4 A B C D E	54 A B C D E	104 A B C D E
5 A B C D E	55 A B C D E	105 A B C D E
6 A B C D E	56 A B C D E	106 A B C D E
7 A B C D E	57 A B C D E	107 A B C D E
8 A B C D E	58 A B C D E	108 A B C D E
9 A B C D E	59 A B C D E	109 A B C D E
10 A B C D E	60 A B C D E	110 A B C D E
11 A B C D E	61 A B C D E	111 A B C D E
12 A B C D E	62 A B C D E	112 A B C D E
13 A B C D E	63 A B C D E	113 A B C D E
14 A B C D E	64 A B C D E	114 A B C D E
15 A B C D E	65 A B C D E	115 A B C D E
16 A B C D E	66 A B C D E	116 A B C D E
17 A B C D E	67 A B C D E	117 A B C D E
18 A B C D E	68 A B C D E	118 A B C D E
19 A B C D E	69 A B C D E	119 A B C D E
20 A B C D E	70 A B C D E	120 A B C D E
21 A B C D E	71 A B C D E	121 A B C D E
22 A B C D E	72 A B C D E	122 A B C D E
23 A B C D E	73 A B C D E	123 A B C D E
24 A B C D E	74 A B C D E	124 A B C D E
25 A B C D E	75 A B C D E	125 A B C D E
26 A B C D E	76 A B C D E	126 A B C D E
27 A B C D E	77 A B C D E	127 A B C D E
28 A B C D E	78 A B C D E	128 A B C D E
29 A B C D E	79 A B C D E	129 A B C D E
30 A B C D E	80 A B C D E	130 A B C D E
31 A B C D E	81 A B C D E	131 A B C D E
32 A B C D E	82 A B C D E	132 A B C D E
33 A B C D E	83 A B C D E	133 A B C D E
34 A B C D E	84 A B C D E	134 A B C D E
35 A B C D E	85 A B C D E	135 A B C D E
36 A B C D E	86 A B C D E	136 A B C D E
37 A B C D E	87 A B C D E	137 A B C D E
38 A B C D E	88 A B C D E	138 A B C D E
39 A B C D E	89 A B C D E	139 A B C D E
40 A B C D E	90 A B C D E	140 A B C D E
41 A B C D E	91 A B C D E	141 A B C D E
42 A B C D E	92 A B C D E	142 A B C D E
43 A B C D E	93 A B C D E	143 A B C D E
44 A B C D E	94 A B C D E	144 A B C D E
45 A B C D E	95 A B C D E	145 A B C D E
46 A B C D E	96 A B C D E	146 A B C D E
47 A B C D E	97 A B C D E	147 A B C D E
48 A B C D E	98 A B C D E	148 A B C D E
49 A B C D E	99 A B C D E	149 A B C D E
50 A B C D E	100 A B C D E	150 A B C D E

TEST II

1 A B C D E	51 A B C D E	101 A B C D E
2 A B C D E	52 A B C D E	102 A B C D E
3 A B C D E	53 A B C D E	103 A B C D E
4 A B C D E	54 A B C D E	104 A B C D E
5 A B C D E	55 A B C D E	105 A B C D E
6 A B C D E	56 A B C D E	106 A B C D E
7 A B C D E	57 A B C D E	107 A B C D E
8 A B C D E	58 A B C D E	108 A B C D E
9 A B C D E	59 A B C D E	109 A B C D E
10 A B C D E	60 A B C D E	110 A B C D E
11 A B C D E	61 A B C D E	111 A B C D E
12 A B C D E	62 A B C D E	112 A B C D E
13 A B C D E	63 A B C D E	113 A B C D E
14 A B C D E	64 A B C D E	114 A B C D E
15 A B C D E	65 A B C D E	115 A B C D E
16 A B C D E	66 A B C D E	116 A B C D E
17 A B C D E	67 A B C D E	117 A B C D E
18 A B C D E	68 A B C D E	118 A B C D E
19 A B C D E	69 A B C D E	119 A B C D E
20 A B C D E	70 A B C D E	120 A B C D E
21 A B C D E	71 A B C D E	121 A B C D E
22 A B C D E	72 A B C D E	122 A B C D E
23 A B C D E	73 A B C D E	123 A B C D E
24 A B C D E	74 A B C D E	124 A B C D E
25 A B C D E	75 A B C D E	125 A B C D E
26 A B C D E	76 A B C D E	126 A B C D E
27 A B C D E	77 A B C D E	127 A B C D E
28 A B C D E	78 A B C D E	128 A B C D E
29 A B C D E	79 A B C D E	129 A B C D E
30 A B C D E	80 A B C D E	130 A B C D E
31 A B C D E	81 A B C D E	131 A B C D E
32 A B C D E	82 A B C D E	132 A B C D E
33 A B C D E	83 A B C D E	133 A B C D E
34 A B C D E	84 A B C D E	134 A B C D E
35 A B C D E	85 A B C D E	135 A B C D E
36 A B C D E	86 A B C D E	136 A B C D E
37 A B C D E	87 A B C D E	137 A B C D E
38 A B C D E	88 A B C D E	138 A B C D E
39 A B C D E	89 A B C D E	139 A B C D E
40 A B C D E	90 A B C D E	140 A B C D E
41 A B C D E	91 A B C D E	141 A B C D E
42 A B C D E	92 A B C D E	142 A B C D E
43 A B C D E	93 A B C D E	143 A B C D E
44 A B C D E	94 A B C D E	144 A B C D E
45 A B C D E	95 A B C D E	145 A B C D E
46 A B C D E	96 A B C D E	146 A B C D E
47 A B C D E	97 A B C D E	147 A B C D E
48 A B C D E	98 A B C D E	148 A B C D E
49 A B C D E	99 A B C D E	149 A B C D E
50 A B C D E	100 A B C D E	150 A B C D E

Review for USMLE Step 3 Answer Sheet

TEST III

1 A B C D E	51 A B C D E	101 A B C D E
2 A B C D E	52 A B C D E	102 A B C D E
3 A B C D E	53 A B C D E	103 A B C D E
4 A B C D E	54 A B C D E	104 A B C D E
5 A B C D E	55 A B C D E	105 A B C D E
6 A B C D E	56 A B C D E	106 A B C D E
7 A B C D E	57 A B C D E	107 A B C D E
8 A B C D E	58 A B C D E	108 A B C D E
9 A B C D E	59 A B C D E	109 A B C D E
10 A B C D E	60 A B C D E	110 A B C D E
11 A B C D E	61 A B C D E	111 A B C D E
12 A B C D E	62 A B C D E	112 A B C D E
13 A B C D E	63 A B C D E	113 A B C D E
14 A B C D E	64 A B C D E	114 A B C D E
15 A B C D E	65 A B C D E	115 A B C D E
16 A B C D E	66 A B C D E	116 A B C D E
17 A B C D E	67 A B C D E	117 A B C D E
18 A B C D E	68 A B C D E	118 A B C D E
19 A B C D E	69 A B C D E	119 A B C D E
20 A B C D E	70 A B C D E	120 A B C D E
21 A B C D E	71 A B C D E	121 A B C D E
22 A B C D E	72 A B C D E	122 A B C D E
23 A B C D E	73 A B C D E	123 A B C D E
24 A B C D E	74 A B C D E	124 A B C D E
25 A B C D E	75 A B C D E	125 A B C D E
26 A B C D E	76 A B C D E	126 A B C D E
27 A B C D E	77 A B C D E	127 A B C D E
28 A B C D E	78 A B C D E	128 A B C D E
29 A B C D E	79 A B C D E	129 A B C D E
30 A B C D E	80 A B C D E	130 A B C D E
31 A B C D E	81 A B C D E	131 A B C D E
32 A B C D E	82 A B C D E	132 A B C D E
33 A B C D E	83 A B C D E	133 A B C D E
34 A B C D E	84 A B C D E	134 A B C D E
35 A B C D E	85 A B C D E	135 A B C D E
36 A B C D E	86 A B C D E	136 A B C D E
37 A B C D E	87 A B C D E	137 A B C D E
38 A B C D E	88 A B C D E	138 A B C D E
39 A B C D E	89 A B C D E	139 A B C D E
40 A B C D E	90 A B C D E	140 A B C D E
41 A B C D E	91 A B C D E	141 A B C D E
42 A B C D E	92 A B C D E	142 A B C D E
43 A B C D E	93 A B C D E	143 A B C D E
44 A B C D E	94 A B C D E	144 A B C D E
45 A B C D E	95 A B C D E	145 A B C D E
46 A B C D E	96 A B C D E	146 A B C D E
47 A B C D E	97 A B C D E	147 A B C D E
48 A B C D E	98 A B C D E	148 A B C D E
49 A B C D E	99 A B C D E	149 A B C D E
50 A B C D E	100 A B C D E	150 A B C D E

TEST IV

1 A B C D E	51 A B C D E	101 A B C D E
2 A B C D E	52 A B C D E	102 A B C D E
3 A B C D E	53 A B C D E	103 A B C D E
4 A B C D E	54 A B C D E	104 A B C D E
5 A B C D E	55 A B C D E	105 A B C D E
6 A B C D E	56 A B C D E	106 A B C D E
7 A B C D E	57 A B C D E	107 A B C D E
8 A B C D E	58 A B C D E	108 A B C D E
9 A B C D E	59 A B C D E	109 A B C D E
10 A B C D E	60 A B C D E	110 A B C D E
11 A B C D E	61 A B C D E	111 A B C D E
12 A B C D E	62 A B C D E	112 A B C D E
13 A B C D E	63 A B C D E	113 A B C D E
14 A B C D E	64 A B C D E	114 A B C D E
15 A B C D E	65 A B C D E	115 A B C D E
16 A B C D E	66 A B C D E	116 A B C D E
17 A B C D E	67 A B C D E	117 A B C D E
18 A B C D E	68 A B C D E	118 A B C D E
19 A B C D E	69 A B C D E	119 A B C D E
20 A B C D E	70 A B C D E	120 A B C D E
21 A B C D E	71 A B C D E	121 A B C D E
22 A B C D E	72 A B C D E	122 A B C D E
23 A B C D E	73 A B C D E	123 A B C D E
24 A B C D E	74 A B C D E	124 A B C D E
25 A B C D E	75 A B C D E	125 A B C D E
26 A B C D E	76 A B C D E	126 A B C D E
27 A B C D E	77 A B C D E	127 A B C D E
28 A B C D E	78 A B C D E	128 A B C D E
29 A B C D E	79 A B C D E	129 A B C D E
30 A B C D E	80 A B C D E	130 A B C D E
31 A B C D E	81 A B C D E	131 A B C D E
32 A B C D E	82 A B C D E	132 A B C D E
33 A B C D E	83 A B C D E	133 A B C D E
34 A B C D E	84 A B C D E	134 A B C D E
35 A B C D E	85 A B C D E	135 A B C D E
36 A B C D E	86 A B C D E	136 A B C D E
37 A B C D E	87 A B C D E	137 A B C D E
38 A B C D E	88 A B C D E	138 A B C D E
39 A B C D E	89 A B C D E	139 A B C D E
40 A B C D E	90 A B C D E	140 A B C D E
41 A B C D E	91 A B C D E	141 A B C D E
42 A B C D E	92 A B C D E	142 A B C D E
43 A B C D E	93 A B C D E	143 A B C D E
44 A B C D E	94 A B C D E	144 A B C D E
45 A B C D E	95 A B C D E	145 A B C D E
46 A B C D E	96 A B C D E	146 A B C D E
47 A B C D E	97 A B C D E	147 A B C D E
48 A B C D E	98 A B C D E	148 A B C D E
49 A B C D E	99 A B C D E	149 A B C D E
50 A B C D E	100 A B C D E	150 A B C D E

Review for USMLE Step 3 Answer Sheet

TEST V

1 A B C D E	51 A B C D E	101 A B C D E
2 A B C D E	52 A B C D E	102 A B C D E
3 A B C D E	53 A B C D E	103 A B C D E
4 A B C D E	54 A B C D E	104 A B C D E
5 A B C D E	55 A B C D E	105 A B C D E
6 A B C D E	56 A B C D E	106 A B C D E
7 A B C D E	57 A B C D E	107 A B C D E
8 A B C D E	58 A B C D E	108 A B C D E
9 A B C D E	59 A B C D E	109 A B C D E
10 A B C D E	60 A B C D E	110 A B C D E
11 A B C D E	61 A B C D E	111 A B C D E
12 A B C D E	62 A B C D E	112 A B C D E
13 A B C D E	63 A B C D E	113 A B C D E
14 A B C D E	64 A B C D E	114 A B C D E
15 A B C D E	65 A B C D E	115 A B C D E
16 A B C D E	66 A B C D E	116 A B C D E
17 A B C D E	67 A B C D E	117 A B C D E
18 A B C D E	68 A B C D E	118 A B C D E
19 A B C D E	69 A B C D E	119 A B C D E
20 A B C D E	70 A B C D E	120 A B C D E
21 A B C D E	71 A B C D E	121 A B C D E
22 A B C D E	72 A B C D E	122 A B C D E
23 A B C D E	73 A B C D E	123 A B C D E
24 A B C D E	74 A B C D E	124 A B C D E
25 A B C D E	75 A B C D E	125 A B C D E
26 A B C D E	76 A B C D E	126 A B C D E
27 A B C D E	77 A B C D E	127 A B C D E
28 A B C D E	78 A B C D E	128 A B C D E
29 A B C D E	79 A B C D E	129 A B C D E
30 A B C D E	80 A B C D E	130 A B C D E
31 A B C D E	81 A B C D E	131 A B C D E
32 A B C D E	82 A B C D E	132 A B C D E
33 A B C D E	83 A B C D E	133 A B C D E
34 A B C D E	84 A B C D E	134 A B C D E
35 A B C D E	85 A B C D E	135 A B C D E
36 A B C D E	86 A B C D E	136 A B C D E
37 A B C D E	87 A B C D E	137 A B C D E
38 A B C D E	88 A B C D E	138 A B C D E
39 A B C D E	89 A B C D E	139 A B C D E
40 A B C D E	90 A B C D E	140 A B C D E
41 A B C D E	91 A B C D E	141 A B C D E
42 A B C D E	92 A B C D E	142 A B C D E
43 A B C D E	93 A B C D E	143 A B C D E
44 A B C D E	94 A B C D E	144 A B C D E
45 A B C D E	95 A B C D E	145 A B C D E
46 A B C D E	96 A B C D E	146 A B C D E
47 A B C D E	97 A B C D E	147 A B C D E
48 A B C D E	98 A B C D E	148 A B C D E
49 A B C D E	99 A B C D E	149 A B C D E
50 A B C D E	100 A B C D E	150 A B C D E